Black and minority
ethnic groups in England:
the second health and lifestyles survey

Black and minority ethnic groups in England:
the second health and lifestyles survey

Acknowledgements

In an extended research programme such as this, there are many people who have been involved and offered guidance, advice and expertise. We wish to thank, first and foremost, all those who took the time and effort to complete the questionnaire. Our thanks are extended also to all the organisations and individuals involved in this project.

About the authors

This report was written for the Health Education Authority by Dr Mark R.D. Johnson, Reader in Primary Care in the School of Nursing and Midwifery, Mary Seacole Research Centre, De Montfort University; Dr David Owen, Director of the National Ethnic Minority Data Archive at the Centre for Research in Ethnic Relations, University of Warwick; and Clare Blackburn, Senior Research Fellow in the Department of Social Policy and Social Work, University of Warwick.

The introduction was written by Dr James Nazroo – Department of Epidemiology and Public Health, University College London.

The field work was carried out by MORI.

The research was managed by Hamid Rehman, Head of Ethnic Minority Health at the Health Education Authority.

Authors' note

In order to avoid the traditional order of male norm, female deviation, the authors have consistently reported female data before male data.

© Health Education Authority 2000

Health Education Authority
Trevelyan House
30 Great Peter Street
London SW1P 2HW

www.hea.org.uk

Cover design by Crescent Creative
Text design by Foster and Lisle
Typesetting by Type Generation
Printed by Bell & Bain Ltd., Glasgow
1m 3/00 01

ISBN 0 7521 1577 4

Contents

Foreword

Reducing inequalities in health is a key aim of the Government's public health policy. The Acheson report (1998), provides evidence to show that social and economic factors affect health and illness. There are systematic patterns underlying ill-health: some groups within society experience poorer health because of their socio-economic status, gender or ethnicity, since these tend to be correlated with low income, poorer education and poorer material environment. The report recommends a broad range of policies to reduce inequalities, with particular emphasis on improving the health of the 'least well off in society'.

The Government has initiated a number of key policies to tackle some of the most pressing sources of inequalities. New national policies on education, the 'Welfare to Work' programme, and the introduction of the national minimum wage, for instance, are but some of the strategies currently being implemented to improve both the material conditions and the social capital of the most disadvantaged groups in British society. In addition, targeted programmes such as Health Action Zones, Education Action Zones, Sure Start and the New Deal for Communities aim to tackle social exclusion in particularly deprived areas. These programmes are all expected to have significant positive effects on the health of the least well off in society and are the backdrop to the public health strategy, *Our Healthier Nation*, which places particular emphasis on the healthy neighbourhood as a focus for action on health inequalities. They are essential: targeting the structural factors that underpin inequalities is crucial if the present health differentials are to be eradicated.

Black and ethnic minority groups are at a clear and unjustifiable disadvantage in terms of their actual health condition, of their knowledge about health issues, and of their access to appropriate health services. They are affected in much larger proportions than the white population by certain conditions. They tend to live in poorer material conditions. They experience stress and often live in fear of racial harassment.

The situation of black and minority ethnic groups can be significantly improved. The Government initiatives outlined above are a major step towards this aim. They can make a radical contribution to improving the social and economic circumstances of the more deprived communities of this country, regardless of their ethnic status. However, unless ethnic minority needs are specifically targeted, such programmes and initiatives will fail to alleviate the burden of ill-health experienced by ethnic minorities. In particular, they will fail to reach those who cannot speak English, who have limited knowledge about the nature and value of certain services, who find the information presented to them inappropriate or irrelevant, who have no means of access to services, or who are systematically dissatisfied by their experiences of health services.

In this context, health education has a key role to play, both with respect to health professionals – in sensitising them to the needs of their communities – and to lay people – in making them more knowledgeable of risk factors associated with health, in diffusing culturally relevant information, and in raising awareness of the provisions available to them.

The HEA research presented here demonstrates that health messages often fail to reach these groups. Strategies to improve ethnic health include the development of specific health promotion policies and strategies at national, regional and local level and the development of health messages and health promotion activities for each community, in line with its own health needs and culture and with the full involvement of that community.

Hamid Rehman
Head of Ethnic Minority Health
Health Education Authority

Introduction
An overview of minority ethnic groups and health in Britain

This report presents the findings of the second Health Education Authority survey on the health and lifestyles of black and minority ethnic groups in Britain. The first survey, reported in 1994, provided information about variations in health both within and between the different minority ethnic groups which together make up over 5% of the British population. While the first survey covered a range of key areas, including aspects of ethnic identity, and focused particularly on smoking, the second survey provides further information on the characteristics of black and minority ethnic people in Britain, featuring more detailed analyses of demography, language and religion. Issues relevant to circulatory disorders (including diabetes) are highlighted, both because these have been shown to be prime concerns of people of minority ethnicity, and also because they are major causes of morbidity and mortality among these populations.

This chapter will provide an overview of key dimensions of the experiences of ethnic minority people in Britain, in order to set the context for the remainder of this volume. This will include a discussion of the epidemiological literature on ethnic inequalities in health and health experience across different ethnic groups. But, perhaps more importantly, this chapter will begin with a review of the socio-demographic profile of the ethnic minority groups covered by this survey.

Ethnic minority groups in Britain

Most of what we know about the social and economic circumstances of the ethnic minority population of Britain comes from two sources, the 1991 Census[1] and the 1993/4 Fourth National Survey of Ethnic Minorities.[2] Unfortunately, both data sources contain significant limitations, most notably that they had restricted coverage of some ethnic minority groups, such as white minority groups and mixed ethnicity. The data from these sources needs to be renewed, but we will have to wait until findings from the 2001 Census become available to address these problems.

Ethnic group	Number	Percentage	Percentage born in UK
White	51 873 794	94.5	95.8
All ethnic minorities	3 015 050	5.5	46.8
All black	890 727	1.6	55.7
Black-Caribbean	499 964	0.9	53.7
Black-African	212 362	0.4	36.4
Black-other[1]	178 401	0.3	84.4
All South Asian	1 479 645	2.7	44.1
Indian	840 255	1.5	43.0
Pakistani	476 555	0.9	50.5
Bangladeshi	162 835	0.3	36.7
Chinese and others	644 678	1.2	40.6
Chinese	156 938	0.3	28.4
Other-Asian	197 534	0.4	21.9
Other-other[2]	290 206	0.5	59.8

Notes:

[1]The 'black-other' group contains people recorded as 'black' with no further details, those identifying themselves as black-British', and people with ethnic origins classified as mixed black/white and black/other ethnic group. It seems that most of the 'black-other' group had Caribbean family origins, but were born in Britain.

[2]The 'other-other' group contains North Africans, Arabs, Iranians, together with people of mixed Asian/white, mixed black/white and 'other mixed categories.[3]

Figure 1: Ethnic composition of the UK population at the 1991 Census

The 1991 Census included questions on country of birth and, for the first time in a British census, ethnic group. Previously the census had asked only about nationality and country of birth. In 1991 respondents were asked to indicate which ethnic group they belonged to from a fixed range of choices that encompassed both skin colour and country of origin. The original fixed-choice categories covered 'White; Black-Caribbean; Black-African; Black-Other; Indian; Pakistani; Bangladeshi; Chinese; Any other Ethnic Group'. For those with 'mixed descent', respondents were instructed to use the category that was most appropriate or the 'Any other

Ethnic Group' category together with a description. Responses to the ethnic group question, 'recoded' into ten categories, are shown in Figure 1 along with the percentage in each group who were born in Britain. The figure shows that in 1991 5.5% of the population (just over 3 million people) identified themselves as belonging to one of the listed ethnic minority groups. Almost half of these people were born in Britain.

The figure also shows the diversity of the origins of ethnic minority people in Britain, with the largest group, Indians, making up only just over a quarter of ethnic minority people and some of the groups, including Indians, very obviously encompassing quite diverse sub-groups. It is important to note that undercounting at the 1991 Census varied by ethnic group in addition to age and gender. The undercount appeared to be greatest for young ethnic minority men; published adjustment tables suggest that for 25–29-year-old ethnic minority men the undercount was in the range of 13–17%.[4]

Analysis of the 1991 Census has also shown that there were important differences in the geographical locations of different ethnic groups. The ethnic minority population is largely concentrated in England and mainly in the most populous areas. Owen's analysis[5] of the 1991 Census data showed that:

■ More than half (56.2%) of the ethnic minority population lived in South East England, where less than a third (31.3%) of the total population lived.

■ Greater London contained 44.8% of the ethnic minority population but only 10.3 per cent of the total population.

■ The West Midlands, West Yorkshire and Greater Manchester contained the highest relative concentrations of people from ethnic minorities outside Greater London.

■ Almost 70% of ethnic minority people lived in Greater London, the West Midlands, West Yorkshire and Greater Manchester, compared with just over 25% of all people.

■ There are even greater differences when smaller areas are considered. More than half of ethnic minority people lived in areas where the total ethnic minority population exceeds 44%, compared with the 5.5% national average.

There are also important differences between the geographical locations of different ethnic minority groups. For example, among South Asian people Indians are more concentrated in London and the West Midlands, Pakistanis are more concentrated in West Yorkshire, Greater Manchester and the West Midlands, and Bangladeshis are strongly concentrated in London, Birmingham and Greater Manchester.

OPCS classification	White	All ethnic minorities	All black groups	South Asian
Established high status	14.0	17.1	14.1	16.6
Higher status growth	9.4	3.1	2.8	2.3
More rural areas	13.1	1.6	1.4	0.6
Resort and retirement	5.4	1.1	0.8	0.6
Mixed town and country, some industry	23.3	8.3	5.7	9.3
Traditional manufacturing	8.4	27.8	20.0	39.2
Service centres and cities	13.7	11.3	12.1	9.5
Areas with much local authority housing	8.4	4.2	2.5	5.2
Parts of Inner London	3.2	21.8	35.8	14.9
Central London	1.0	3.8	5.2	1.8

Figure 2: Types of areas where ethnic minority and white people live (percentages)

Figure 2 drawn from Owen,[6] uses an OPCS classification to characterise local authorities and shows the percentage of different ethnic groups living in each type. It clearly shows the higher concentration of the white population in rural and suburban areas and the higher concentration of ethnic minority people in industrial areas and London.

The 1991 Census also showed the relative youth of ethnic minority groups.[7] Children formed a third of the ethnic minority population, compared with under a fifth of the white population. In contrast, while 16% of the population as a whole were aged over 65, only just over 3% of the ethnic minority population fell within this age group. Differences in age profiles are summarised in Figure 3, which also suggests differences in the age structures of particular ethnic minority groups (for example, the South Asian group has a high proportion of people in the 5–15 age range). In summary, among the ethnic minority groups, Black-Caribbeans, Chinese, Indians and Other Asians tended to be older, while Bangladeshis, Pakistanis and, not surprisingly, Black-others, were younger.

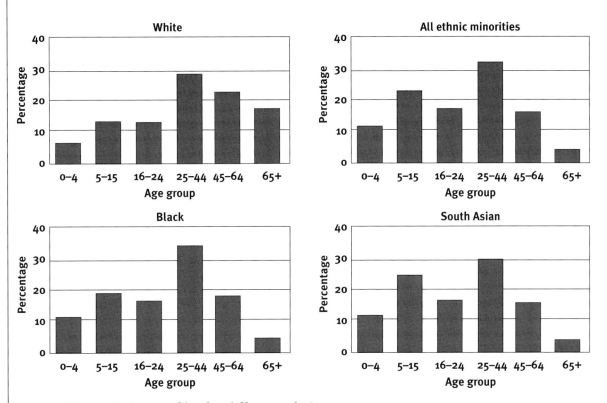

Figure 3: Age profiles for different ethnic groups

Differences in family formation, household structure and household size across ethnic groups in Britain also exist. Analysis of the 1991 Census[8] and the *Fourth National Survey*[9] showed that white, Caribbean, Indian and Chinese families had similar numbers of children, while Pakistani and Bangladeshi families had more. The analysis of the *Fourth National Survey*, which took into account life-stage, suggested that most white families would have one or two children and more than 90% of them had no more than three children. In contrast, most Pakistani and Bangladeshi families had four or more children and 85% of them had three or more children. South Asian households were also larger because of the number of adults they contained. Half of Pakistani and Bangladeshi households had three or more adults in them compared with two-fifths of Indian and Chinese households, and less than one-fifth of white and Caribbean households. Caribbean households were more likely than others to contain one adult with children, that is, were 'lone parent' households: about one in six Caribbean households had this structure, compared with less than one in twenty of other households.

Both the 1991 Census and the *Fourth National Survey* also provided detailed information on the socio-economic profiles of different ethnic minority groups. The following is a summary of key points from the *Fourth National Survey*,[10] which are largely supported by data from the 1991 Census.[11]

In terms of economic activity, the most striking findings concerned women: 80% of Bangladeshi and 70% of Pakistani women described themselves as looking after the home or family compared with about 30% of white and Indian women, and only 13% of Caribbean women. In contrast, most pre-retirement age men in all of the ethnic groups were in the labour market. Differences here were largely due to different rates of unemployment, which were very high among Pakistani and Bangladeshi men (almost four times that among the white population) and also high among Caribbean men (more than twice the white rate). Detailed analyses showed that these higher rates of unemployment for Caribbean, Pakistani and Bangladeshi men persisted regardless of geographical location or qualifications, although the size of the differences varied.[12]

The *Fourth National Survey* included several indicators of socio-economic position, and a summary indicator, equivalised household income, is shown in Figure 4.[13] This shows the distribution of households according to average incomes and the great extent of poverty among Pakistani and Bangladeshi households. More than four-fifths of Pakistani and Bangladeshi households had below half average income, a profile that is worse than that of white lone parents and white people of post-retirement age. Two-fifths of Caribbean and Indian households were also in this position, compared with a third of Chinese and less than a third of white households.

	White	Caribbean	Indian	Pakistani	Bangladeshi	Chinese
More than 1½ times average	23	12	14	1	2	22
½ to 1½ times average	49	47	45	17	14	44
Below ½ of the average	28	41	42	82	84	34

Figure 4: Household incomes and ethnicity (percentages)

Finally, no description of the lives of ethnic minority people in Britain would be complete without coverage of experiences of racism. A central element of the *Fourth National Survey* was an attempt to assess the degree to which the lives of ethnic minority people were directly affected by racism. As part of this, white respondents were asked if they were prejudiced against certain ethnic minority groups. As many as one in five of the white respondents said that they were racially prejudiced against Caribbeans, while as many as one in four said that they were racially prejudiced against South Asians (slightly more for men and slightly less for women).[14] In interpreting this figure, the author suggested that the crudeness of the question and under-reporting probably meant that this was an underestimate of the extent of racial prejudice, but that the findings nevertheless indicated that 'a current of racist beliefs is clearly evident among a significant proportion of the white population'.[15]

This was reflected in the widespread belief among the ethnic minority respondents to the *Fourth National Survey* that employers discriminated against ethnic minority applicants for jobs and their reporting of widespread experience of such discrimination.[16] There was also widespread experience of racial harassment reported in response to questions asking about being physically attacked, having property damaged or being insulted for reasons to do with 'race' or colour. More than one in eight ethnic minority people reported having experienced some form of racial harassment in the past year.[17] Most of these incidents involved racial insults, many of the respondents reported repeated victimisation and a quarter of the ethnic minority respondents reported being fearful of racial harassment. The degree to which racial harassment is rooted in white British culture is indicated by the fact that the perpetrators of such incidents ranged from neighbours to people in shops, though they were predominantly strangers, and that the incidents occurred in almost all areas of the respondents' lives, including work.

Ethnic inequalities in health

Since the early 1970s ethnic inequalities in health have become an increasing focus of research in Britain.[18] More recently there have been national surveys of variations in morbidity rates by ethnic group[19] and the tradition of analysing differences in mortality rates by country of birth has continued.[20] A number of key points have emerged from these recent morbidity and immigrant mortality data.

1 Ethnic minority groups are not uniformly at greater risk of mortality or poor health. For example, both mortality and morbidity data suggest that Indians have reasonably good overall health.[21]

2 For some outcomes ethnic minority groups appear to be significantly better off than the ethnic majority (e.g. respiratory symptoms/disease and lung cancer).

3 Particular ethnic groups appear to be particularly disadvantaged by different diseases. For example, Caribbeans have high rates of stroke/hypertension and South Asians have high rates of CHD/severe chest pain. But all ethnic minority groups have higher rates of diabetes than white groups, and the white population have higher rates of respiratory diseases.[22]

4 Ethnic inequalities in socio-economic position make a significant contribution to ethnic inequalities in health.[23]

This final point is worth discussing in some detail. Analyses of immigrant mortality data from the 1970s showed no occupational class gradient for men born in the Indian subcontinent, a reversed gradient for men born in the Caribbean, and that class difference effects made no contribution to the reported ethnic variations in mortality rates.[24] This led many commentators to conclude that socio-economic differences made no contribution to ethnic differences in health. However, analysis of the more recent data on immigrant mortality rates has shown a clear relationship between occupational class and mortality rates for all migrant groups.[25] Considering deaths from all causes, men in manual classes had markedly higher rates of mortality than those in non-manual classes in each migrant group, except those born in West/South Africa where the difference, although present, was smaller. This pattern was repeated, with only a few exceptions, for each migrant group for specific causes of death. A similar pattern of findings was present in the *Fourth National Survey* morbidity data.[26] These showed a clear class gradient for reporting fair or poor health in each ethnic group and, again with only a very few exceptions, this pattern was clearly repeated for specific diseases. These data have now clearly established the presence of socio-economic gradients in health within ethnic minority groups.

Despite this, like the earlier analysis of immigrant mortality data, the most recent analysis has suggested that socio-economic differentials make minimal contributions to ethnic variations in health – for men in most migrant groups adjusting for occupational class differences did not alter their higher mortality rates compared with those born in Britain.[27] However, it is likely that this is a consequence of the difficulties in adjusting for socio-economic effects across ethnic groups.[28] In the *Fourth National Survey* morbidity data, adjusting for a more sensitive index of socio-economic position than occupational class gives a large reduction in relative risk for adverse health outcomes for all ethnic minority groups,[29] providing convincing evidence of the socio-economic basis of ethnic inequalities in health.[30]

Of course other factors may also play an important role in contributing to ethnic inequalities in health and health experience. Inequalities in access to health services have been well established in a number of studies. Although ethnic minority people are at least as likely as white people to consult with their GP, they are less likely than whites to leave the surgery with a follow-up appointment,[31] or to receive follow-up services, such as a district nurse.[32] South Asian people with CHD wait longer for referral to specialist care than white people,[33] despite being more likely to seek immediate care.[34] And in one study they were less than half as likely to receive grafts for triple-vessel disease, despite having further progressed disease.[35]

None of these studies have been able to explore reasons for these possible differences in quality of care. But it has been shown that ethnic minority people are more likely than whites to find physical access to their GP difficult; have longer waiting times in the surgery; feel that the time their GP had spent with them was inadequate; and to be unhappy with the outcome of the consultation.[36] Part of this might be related to communication problems. In terms of language, a significant number of South Asians (particularly Bangladeshi women) and Chinese people find it difficult to communicate with their GP.[37] There may be cultural differences in the expression of symptoms, making the use of western diagnostic approaches inappropriate for some groups, especially as far as mental illness is concerned.[38] Many ethnic minority women prefer to consult with female doctors and, in order to overcome communication difficulties, female doctors with the same ethnic minority background as themselves.[39]

Indicators of socioeconomic position only partially account for the social disadvantage faced by ethnic minority groups. Other forms of social disadvantage might also affect their health. As described above, racism is a common feature of the lives of ethnic minority people. As well as having an indirect effect on health by influencing socioeconomic position, racism could affect health in two further ways. First, ethnic minority people will have a clear recognition of the relative disadvantage they face as a result of the discrimination and racism they experience. This sense of relative disadvantage might have a significant impact on health.[40] Second, experiencing racism and harassment might have a direct effect on health.[41]

The specific geographical locations of ethnic minority people might also be an important source of relative social disadvantage and contribute to ethnic inequalities in health. There is a growing body of evidence showing the importance of geographical effects and how they might operate,[42] and, as described above, it is also clear that ethnic minority people are more likely to be found in the most 'unhealthy' areas of England. However, the concentration of ethnic minority people in particular areas might also be protective of health, by improving levels of social support and a sense of community.[43]

Genetic differences between ethnic groups may also be important. Some diseases, such as haemoglobinopathies, are clearly related to genetic factors that vary across, but are not exclusive to, particular ethnic groups. There are also research programmes investigating whether more common diseases, such as diabetes, CHD and hypertension, are influenced by genetic factors that vary across ethnic groups.[44] Although biological markers have been found, such as insulin resistance syndrome and waist-to-hip ratios, it is not clear whether these are a consequence of genetic differences or environmental effects.

Finally, of course, cultural differences might contribute to ethnic variations in health in a number of ways, but most importantly through influencing health-related behaviours. Patterns of smoking and drinking have been shown to vary across ethnic groups, and the differences in patterns of smoking have been shown to make a major contribution to ethnic differences in the reporting of respiratory symptoms.[45] Unfortunately, beyond smoking and drinking, there has been very little coverage of health behaviours and beliefs in the epidemiological data. This is largely because of the limitations of available data sources, which will be discussed in the next section. Consequently, to date, discussion of ethnic variations in these factors have been largely based on speculation. Health behaviours and beliefs are, of course, the focus of this volume, but it is important to remember that culture is not static, and that health behaviours are influenced by other factors as well, such as gender and class.[46]

Sources of data on ethnicity and health

The dominance of the descriptive epidemiological approach to work on ethnic health differences must be understood in the light of the type of data that has, to date, been available to researchers. The most influential work has been based on immigrant mortality statistics derived from national data sets. Country of birth is recorded on death certificates and has also been recorded in the decennial census, allowing an investigation of differences in mortality rates by both cause of death and country of birth.[47] Of course there are some problems with the interpretation of these data,[48] not least that they contain no explanatory variables beyond occupational class as recorded on death certificates so they can do little more than describe variations in mortality rates. Also, if our concern is with the health of the population, mortality rates are a very crude indication of this complex multi-dimensional concept.

More recently, additional sources of data that contain more explanatory power to explore ethnic inequalities in health have become available. The 1991 Census, in addition to the question on self-assigned ethnic group, also included a question on the presence of a long-standing limiting illness. So far there has been little analysis of these data, although some is presented in one report.[49] Nevertheless, the Sample of Anonymised Records, which contains full Census data for 2% of the population, allows for a detailed investigation of responses to the question on long-standing limiting illness. The main limitation of these data is their restriction to only one assessment of health. This may be partly overcome by the routine and systematic collection of data on the ethnicity of patients admitted to hospital, introduced on 1 April 1996, which can be related back to population data derived from the Census, although there may be some problems with this process.[50] Additional problems with such data are that they reflect only the small hospital-treated proportion of those who are ill, a proportion that may well vary according to ethnicity. In addition, other factors of possible interest, such as socio-economic position, are not being collected alongside ethnicity.

There have also been three national surveys containing data on the health of ethnic minority people, and a fourth, the Health Survey for England 1999, is currently under-way. Among these surveys the *Fourth National Survey*[51] and the forthcoming Health Survey for England have retained a traditional focus on disease and illness. As such they supplement existing mortality data with their focus on morbidity and by containing more material on possible explanatory factors. However, they still contain limited data on health behaviours and beliefs. So, while they can tell us much about the epidemiology of particular diseases and associated risk factors, they tell us little or nothing about health beliefs and health behaviours, and only a little about the use of health services.

In contrast, the two Health Education Authority surveys on the health and lifestyles of black and minority ethnic groups, together with the Health Education Authority survey of Chinese people,[52] uniquely cover such topics as diet, exercise and both the smoking and chewing of tobacco. They thus provide us with crucial and unique information on a range of health behaviours, health beliefs, health promotion issues and health care use for several ethnic minority groups in Britain. This volume reports on the initial analysis of the second Health Education Authority survey of black and minority ethnic groups. The data provided help us take an important step forward in addressing the need to explore the potentially complex interrelationships between the structural, cultural and biological factors involved in the aetiology of particular diseases.

Notes

1. D. Coleman and J. Salt, *Ethnicity in the 1991 Census: volume 1, Demographic characteristics of the ethnic minority populations* (HMSO, London, 1996); C. Peach, *Ethnicity in the 1991 Census: volume 2, The ethnic minority populations of Great Britain* (HMSO, London, 1996); P. Ratcliffe, *Ethnicity in the 1991 Census: volume 3, Social geography and ethnicity in Britain: geographical spread, spatial concentration and internal migration* (HMSO, London, 1996); V. Karn, *Ethnicity in the 1991 Census: volume 4, Employment, education and housing among the ethnic minority populations of Britain* (HMSO, London, 1997).

2. T. Modood, R. Berthoud, and J. Lakey *et al.*, *Ethnic minorities in Britain: diversity and disadvantage* (Policy Studies Institute, London, 1997).

3. Peach, *The ethnic minority populations of Great Britain*.

4. Office of Population Censuses and Surveys, *Undercoverage in Great Britain (census user guide no. 58)* (HMSO, London, 1994); Peach, *The ethnic minority populations of Great Britain* (HMSO, London, 1996).

5. D. Owen, 'Ethnic minorities in Great Britain: settlement patterns', *National Ethnic Minority Data Archive 1991 Census Statistical Paper no. 1* (Centre for Research in Ethnic Relations, University of Warwick, 1993); D. Owen, 'Spatial variations in ethnic minority groups populations in Great Britain', *Population Trends* 78 (1994): 23–33.

6. Owen, 'Ethnic minorities in Great Britain: settlement patterns'.

7. D. Owen, 'Ethnic minorities in Britain: age and gender structure', *National Ethnic Minority Data Archive 1991 Census Statistical Paper no. 2* (Centre for Research in Ethnic Relations, University of Warwick, 1992).

8. Coleman and Salt, *Demographic characteristics of the ethnic minority populations*.

9. R. Berthoud and S. Beishon, 'People, families and households', in T. Modood, R. Berthoud and J. Lakey *et al.*, *Ethnic minorities in Britain: diversity and disadvantage* (Policy Studies Institute, London, 1997).

10. Modood, Berthoud and Lakey *et al.*, *Ethnic minorities in Britain*.

11. Peach, *The ethnic minority populations of Great Britain*.

12. Modood, 'Employment', in Modood, Berthoud and Lakey *et al.*, *Ethnic minorities in Britain*.

13. R. Berthoud, 'Income and standards of living', in Modood, Berthoud and Lakey *et al.*, *Ethnic minorities in Britain*.

14. S. Virdee, 'Racial harassment', in Modood, Berthoud and Lakey *et al.*, *Ethnic minorities in Britain*.

15. Virdee, 'Racial harassment', p. 278.

16. Modood, 'Employment', in Modood, Berthoud and Lakey *et al.*, *Ethnic minorities in Britain*.

17. Virdee, 'Racial harassment'.

18. Summaries of current work can be found in R. Balarajan and V. Soni Raleigh, *Ethnicity and health in England* (HMSO, London, 1995), which relates work on ethnic variations in health to the then Health of the Nation targets; C. Smaje, *Health, race and ethnicity: making sense of the evidence* (King's Fund Institute, London, 1995), which provides a comprehensive overview of the existing state of affairs in research on health and ethnicity; W.I.U. Ahmad, *Race and health in contemporary Britain* (Open University Press, Buckingham, 1993), and D. Kelleher and S. Hillier, *Researching cultural differences in health* (Routledge, London, 1996), both edited volumes that give a critical perspective on several of the key issues in this area; and M.G. Marmot, A.M. Adelstein, L. Bulusu, *Immigrant mortality in England and Wales, 1970–78: causes of death by country of birth* (HMSO, London, 1984), a classic epidemiological study of ethnicity and health that has provided the model followed by many others.

19. K. Rudat, *Health and lifestyles: black and minority ethnic groups in England.* (Health Education Authority, London, 1994); J.Y. Nazroo, *The health of Britain's ethnic minorities: findings from a national survey* (Policy Studies Institute, London, 1997); J.Y. Nazroo, *Ethnicity and mental health: findings from a national community survey* (Policy Studies Institute, London, 1997).

20. For example, S. Harding and R. Maxwell, 'Differences in mortality of migrants', in F. Drever and M. Whitehead (eds.), *Health inequalities: decennial supplement series DS No. 15* (Stationery Office, London, 1997); S. Wild and P. McKeigue, 'Cross sectional analysis of mortality by country of birth in England and Wales', *British Medical Journal* 314 (1997): 705–10.

21. Harding and Maxwell, 'Differences in mortality of migrants'.

22. For a comprehensive review of ethnic variations in disease, see Balarajan and Soni Raleigh, *Ethnicity and health in England*; and C. Smaje, *Health, race and ethnicity*.

23. See also J.Y. Nazroo, 'Genetic, cultural or socio-economic vulnerability? Explaining ethnic inequalities in health', *Sociology of Health and Illness* 20(5) (1998): 710–30.

24. Marmot, Adelstein and Bulusu, *Immigrant mortality in England and Wales, 1970–78*.

25. Harding and Maxwell, 'Differences in mortality of migrants'.

26. Nazroo, *The health of Britain's ethnic minorities*.

27. Harding and Maxwell, 'Differences in mortality of migrants'.

28. Nazroo, 'Genetic, cultural or socio-economic vulnerability?'.

29. Nazroo, *The health of Britain's ethnic minorities*.

30. Nazroo, 'Genetic, cultural or socio-economic vulnerability?'.

31. S.J. Gilliam, B. Jarman, P. White and R. Law, 'Ethnic differences in consultation rates in urban general practice', *British Medical Journal* 299 (1989): 953–7.

32. F. Badger, K. Atkin and R Griffiths, 'Why don't general practitioners refer their disabled Asian patients to district nurses', *Health Trends* 21 (1989): 31–2.

33. N. Shaukat, D.P. de Bono and J.K Cruikshank, 'Clinical features, risk factors and referral delay in British patients of Indian and European origin with angina', *British Medical Journal* 307 (1993): 717–18.

34. Y. Ben Shlomo, H. Rai and N. Chaturvedi, 'Lay diagnosis and health care seeking behaviour for chest pain in South Asians and Europeans in London', *Journal of Epidemiology and Community Health* 5 (1997), abstract.

35. N. Shaukat, J. Lear, S. Fletcher, D.P. de Bono and K.L. Woods, 'First myocardial infarction in patients of Indian subcontinent and European origin: comparison of risk factors, management and long term outcome', *British Medical Journal* 314 (1997): 639–42.

36. Rudat, *Health and lifestyles: black and minority ethnic groups in England.*

37. Nazroo, *The health of Britain's ethnic minorities;* Rudat, *Health and lifestyles: black and minority ethnic groups in England.*

38. Nazroo, *Ethnicity and mental health.*

39. Nazroo, *The health of Britain's ethnic minorities;* Rudat, *Health and lifestyles: black and minority ethnic groups in England.*

40. R.G. Wilkinson, *Unhealthy societies: the afflictions of inequality* (Routledge, London, 1996).

41. M. Benzeval, K. Judge and M. Solomon, *The health status of Londoners* (King's Fund Institute, London, 1992).

42. S. MacIntyre, S. MacIver and A. Soomans, 'Area, class and health: should we be focusing on places or people?', *Journal of Social Policy* 22(2) (1993): 213–34; A. Sloggett and H. Joshi, 'Higher mortality in deprived areas: community or personal disadvantage', *British Medical Journal* 309 (1994): 1470–74.

43. D. Halpern, 'Minorities and mental health', *Social Science and Medicine* 36(5) (1993): 597–607; C. Smaje, 'Ethnic residential concentration and health: evidence for a positive effect?', *Policy and Politics* 23(3) (1995): 251–69.

44. Wild and McKeigue, 'Cross sectional analysis of mortality by country of birth in England and Wales'.

45. Nazroo, *The health of Britain's ethnic minorities*; Rudat, *Health and lifestyles: black and minority ethnic groups in England*.

46. Nazroo, 'Genetic, cultural or socio-economic vulnerability?'.

47. Marmot, Adelstein and Bulusu, *Immigrant mortality in England and Wales, 1970–78*; R. Balarajan and L. Bulusu, 'Mortality among immigrants in England and Wales, 1979–83', in M. Britton (ed.), *Mortality and geography: a review in the mid-1980s, England and Wales* (OPCS, London, 1990); R. Balarajan, 'Ethnicity and variations in the nation's health', *Health Trends* 27(4) (1996): 114–19; Harding and Maxwell, 'Differences in mortality of migrants'; Wild and McKeigue, 'Cross sectional analysis of mortality by country of birth in England and Wales'.

48. Nazroo, 'Genetic, cultural or socio-economic vulnerability?'.

49. K. Dunnell, *Sources and nature of ethnic health data* (North East and North West Thames RHA, London, 1993).

50. P. Aspinall, 'Department of Health's requirements for mandatory collection of data on ethnic group inpatients', *British Medical Journal* 311 (1995): 1006–9.

51. Nazroo, *The health of Britain's ethnic minorities*; Nazroo, *Ethnicity and mental health*.

52. K. Sprotson, L. Pitson, G. Whitfield and E. Walker, *Health and lifestyles of the Chinese population in England* (Health Education Authority, London, 1999).

1   Background to the survey

Since the inception of the National Health Service in 1948, the practice of medicine and the role of health promotion services, has changed dramatically. So indeed has the state of the nation's health and the priorities attached to it. In the same period, and connected in some ways to these changes, there has been a significant shift in the cultural and demographic profile of the nation. The presence of significant numbers of people whose parents and families trace their recent personal histories to Asia, Africa and the Caribbean have consequences for health policy, and for the practice of health promotion.[1] However, as Bhopal has observed, while there has been in Britain as in America and elsewhere a blossoming of the study of 'ethnic health issues', few of these have led to significant benefits to members of the black and minority ethnic groups living in British communities.[2]

More recently, there has been a growing recognition that, for the majority of the black and minority ethnic population, 'common diseases occur commonly', and that they have similar health needs to those of the majority population – but often expressed or mediated in distinctive ways. Furthermore, even where those differences are *not* apparent, there is sometimes an assumption that difference must exist, and therefore their needs go unrecognised and unmet, awaiting 'special provision'.[3] It should not be necessary to demonstrate inequality (or variation) in health before attention is paid to the needs of people from minority ethnic backgrounds. It was therefore significant that the 1991 report of the chief medical officer[4] laid stress on the variations in disease patterns found in differing ethnic groups, and commented on the need for an information base on which to built an appropriate evidence-based practice of medicine. This signalled the start of a wider initiative in the early 1990s under the banner of the 'Health of the Nation', which, while concentrating upon five key areas of national importance, did take pains to spell out and subsequently to explore in greater detail the relevance of these key areas for minority ethnic groups.[5] Subsequent attention has been focused upon the existence of health inequalities. Associated with the drive towards a more scientific practice of both curative and preventive health work was the conduct of a number of studies – notably the Allied Dunbar national survey of health and fitness (ADNFS[6]) and the Health Survey for England (HSE[7]). However, the former, while collecting a unique picture of the average Briton's physical fitness and activity levels, was conducted in constituencies of which possibly only one had more than the national average proportion of minority ethnic adults. It was unable to present any analyses of its data by 'ethnic group'. Similarly, the series of surveys conducted under the rubric of the HSE has so far also been notable for its failure to present such analyses.

Subsequently, the Health Education Authority (HEA) has taken steps to remedy the lacunae in its information base, both through the setting up of databases on health-related resources for black and minority ethnic groups, conducting workshops and specific research relating to particular health issues, and a major survey of health and lifestyle information linked to and complementing its own general population surveys. These specialised surveys have confirmed the existence of significant inequalities in health and access to health provision, and provide a major tool for the assault upon those inequalities. An earlier volume[8] reported on the first of these, which concentrated mostly upon the key areas of health information knowledge and attitudes towards lifestyle change, smoking and sexual health, cancer and psycho-social health, and service use. Particular attention was paid to establishing people's priorities, their experience of health promotion activity and relevant social and environmental data, including of course their education, language, literacy, religion and other materials relevant to an understanding of the 'meaning' of ethnic identity. The main area of 'health behaviour' investigated was that of smoking: there was relatively little attention in that study to issues of physical activity.

This volume reports on a second national survey of black and minority ethnic groups that was conducted in 1994 and designed to complement the first. It concentrated on issues relevant to circulatory disorders (including diabetes) which have been shown to have the major effect on morbidity and mortality among these populations, and to be prime concerns of people in these groups. The survey also provides further information on the characteristics of the people who make up the black and minority ethnic group communities of Britain. In particular, we are able to give more detailed analysis of issues of demography, language and religion, in keeping with the findings of the Policy Studies Institute that more attention needs to be given to differences between minority ethnic groups. It should be noted that these are changing, as indeed the data demonstrate, particularly by reference to the only previous national source of relevant data in the

1991 national census of population. Also, we should insist that, while there may be certain groups which do form distinctive communities, the reality is that even within a carefully defined 'ethnic group', such as Bangladeshi or 'African-Caribbean', there are a series of communities with their own priorities and networks. This point is well explored in the only other comparable set of survey-based analyses, deriving from the fourth national survey of the Policy Studies Institute in 1993–4. Previous rounds of that exercise did not collect information on health, but concentrated on the then more pressing issues of employment and housing. The most recent, however, reports on health and welfare issues in much greater detail than its predecessors, and should be seen as complementing the work of the HEA in this study.[9] The survey did not include a 'white comparison' sample, and we have not in general attempted to compare these data with that for the general population, because of the dangers inherent in attempting to compare data collected in different ways. Like should be compared with like, in methodological terms, since differences in sampling, phrasing or context can create artefactual differences in the pattern of replies to any survey questions.

1.1 A note on terminology

 There is an extensive literature debating issues and terminology relating to 'race', ethnicity and culture. We have chosen to use the term 'minority ethnic group' as a shorthand phrase that encapsulates the experience of social differentiation on the grounds of 'race', cultural difference and religion. In general this refers to black and minority ethnic communities and groups largely of African-Caribbean and Asian origin, including also those of South-East Asian origin. Where appropriate, the more specific term is used, using the 1991 Census 'ethnic group question' definitions as a standard. In general, we have accepted the terminology used in the survey, when respondents were asked, 'How would you describe your race or ethnic origin' (Q197) and the answers were recorded and coded as given. For clarity of analysis, however, we have used somewhat fewer categories, grouping these responses in such a way as to resemble more closely the groups used in the 1991 Census. We recognise that there is considerable heterogeneity within any such socio-political grouping, although minority ethnic group concerns are generally considered together because of shared experiences of racism, labelling or marginalisation. Equally, the 'white' sector of society is marked by diversity and contains groups who may suffer discrimination or have particular cultural and linguistic needs: Welsh and Irish concerns have been explicitly noted. The term 'minority' perhaps refers more to an overall societal situation: in certain local cases black or Asian groups may form a majority, but they rarely enjoy political or institutional control. We use the term 'culture' to refer to the combination of a number of 'rules for living' or means of expressing identity, which may be related to a variety of elements, including language, diet, religion and a shared heritage of 'common knowledge'.

Notes

1. M.R.D. Johnson, 'Towards racial equality in health and welfare: what progress?', *New Community* 15(1) (1987): 128–35.

2. R.S. Bhopal, 'Future research on the health of ethnic minorities: back to basics', *Ethnic Minorities Health: A Current Awareness Bulletin* 1(3) (1990): 1–3.

3. M. Cross, M. Johnson and B. Cox, *Black welfare and local government* (Centre for Research in Ethnic Relations, University of Warwick, Coventry, 1988).

4. K. Calman, *On the state of the public health: the annual report of the Chief Medical Officer of the Department of Health for the year 1991* (HMSO, London, 1992).

5. R. Balarajan and V.S. Raleigh, *Ethnicity and health: a guide for the NHS* (Department of Health, London, 1993).

6. Health Education Authority and Sports Council, *Allied Dunbar National Fitness Survey* (London, 1992).

7. Joint Health Surveys Unit, Social and Community Planning Research, Department of Epidemiology and Public Health, University College London, *Health Survey for England 1994* (London, 1996). The one element (Table 7.2) in this report of the 1993–4 surveys which does distinguish between 'white' and 'non-white' respondents amalgamates the rich diversity of South Asian, African-Caribbean and other cultures and culinary traditions to examine possible variation in eating habits.

8. K. Rudat, *Health and lifestyles: black and minority ethnic groups in England.* (Health Education Authority, London, 1994).

9. C. Brown, *Black and white Britain* (Policy Studies Institute, London, 1984); T. Modood *et al.*, *Ethnic minorities in Britain: diversity and disadvantage* (Policy Studies Institute, London, 1997). Note especially Chapter 7 by James Nazroo, pp. 224–58; J.Y. Nazroo, *The health of Britain's ethnic minorities* (Policy Studies Institute, London, 1997).

...development work undertaken by the fieldwork company ...before the first HEA survey of black and minority ethnic groups in England are laid out in the 1994 report of that work.[1] Much of the experience gained on that exercise was also utilised in the second survey reported here. In particular the value of the community consultation and qualitative input to the design of the survey should not be underestimated. It was clear that there were many issues of concern to members of the communities with whom these discussions took place, and equally that it was impossible to cover all of them in sufficient depth in a single survey. The HEA therefore decided to commission a second, complementary survey to address these issues in the light of appropriate epidemiological and clinical evidence. In particular, the second survey focuses more upon issues of 'healthy behaviour' and physical activity rather than on 'health beliefs' and use of health care services. Some questions on health beliefs and knowledge were involved, insofar as they related to physical activity, diet and heart disease. We have not included the full details of the survey methodology here, but these are available from the HEA, and the questionnaire is provided in the appendix. Chapter 3 gives more details of the socio-economic profile of the population: details on the sampling and response rate are given at the end of this chapter. Information on the weights applied to the sample described in Section 3.2, on p.21.

2.1 The areas of enquiry

It is well established that there are higher rates of diabetes and coronary heart disease amongst people of South Asian origin living in Britain. During the qualitative consultative phase of the first survey, it became clear that this fact was both known and a matter of concern to members of those groups. However, there is some interest from a clinical perspective, since at least certain research investigations at local or small scale have suggested that different factors affect the prevalence of these conditions amongst people of Asian origin, when compared to the white majority. The importance of heart disease and related conditions was highlighted at the time, in the context of the 'Health of the Nation' initiative.[2] There is also growing evidence that not only are the 'types' of disease different between ethnic groups (for example, the prevalence of non-insulin dependent diabetes mellitus [NIDDM]) but the course and specific risk factors associated with a disease may differ also between ethnic groups.[3] In particular, it is well known that the principal risk factors for these conditions generally include the amount of fat (particularly saturated fats) in the diet, cigarette smoking, physical activity and being 'overweight'. Given the religious prohibition of smoking among Sikhs, and possibly other cultural predispositions, it has not been surprising to observe relatively low levels of smoking in Asian populations overall, as was indeed shown in the 1991–2 survey. However, there was virtually no firm evidence on the levels of fat in the diet beyond the anecdotal and possibly flawed observation of 'public' eating in restaurants and at community or family festival occasions.

Similarly, although there may be some conclusions drawn from the occupational profile of minority ethnic groups about the probability of their working in demanding physical occupations,[4] there was at that stage no data which could inform a discussion about levels of physical activity and exercise. Many of these observations also apply to the African-Caribbean population, which also displays a high risk of NIDDM, much higher mortality from stroke and raised levels of hypertension. It was therefore seen as appropriate that the second survey should focus upon the risk factors most closely associated with these conditions and on collecting data that would complement the information on physical activity and exercise contained in the Allied Dunbar and HSE surveys. These would cover not only 'behaviour' but also knowledge and attitudes, to facilitate the design and use of suitable strategies and materials for intervention to tackle the known clinical problems. It was intended that this information would feed into policy and practice at all levels and also be useful for individual practitioners as well as those responsible at a more strategic level for commissioning and purchasing health care and health education. The decision was also taken that the survey would confine itself to the main groups identified and covered by the first survey, rather than seeking to extend its coverage to smaller groups, such as those of Chinese, Vietnamese or more recent refugee origins.

2.2 Defining terms and information to be (

One of the main problems experienced by   ·he
issues of 'race' and ethnicity is the selection   ies
which are meaningful and acceptable to those ᵥ   ... who have to apply
the findings.⁵ Frequently this requires the application of a number of compromises, not the least
because of the need to map the findings of the research to those of other data sources, including
the national census. That, based on extensive pre-consultation and piloting, adopted a relatively
simple (though not uncontested) set of categories, which mixed 'race' (in the sense of colour of
skin or phenotypical appearance, e.g. 'White'), nationality ('Bangladeshi') and geographical area
of origin ('African-Caribbean', relating, in most cases, to family origins rather than individuals).
The second HEA survey, however, adopted the strategy of recognising that such a taxonomy
accounts for only part of a person's identity and cultural repertoire, and additional questions
explored such issues as religion, language and birthplace. While the majority of the description in
this report is performed using the standard 'ethnic group' category, data relating to the other
dimensions are available for further analysis, and have been reported on when they can be seen
to have particular relevance to the analyses described.

Ethnic groups

Following established 'best practice', all respondents were asked to indicate their own personal
definition of their ethnic origin, and these were recorded without prompting, using precodes
derived from earlier fieldwork (such as Black British, Sylheti and East African Asian) or writing
in the verbatim replies of any not covered by one of these. Subsequently, for the purposes of
comparison, these have been mapped back on the basis of internal evidence to one of the four
major groupings recognised by the census and used in most published analyses. In this, we have
followed as far as possible the procedures adopted by the census.⁶ When used in this report,
therefore, the terms carry no implications for nationality and are used in the inclusive sense
adopted for the Office of National Statistics.⁷ African-Caribbean people are those who were born
in, or have recent family forebears in, the West Indies (including mainland territories, such as
Guyana) and more distant connections with the African continent, but excludes the (significant)
number of people of European ('White') or Asian origins with similar migration histories as well
as those whose families may have come more directly to Britain from Africa. Equally, Indian,
Pakistani and Bangladeshi are terms used to describe people who have recognisable connections
with the Indian subcontinent, including those who may have described themselves as of 'East
African' origin, such as those whose families left Tanzania, Kenya and Uganda following the
events associated with decolonisation and 'Africanisation': the 'twice migrants'.⁸

Physical measurements

Since a primary focus of the study was on conditions associated with physique ('overweight' and
'fitness'), it was clearly necessary to incorporate a number of physical measurements of the
respondents as well as questions on exercise, activity level and 'body image'. Where possible,
discussion was held with those responsible for the ADNFS and terms and questions used which
were compatible with those datasets. In particular, attention was paid to selecting suitable
measurements of respondents bodies which could be carried out without extensive specialised
training (the ADNFS used mobile clinics with nursing staff) and which would not be offensive to
the survey populations, but would give useful information. Epidemiological evidence has
established that it is not simply the weight of an individual, but also the relationship of this to
height, and the disposition of fat on the body, which affect propensity to coronary heart disease.
The standard method of assessing obesity or degree of overweight is the formula used to derive
'Body Mass Index' (BMI) – the weight (in kilograms) divided by the square of the height (in
metres). However, while this is useful, particularly for comparative purposes, it was felt not to be
adequate. Researchers⁹ have observed a distinctive pattern of weight gain found in many people
of South Asian origin, termed 'central pattern obesity', where excess body fat is accumulated
around the waist rather than on the hips and thighs. This is thought to be associated with the
variation observed in heart disease. Similarly, the ratio of waist measurement to hip circumference
is also noted to relate to CHD risk levels. Other possible measures, such as respiratory and
exercise tests, were felt to be excessively intrusive and costly to replicate in this survey and were
therefore excluded. Details of the measurements taken, and the method used to standardise them,
are given in Section 2.4.

Consistency with the first HEA survey

As stated, a primary concern of the study was to ensure comparability and consistency. This meant that in most respects the methodology, including the training of the field force interviewers, followed the same principles established for the previous HEA study, whose fieldwork was carried out in 1991–2, before the results of the 1991 Census were available. As in that survey, it was felt necessary to provide translated versions of the questionnaires, and this time it was also possible to draw upon the experience and data collected in that exercise. The languages selected for translation were again Gujerati, Punjabi in the Gurmukhi script,[10] Bengali and Urdu, paying attention to the need to distinguish between classical versions of these latter languages and the spoken varieties in use by most communities in the UK. Most people of Bangladeshi origin in the UK (but not all) speak Sylheti, which resembles but is different from the Bengali spoken in India and Dhaka. Sylheti does not have a written form, although many people educated in Bangladesh (less often their children brought up in the UK) are familiar with the standard variety. Advice was taken to ensure that the translated questionnaires used terms which would be familiar to Sylheti speakers, but which could also be understood by people from the Indian state of West Bengal. In the homes of Pakistani Punjabis (sometimes referred to as Kashmiris[11]) interviewers supplemented the Urdu version of the questionnaire with Punjabi as required. Translations were cross-checked between agency and community-based agencies. While the use of Patois and Caribbean dialects was allowed for in the information-gathering exercise, it was assumed that, as in the previous survey, people of African-Caribbean origin would be happy to be interviewed in English.

Questions included in the survey were also, when possible, chosen to be comparable with those asked in other national surveys, such as the ADNFS and HSE. These do not always exactly correspond with each other, and, where there was a choice of questions, compatibility with the previous HEA Health and Lifestyle Survey was given priority.

2.3 Piloting

The questionnaires were piloted in various locations among all the target ethnic groups. Separate versions of the questionnaires had to be drawn up for African-Caribbean and South Asian groups, since certain questions (notably on language and diet) needed to be more closely focused in each major sub-category. For the majority of questions, almost identical coding schemes were adopted to facilitate comparison of the two datasets. It would, however, have been cumbersome to have attempted to phrase such questions as, 'It is too much trouble to try to cook traditional West Indian foods all the time' (Q62) in a totally inclusive fashion: other habits, such as the habitual use of 'betel' or 'paan' (see Chapter 6), are effectively confined to people of South Asian origin.

Two pilots were conducted, the first one in January 1994 and a supplementary one in March of the same year, to check the effectiveness of the alterations made. The main pilot tested both the appropriateness of question wording and respondent understanding of technical, clinical or medical terms, and also the time taken to conduct the interviews. Measurement of height, weight, hip and waist was also piloted for acceptability and to test the suitability and functioning of the equipment. Pilots were carried out in areas indicated by the 1991 Census as likely to contain high concentrations of the target ethnic groups, the interviewers themselves screening addresses to find suitable respondents matched by gender. The Gujerati and Bengali versions were tested in London and Birmingham, the Punjabi in the Leeds–Bradford conurbation, and the Urdu there and in Birmingham. Parallel tests in all these areas were conducted for the English version of the 'Asian' questionnaire, while the 'African-Caribbean' questionnaire was tested in London and Birmingham. The translated versions were produced as bilingual instruments with both the English and the translated language shown: show cards were also translated.

Results of the pilot exercise

A number of significant points did emerge from the pilots and were taken account of in the conduct of the main survey. In particular, show cards (displaying possible responses) were not a successful way of asking questions in communities where few respondents were able to read them. Literacy (in either English or 'mother tongue') could not be assumed, as noted in the first HEA survey. Where used, show cards had to be restricted to a short list of items (no more than eight). Equally, a number of technical medical terms were not widely understood, most notably by South Asian respondents. Many did not know the difference between a heart attack and a stroke, which have distinctive clinical patterns and causes, and equally the terms 'heart disease' and 'angina' were not widely understood. It should be remarked that these problems may not be confined to non-European minority ethnic groups: French-speaking students in Britain confuse 'angina' with the term 'l'angine' (the tonsil), and we have no data on the comprehension of these terms with a reference white group for England. Dietary terms, such as 'saturated fat' and 'dietary fibre', are equally problematic, even if increasingly used on packaging and in school home economics classes. Many such terms, which health educators and researchers use widely are understood only hazily and are difficult to translate into terms which would be widely understood in the relevant Asian languages.

2.4   Taking measurements

The issue of taking measurements met with a number of problems, notably the fact that the request came at the end of a long interview. Issues of modesty and embarrassment were encountered, especially when there were other people present in the room. It was felt that presenting people with reasons for the measurements, as well as shortening the interview, would help to overcome many of these barriers, although nothing much could be done about those who were sensitive about their weight or dimensions. Extra training was also given to interviewers to ensure that measurements were as standardised as possible, using the same equipment as the National Child Development Study and the procedures described for the HSE, with the difference that it was not possible to request respondents to modify the garments they were wearing (which might, indeed, have led to cultural problems). Interviewers, while not professional nurses (as in the HSE and ADNFS) were trained in the appropriate procedures by nurses and observed practising in groups (gender-matched, as in the case of all recorded measurements during the survey). Certain categories of respondent were excluded from measurement, notably those who were chair-bound or unsteady on their feet (their judgement being taken on this issue), and those who were pregnant or had a colostomy bag were also excluded from measurement of waist and hips (and weight, in the case of pregnancy).

Interviewers were instructed to take measurements on level, uncarpeted floors if possible or at least on the thinnest carpet available. Where this was not the case, a note was taken, and if the measurements were likely to be unreliable in the interviewer's judgement, the data has been excluded. Weight was measured using portable electronic scales (to the nearest 0.1 kg); height with a portable baseless stadiometer and sliding headpiece. Waist and hip measurements were taken using a plastic tape on a metal reel, and people wearing either very tight or baggy clothing were not included, although, if possible, respondents were asked to remove outer layers, such as jackets and jumpers, or restrictive items, such as belts and corsets. The definition of 'waist' used was standardised as the midpoint between lowest rib and top of hipbone: the hip as the widest circumference over the buttocks and below the hipbone. Both measurements were taken twice and an average struck.

2.5   Sampling

The survey could not be conducted using traditional random sampling techniques, since it is known that the residential patterns of minority ethnic groups in England are quite distinctive from those of the majority white population.[12] Given the difficulty of locating a representative sample of any minority population through standard sampling procedures, a multi-stage approach was adopted, as has been followed by the majority of national studies of minority ethnic groups.

Geographical sampling

All interviews were conducted at pre-selected addresses drawn at random from the 'Small Users Postcode Address File' (PAF) in those areas where the 1991 Census 'Small Area Statistics' identified the Enumeration District (ED) level data as containing 10% or more of the population from one of the target ethnic groups identified for the survey, that is, 'Black' (African-Caribbean) or 'Asian' (Indian, Pakistani, Bangladeshi or East African Asian). Four interlocking samples were drawn from this overall universe, one for each of the target ethnic groups. Each was based primarily on EDs where at least 10% of enumerated residents were from that ethnic group, but with varying penetrations of the other target ethnic groups. While some surveys in the past have used electoral registration files as a source of names and/or addresses, this technique has been superseded by the availability of the PAF data. Hence problems of electoral non-registration, believed to be greatest amongst ethnic minority and inner city populations, are thereby avoided.[13]

The overall sample consisted of 510 sampling points (post code areas). In each, a fixed number of addresses were derived at random: 75 addresses in 'points' within the 4 'Thames' regional health authorities (i.e. around Greater London) and 65 addresses from each of the other sampling point locations. All sampled addresses were then screened by MORI interviewers, who immediately eliminated all those identified as invalid for reasons of being non-residential, vacant or demolished. If no one could be contacted at an address, repeat calls were made at different times and on different days of the week over a period of time to ensure people who were away for short holidays or on business were not excluded.

Selection of households and individual respondents

Where multiple households were located at a single address, a standard random selection procedure (a Kish grid[14]) was used to select one of these. Selected households were subsequently screened for 'ethnicity'. The informant was asked whether the household contained people who were Caribbean/West Indian (including Guyanese), Indian, Pakistani, Bangladeshi, East African Asian or Sikh. Those described as 'Kenyan Asian' or 'Ugandan Asian' were included within the category of East African Asian. If the informant referred to people who were Black British, British Asian or of 'mixed race', interviewers were asked to probe further by asking if the parents of these individuals were from one of the ethnic groups listed, and the relevant parental origin was coded.

Where the household contained only people of European or other ethnic origins, the screening process was terminated. If households contained people from one or more of the target ethnic groups, a listing of all adults eligible to take part in the survey was compiled. These were defined as being 'household members aged 16–74, normally resident at the address and belonging to one of the target ethnic groups'. Households containing only people aged 75 or more were also eliminated from the survey. Respondents were then selected from those remaining, by use of a Kish grid (randomised) technique.

The identified respondent was asked to nominate their preferred language for interview. If these matched the skills of the interviewer (and the gender of respondent and interviewer also matched) an interview was conducted at that time, if the respondent agreed. If the respondent selected and the interviewer were of different genders, the interview could only proceed if they were accompanied by a supervisor of the appropriate gender, and the supervisor would then take the body measurements. Otherwise, a suitable time was noted for another interviewer to return and conduct the interview: these revisits were subjected to a secondary sampling process, in that when the target number of interviews was achieved within a health region (RHA), no further addresses for that category of language, ethnic group and/or gender were issued.

Of the 37,278 addresses which were drawn, a number had to be excluded from the survey either because there was no one living at the address (voids), no contact with a household member could be established or information was refused. Thus just over one in four addresses (27%) were rejected. Where households definitely contained at least one member of a target ethnic group, they were subject to the secondary sampling noted above, but might also be excluded on grounds of age or because key information was refused. As some respondents were ill, or had moved away when the interviewer returned, it was therefore impossible to establish their eligibility. Even when selected, households might be lost to the sample through refusal, ill health or other problems in making contact.

Addresses drawn		37 278	*Initial sample*
'Voids' (unoccupied)		4 752	13%
'No contact'		3 677	10%
Information refused		1 692	5%
Definitely contained one member of target ethnic group		9 436	25%
After secondary sampling		**6 683**	*Main sample*
Also excluded	All over 75	74	
	Information refused	135	
	No contact/ill	301	
Valid sample		**6 173**	*Final sample*
Interview refused		1 031	17%
No contact		689	11%
Successful interview		**4 452***	72%

*Eight cases were deleted in processing, due to incomplete data.

Figure 2.1: The sampling process

Breakdown of the sample and response rates

Interviews were conducted with 4452 respondents (at 72% of valid screened addresses): these comprised 1071 (60% of identified) African-Caribbean, 1063 (71%) Indian (including East African Asian), 1145 (79%) Pakistani, and 1173 (81%) Bangladeshi individuals. These figures, and other relevant data relating to the screening and interviewing process, are given in Figures 2.1 and 2.2. It can be seen that one reason for the apparent lower success rate in African-Caribbean households is the greater age of this population: while also slightly more likely to refuse household type information, they were no more likely than Indian (but twice as likely as Bangladeshis) to refuse to take part. They were, however, also very much more likely to be uncontactable, which again may be related to work patterns, although this is only speculation based upon previous research data on employment.[15] It will also be noted that two-thirds of interviews with Bangladeshi respondents, but only a third of those classified as 'Indian', were conducted in the 'mother tongue' of the respondent.

	African-Caribbean	Indian/East African	Pakistani	Bangladeshi
Identified	1 990	1 608	1 552	1 533
All over 75	46	14	4	10
Information on household type refused	70	26	24	15
Refused, ill, away or moved after initial contact	83	75	75	68
Valid address	1 791	1 493	1 449	1 440
Refusal	378	301	207	145
Non-contact	342	129	96	122
Successful interview	1 071	1 063	1 145	1 173
As percentage of available and eligible pursued	60%	71%	79%	81%
Conducted in language other than English	na	32%	49%	67%

Figure 2.2: Response rates and numbers of identified potential respondents

Notes

1. K. Rudat K, *Health and lifestyles: black and minority ethnic groups in England.* (Health Education Authority, London, 1994).

2. R. Balarajan and V.S. Raleigh, *Ethnicity and health: a guide for the NHS* (Department of Health, London, 1994). See also Chapter 5 of K. Calman, *On the state of the public health: the annual report of the Chief Medical Officer of the Department of Health for the year 1991* (HMSO, London, 1992).

3. C. Smaje, *Health, 'race' and ethnicity* (King's Fund Institute, London, 1995).

4. D. Owen, *Ethnic minorities in Great Britain: economic characteristics* (NEMDA 1991 Census Statistical Paper 3, University of Warwick, Coventry, 1993).

5. P.A. Senior and R. Bhopal, 'Ethnicity as a variable in epidemiological research', *British Medical Journal* 309 (1994): 327–30; K.J. McKenzie and N.S. Crowcroft, 'Race, ethnicity, culture and science', *British Medical Journal* 309 (1994): 286–7.

6. P.J. Aspinall, 'Department of Health's requirement for mandatory collection of data on ethnic group of inpatients', *British Medical Journal* 311 (1995): 1006–9.

7. The Office of National Statistics was formerly known as the Office of Population Census and Statistics (OPCS), responsible not only for the national census but also various specialised surveys.

8. See for example M. Mamdani, *From citizen to refugee: Ugandan Asians come to Britain* (Frances Pinter, London, 1973), or P. Bhachu, *Twice migrants: East African Sikh settlers in Britain* (Tavistock, London).

9. P.M. McKeigue, B. Shah and M.G. Marmot, 'Relation of central obesity and insulin resistance with high diabetes prevalence and cardiovascular risk in South Asians', *Lancet* 337 (1991): 382–6.

10. In this the survey followed the generally accepted practice of M. Stubbs (ed.), *The other languages of England: the linguistic minorities project* (Institute of Education/Routledge, London, 1985).

11. S. Imtiaz and M. Johnson, *Health care provision and the Kashmiri population of Peterborough* (NorthWest Anglia Health Authority and Peterborough Race Equality Council, Peterborough, 1993).

12. P. Ratcliffe, *Geographical spread, spatial concentration and internal migration* (ONS, London, 1996).

13. M.R.D. Johnson and M. Cross, *Surveying service users in multi-ethnic areas* (Centre for Research in Ethnic Relations, Warwick University, Coventry, 1984).

14. L. Kish, *Survey sampling* (John Wiley, Chichester, 1965).

15. T. Modood *et al.*, *Ethnic minorities in Britain: diversity and disadvantage* (Policy Studies Institute, London, 1997).

3 Characteristics of the survey population

Summary of the main findings

- There were 4452 valid observations in the sample, broadly evenly divided among the four ethnic groups.

- The raw data was weighted using a set of factors intended to make the age, sex and geographical distribution of each ethnic group yielded by the survey broadly match the characteristics of 1991 Census data for England.

- All four ethnic groups were on average younger than white people, though South Asian people were younger than African-Caribbean people, amongst whom the percentage of people aged over 50 was greatest.

- Household size was largest for Bangladeshi and Pakistani people and smallest for African-Caribbean people. There were more children present in South Asian, especially Pakistani and Bangladeshi, households than in African-Caribbean households.

- Except in the youngest age group, most South Asian people were married, but African-Caribbean people were more likely to be single, cohabiting or in a 'visiting' relationship.

- Minority ethnic groups were disadvantaged in the labour market, experiencing relatively high unemployment rates. Indian people were least disadvantaged and Bangladeshis most disadvantaged.

- Economic activity was highest for African-Caribbean and Indian people and lowest for Pakistani and Bangladeshi women, many of whom aged over 50 had never worked.

- Long-term unemployment was a severe problem, especially for older Pakistani and Bangladeshi men.

- Indian men were most likely to have high-status occupations. Skilled and semi-skilled manual occupations were the most common occupations across the four ethnic groups, but African-Caribbean women were particularly likely to work in associate professional jobs (such as nursing), while Bangladeshis tended to work in personal service (e.g. restaurant) occupations.

- Indians and Pakistanis displayed a very high level of home ownership, with African-Caribbean and Bangladeshi people more likely to be in social rented housing.

- The level of car ownership was highest for Indian and lowest for Bangladeshi people.

- The ability to speak and read English was greatest among Indians and least among Bangladeshis. Older Bangladeshi women had the lowest levels of ability in English.

- Younger people had a lower level of ability in South Asian languages than older people, and a higher proportion of young people stated that English was the language they understood best.

- Bangladeshi and Pakistani people were most likely to have been born outside the UK.

- Indian people were more likely to be highly qualified than the other three ethnic groups, while Bangladeshi people were least likely to have educational qualifications.

- Patterns of religious affiliation remained fairly stable across age groups within ethnic groups. Nearly all Pakistanis and Bangladeshis were Muslims, while Indians were split between Hinduism, Sikhism and Islam, with the latter greater among young people. African-Caribbeans were mainly Protestant or Catholic, but a larger percentage than for other ethnic groups had no religious faith.

3.1 Introduction

The 1994 HEA survey of black and minority ethnic group health in England yielded data for a total of 4452 individuals, categorised into four broad ethnic groups: African-Caribbean, Indian, Pakistani and Bangladeshi. This chapter describes the age and sex structure of the sample, key features of households and families, economic activity, social structure, country of birth, language ability, education and housing.

3.2 Weighting

The survey was collected using a clustered sampling strategy (rather than random sampling) for reasons of efficiency in contacting the target population. In order to draw inferences from analysis of the data that would have general applicability to the four minority ethnic groups, it was necessary to adjust the data through the application of a 'weight' to each individual case, with the aim of making the characteristics of the surveyed sample approximate to those of the ethnic group as a whole. A set of weights were created which adjusted the survey for bias due to household size, age structure and geographical distribution by calculating the ratio between the percentage breakdown of the sample on these dimensions with the percentage breakdown of the 1991 Census.[1] When producing weighted tabulations from the data, the contribution of each individual to the cell of the table in which it falls is the value of the survey weight (each individual has equal influence in unweighted tables). Since the weights are calculated for each ethnic group separately, the weighted data should not be aggregated across ethnic groups, because their relative sizes differ substantially from the population of England as a whole. Consequently, nowhere in this report are the four ethnic groups added to produce a total.

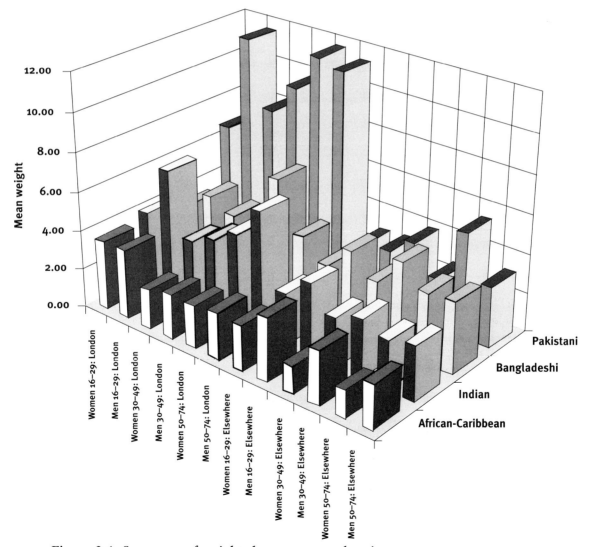

Figure 3.1: Summary of weights by age, sex and region

Figure 3.1 depicts the influence of the weighting procedure upon the survey data in a visual form, while the mean weights are reported in Table 3.1a, 3.1b in the Appendix. The height of the bars represents the mean survey weight for each individual by age group, sex and location within and outside Greater London. Overall, the size of the weights was greatest for the Pakistani ethnic group, and the most striking effect of the weighting procedure is to increase the influence of Pakistani observations in Greater London, indicating that Pakistanis were under-represented in the survey data relative to the census, particularly for men and people aged over 50. Older South Asian women and Indian men were also relatively under-represented in Greater London. The pattern of weights reveals that the sample was also biased towards young South Asian people outside Greater London, but that young people were under-represented in the African-Caribbean ethnic group to a greater degree in Greater London than elsewhere in England.

3.3 Age and sex structure

When weighted, the sample is broadly evenly divided between men and women in each of the four ethnic groups. However, women are in a small majority amongst African-Caribbean people, while the majority of Bangladeshis and Pakistanis interviewed were men. This broadly reflects the census data for these ethnic groups, since in 1991 the ratios of men per 1000 women were 892 for African-Caribbeans, 1003 for Indians, 1068 for Pakistanis and 1106 for Bangladeshis in the age range 16–74 years.

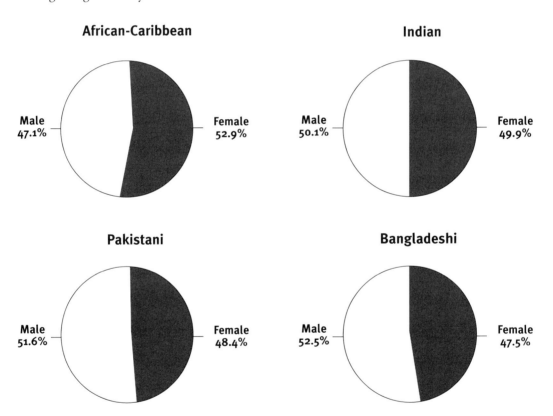

Figure 3.2: Sex breakdown of weighted survey data by ethnic group

The age structure of the weighted data is presented in Table 3.2a and depicted graphically in Figure 3.3. This demonstrates the relative youth of the Pakistani and Bangladeshi ethnic groups, for each of whom over two-fifths of people in the age range 16–74 were aged under 30, compared with just over a third of African-Caribbean and Indian people. In the South Asian ethnic groups, about a fifth of all people in the age range were aged over 50, contrasting with African-Caribbean people, more than a third of whom were aged over 50. This diagram also contrasts the age structure of the four minority ethnic groups with that of white people living in England, revealing that young people were more common and older people less common in the African-Caribbean and South Asian populations than in the white population. Some notable difference by sex are revealed. Women from both the Pakistani and Bangladeshi ethnic groups tended to be younger on average than men, while the percentage of men aged over 50 was particularly high for both the African-Caribbean and Bangladeshi ethnic groups.

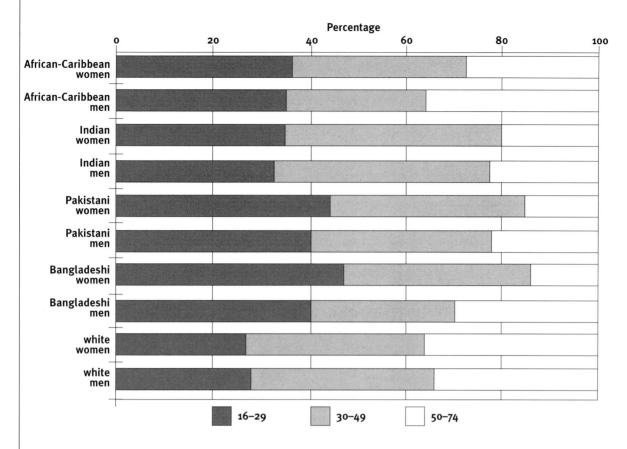

Percentage

| | 16–29 | 30–49 | 50–74 |

Figure 3.3: Age distribution by ethnic group and sex

3.4 Household size and organisation

As shown by Figure 3.4 (and Tables 3.3–3.5), there was a marked contrast in average household size between the African-Caribbean and South Asian ethnic groups, with Bangladeshi households on average containing about twice as many residents as African-Caribbean households. Bangladeshi households contained on average the largest number of residents, with Pakistani households larger than Indian households. South Asian households contained on average around one more adult than African-Caribbean households, and also more children. South Asian households differed in size mainly because of differences in the number of children (aged 0–5) living in a household. On average, there were twice as many children living in Bangladeshi households than were living in Indian households.

On average, younger respondents (both male and female) tended to live in larger households across all ethnic groups, with the oldest age group tending to live in the smallest households. However, older Pakistani and Bangladeshi men tended to live in much larger households than men and women from the other two ethnic groups, possibly indicating that these early migrants were living with other members of their family who had come to join them. The larger average household size for 30–49-year-olds reflects a greater likelihood that these households would contain children.

Contrasts in household size also reflect differences in marital status by sex and ethnic group (Table 3.6). There was a marked difference in the percentage of respondents married and single between African-Caribbean and South Asian people, which was greatest for 30–44-year-olds. Overall, around 70% of South Asians were married, double the corresponding percentage for African-Caribbeans, amongst whom over a third were single, compared with between a fifth and a quarter of South Asians (Figure 3.5). Differences in marital status were least among 16–29-year-olds, for whom the percentage single was very similar across all four ethnic groups (around 70%) for men, while around half of South Asian women, compared with 62% of African-Caribbean women were single. Among 30–44-year-olds, over a third of women and more than a fifth of men from the African-Caribbean ethnic group were still single, while almost no South Asians were single. Most South Asian people were either married or single, but the percentage widowed, separated or divorced increased with age. While very few South Asian men were in these states,

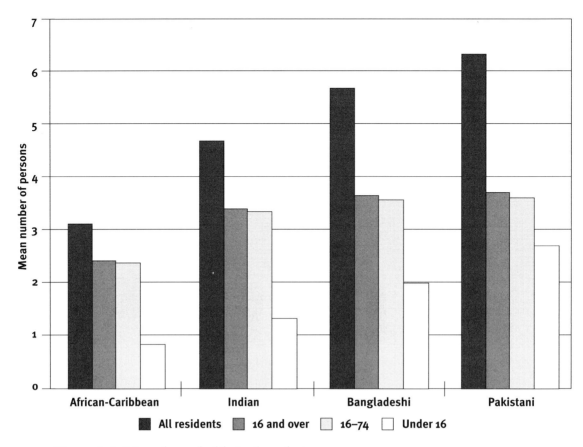

Figure 3.4: Mean household size by ethnic group

more than a fifth of Indian and over a quarter of Bangladeshi women aged over 50 were widows, largely accounting for the smaller percentage of women than men currently married in the oldest age group.

A substantial minority of African-Caribbean people were cohabiting or in a 'visiting' relationship, that is, with a regular partner, but not living with them. These states were more common for younger people, with cohabiting more common for men and visiting relationships more common for women for those aged 16–29 and 30–44. Marriage was more common for men than women amongst those aged 30 and over, while the percentage of single men was smaller than that for women (possibly a reflection of the much smaller number of men contacted by the survey). Marriage was most common for African-Caribbean people in the oldest age group, with over half of women and two-thirds of men married; the bulk of the remainder were widowed or divorced, with cohabitation and visiting relationships relatively rare.

Children were much more likely to be present in South Asian than in African-Caribbean households (Table 3.7), while women in all four ethnic groups were more likely than men to be living in households containing dependent children. The percentage living with dependent children was higher for 30–44-year-olds than 16–29-year-olds, but fell again for people aged over 50, most of whose children would have left the parental home. African-Caribbean and Indian women were less likely than Pakistani and Bangladeshi women to be living in households with dependent children, and African-Caribbean men were less likely than men or women from any of the South Asian ethnic groups to live in households containing dependent children. The percentage of people living with their own children was lowest in the youngest age group, in which most respondents were probably living with younger siblings, this percentage increasing for those aged 30–49, before falling for older people. In the South Asian ethnic groups, about half of women aged 16–29 living in households containing children had their own children, this share being slightly higher for African-Caribbean women, owing to the influence of smaller household size. A larger percentage of Pakistani and Bangladeshi women than African-Caribbean and Indian women lived with their own dependent children. In the youngest age group, dependent children were much more likely to be the offspring of female respondents than male respondents.

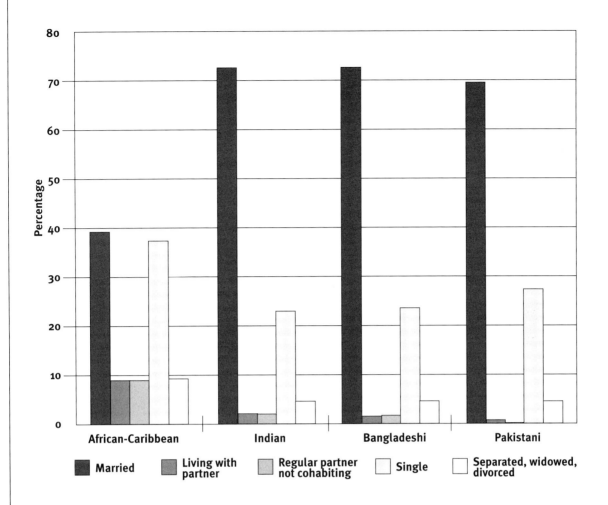

Figure 3.5: Marital status by ethnic group

Of those respondents with their own dependent children, Pakistani and Bangladeshi people had more children than Indian and African-Caribbean people, with 3.2 children per Bangladeshi mother on average, compared with 1.8 children for each African-Caribbean mother (Table 3.8). There was little difference in the mean age of youngest dependent children between ethnic groups (around 5 years of age) but the oldest dependent child was on average about 2 years older for Bangladeshi parents than African-Caribbean parents. Dependent children were on average therefore mainly of primary school age across all four ethnic groups. Bangladeshi and Pakistani women started bearing children earlier than African-Caribbean and Indian women, since women aged 16–29 from these ethnic groups had on average 0.5 more dependent children than women from the other two ethnic groups. People aged 30–49 had the largest number of dependent children, with Bangladeshi women in this age range having an average of about 4 dependent children, around twice as many as African-Caribbean and Indian women and one more than Pakistani women.

About three-quarters of African-Caribbean men were household heads themselves (Table 3.9), compared with nearly two-thirds of men from the South Asian ethnic groups. Nearly all the remaining South Asian men were sons or sons-in-law of the household head, and the percentage of men who reported that they were the partner of the household head was very small in each of the four ethnic groups. Figure 3.6 illustrates the marked contrast between the sexes, with half to two-thirds of South Asian women being partners of the household head, the remainder mainly being daughters or daughters-in-law of the household head, this percentage being much higher for Pakistani and Bangladeshi women than for Indian women. There was a substantial contrast between African-Caribbean and South Asian women, since only 29% of African-Caribbean women were partners of the household head, with half reporting that they were the household head, and a fifth reporting that a parent or parent-in-law was the household head.

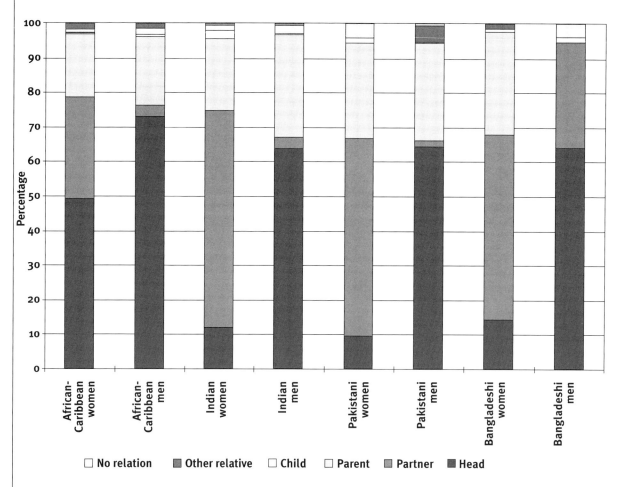

Figure 3.6: Relationship of household head to respondent by ethnic group

Relationship to the household head varies with age of the respondent. Between half and three-quarters of respondents aged 16–29 were the child or child-in-law of the household head, with a further third of African-Caribbeans in this age group themselves being the household head. In the 30–49 age group, the great majority of South Asian men were heads, with a similar percentage of South Asian women the head's partner. However, nearly two-thirds of African-Caribbean women in this age group were household heads. In the oldest age group, nearly all men regarded themselves as the household head, while the percentage of South Asian women who were household heads was larger than in the 30–49 age group, but this percentage fell relative to the younger age group for African-Caribbean women.

3.5   Economic status

Figure 3.7 summarises the economic activity of men and women from the four ethnic groups, classifying the population aged between 16 and 74 into those in work (either employees, self-employed or on government schemes), unemployed (including those waiting to start a job and temporarily sick) and the economically inactive (covering those in full-time education, permanently sick, retired or looking after a home or family full-time). Those in work and those unemployed together represent the economically active population. There were clearly substantial differences between ethnic groups and sexes in the degree to which they participated in the labour market. Indian men were most likely to be in work, and least likely to be economically inactive. Bangladeshi women lay at the other extreme (closely followed by Pakistani women), with a lower percentage in work or economically active than any other ethnic and sex grouping. African-Caribbean and Pakistani men were similar in having a slightly lower rate of economic activity than Indian men, but a much higher level of unemployment. Only about a third of Bangladeshi men were in work. Amongst women, African-Caribbeans displayed the greatest attachment to the labour market, with a higher percentage unemployed than Indian women.

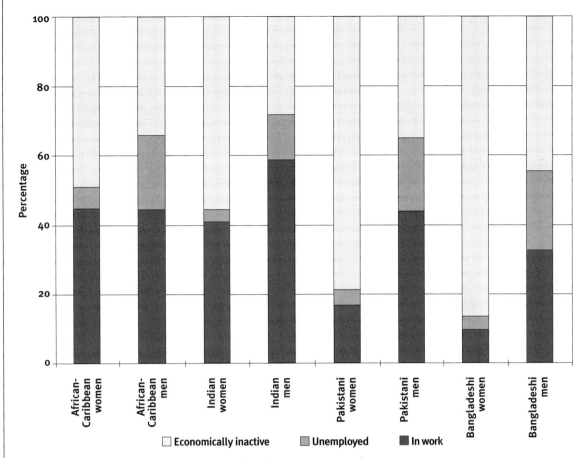

Figure 3.7: Economic status by ethnic group and sex

The unemployment rate (Figure 3.8) measures the percentage of the population who would like to work but cannot find a job. Unemployment rates for minority ethnic groups are typically at least double those for white people, though women from all ethnic groups tend to experience lower unemployment rates than men.[2] Also, young people tend to experience relatively high unemployment rates. Both features are represented in the pattern of unemployment rates by age, sex and ethnic group from the Black and Minority Ethnic Groups Survey (BMEG) data. Unemployment rates for women tended to be lower than those for men in each ethnic group and age group. Unemployment rates also declined with age in the majority of cases, the main exceptions being the exceptionally high unemployment rates faced by Pakistani and Bangladeshi men aged over 50 (of whom two-thirds were unemployed). For both men and women, Indians experienced the lowest unemployment rates, followed by African-Caribbean people, with Bangladeshi people suffering the highest unemployment rates.

The full details of economic activity by ethnic group, age and sex is reported in Table 3.10. This table highlights some important features of economic activity in these four minority ethnic groups. Men from the Indian ethnic group were the most likely to be in full-time work, followed by African-Caribbean men and women. Part-time employment was most important for African-Caribbean and Indian women, though it accounted for a larger share of the small number of Pakistani and Bangladeshi women in work and was relatively uncommon for men. Self-employment was much more common for South Asian than African-Caribbean men, with the South Asian self-employed more likely to have employees. A very small percentage of women were self-employed.

Around a tenth of people in the survey were in full-time education, mostly aged 16–29. Nearly two-fifths of Bangladeshi men and more than a third of Indian men aged 16–29 were students, with African-Caribbean and Pakistani men displaying the lowest rates of participation in full-time education. The percentage of young men who were students was higher than the corresponding percentage for women in all four ethnic groups, of whom between a fifth and a quarter of the age group were in full-time education. Pakistani and Bangladeshi women were distinctive in the high percentages of each age group who were looking after a home or family full-time, and in the high percentage of young women with full-time domestic responsibilities.

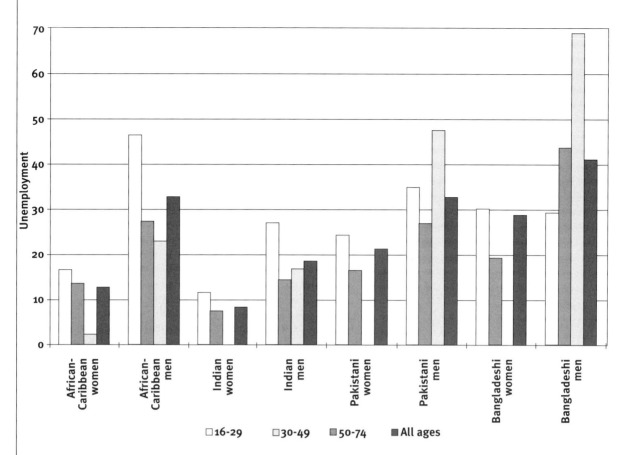

Figure 3.8: Unemployment rates by ethnic group, age and sex

Only a fifth of African-Caribbean and a quarter of Indian women aged 16–29 were looking after the home or family full-time, compared with two-fifths of Pakistani and Bangladeshi women, and a substantial differential also existed in the two older age groups. In contrast with South Asian women, the attachment of African-Caribbean women to the labour market increased with age, with only 16% of those aged 50 and over looking after a home or family full-time. In the oldest age group, retirement was most common in the African-Caribbean and Indian ethnic groups, with very few Pakistani or Bangladeshi women retired. The incidence of permanent sickness increased with age, but was particularly common for Pakistani and Bangladeshi men, with nearly two-fifths of Bangladeshi men aged over 50 economically inactive as a result of permanent sickness. This might reflect the effects of a lifetime in low-skilled employment, but might also be a result of the benefit system's encouragement of long-term unemployed people to register for sickness benefit rather than unemployment benefit.

Table 3.11 suggests the severity of the problem of low income for many ethnic minority families. It presents the percentage of respondents in each of the three age groups by the economic status of the household head. There was a marked contrast between the 42% of Indian men and the 2% of Bangladeshi women who were living in a household whose head is in full-time employment. The percentage of African-Caribbean and Indian people living in household whose head was in work was much higher than that for Pakistani and Bangladeshi people, for whom a higher percentage of respondents lived in households whose head was unemployed, or permanently sick. This problem is confirmed by Table 3.29, which reveals that half of Pakistani people and nearly three-quarters of Bangladeshi women lived in households which received income support, family credit or housing benefit. Over half of Bangladeshi people lived in households receiving income support, compared with two-fifths of Pakistani people, around a third of African-Caribbean people and a quarter of Indian people.

Employment

The type of work in which men and women from the four ethnic groups are engaged in is presented in Table 3.12, in which their jobs are classified into the nine 'major groups' of the Office for National Statistics' Standard Occupational Classification. In the population as a whole, there is a marked 'sexual division of labour', with men more likely to be in managerial and professional jobs and in manual jobs than women, while women's employment is dominated by clerical, sales and personal service (e.g. hairdressing) occupations. There is also an ethnic division of labour, in which ethnic minorities are less likely than white people to have high-status occupations, but are more likely to work in skilled and semi-skilled manual jobs than white people.[3]

This table also reveals a contrast between African-Caribbean and South Asian people in the type of jobs they held. South Asian men (especially Indians) were much more likely than African-Caribbean men to be managers and administrators or to work in professional (e.g. doctors, teachers) occupations, and were much less likely to be unskilled workers (other occupations), while associate professional and technical and craft and skilled manual occupations were more common for African-Caribbean than South Asian men. Over half of Indian and Pakistani men were in manual occupations, but the latter were much more likely to be engaged in semi-skilled work. For Bangladeshis, the importance of the restaurant trade for employment is revealed in the 40% of men working in personal service (e.g. waiters, cooks) occupations. African-Caribbean women were more likely than other women to be employed in the service sector, with the largest occupations being clerical and secretarial, personal and protective services and associate professional and technical jobs (the latter including nursing, traditionally an important source of employment for African-Caribbean women). Clerical and secretarial occupations were an important source of work for Indian women, but as many were employed in skilled and semi-skilled manual jobs, representing such jobs as machinists in the textile and clothing industries. Pakistani women were less likely to be semi-skilled manual workers and more likely to be working in sales or personal service occupations, while the bulk of working Bangladeshi women were in clerical and secretarial jobs, followed by craft and skilled manual and personal service occupations.

This table also highlights the age dimension of occupational specialisation, with younger African-Caribbean women less likely than older women to be in associate professional and technical jobs, and younger African-Caribbean men more likely than older men to work in service sector occupations. The percentage of men in skilled and semi-skilled manual jobs was much greater in the older age groups than the younger, 62% of Pakistani men in work aged over 50 being plant and machine operatives. White-collar jobs were much more common for younger Indian people than for older people, with the exception that a fifth of Indian men aged over 50 were managers and administrators (many running their own businesses). The number of Pakistani and Bangladeshi women in work declined sharply with age, with older women mainly working in clerical and secretarial, personal and protective service and semi-skilled manual (plant and machine operatives) jobs.

The socio-economic group breakdown (Table 3.16) largely reflects the occupational specialisation of respondents, but highlights the large percentages of men and women working in skilled and semi-skilled manual occupations. It also demonstrates that most of those in managerial and professional jobs were mainly in small enterprises (often their own), rather than being in senior positions in the public sector or larger private sector enterprises. The classification highlights the importance of nursing for African-Caribbean women and restaurant jobs for Bangladeshi people (especially those aged 16–29). It also quite strikingly illustrates the greater percentage of African-Caribbean and Indian than Pakistani and Bangladeshi young people in junior non-manual occupations.

Unemployment

Lack of skills makes a person more vulnerable to unemployment, demonstrated by Table 3.13, which presents the occupational distribution of people not in work (unemployed and economically inactive, having previously worked). Across all four ethnic groups and both sexes, the percentage formerly in white-collar jobs was quite low, with much higher percentages of skilled and semi-skilled manual workers. The percentage of plant and machine operatives among older people out of work was particularly high. Amongst those not in work (Table 3.14), a much higher percentage of men than women were seeking work, this percentage being higher for African-Caribbean than South Asian men. The percentage who had never worked was much higher for South Asians than African-Caribbean people, most of whom were in the youngest age group (presumably mainly still in full-time education). A very high percentage of Pakistani and Bangladeshi women in all three age groups had never worked, and nearly all those aged over 50 not in work never having worked.

Long-term unemployment was a serious problem (Table 3.15). Around half of unemployed African-Caribbean people had been out of work for two years or more, with higher rates of very long-term unemployment experienced by Pakistani men. Shorter spells of unemployment (six months or less) were more common for women than men, particularly in South Asian ethnic groups. The incidence of long-duration unemployment was greatest for men aged over 50, particularly for Pakistani men, 91% of whom had been unemployed for two years or more. Amongst those aged 16–29 and 30–49, African-Caribbeans suffered the highest rates of long-term unemployment.

3.6   Social class and living conditions

Variations in the class composition of the four ethnic groups and genders are presented in Tables 3.17 (social class of respondents) and 3.18 (percentage distribution of respondents by social class of household head). Very few people were in the professional class (social class I), this percentage being highest for Indian men. In contrast, the percentage in social class II (intermediate non-manual occupations) was highest for African-Caribbean people, followed by Indian and Pakistani men. The percentage in social class III (non-manual) was highest for African-Caribbean women, while the manual division of this class represented the largest social class for men from all four ethnic groups. Most of the remainder allocated to a social class were in social class IV (partly skilled), but over two-thirds of Pakistani and Bangladeshi women could not be allocated to a social class, having no occupation.

When respondents are classified by the social class of the household head, differences by sex diminish (Figure 3.9). The percentage of respondents living in households with a head from social class I was highest for Indians, while heads from social classes II and III (non-manual) were most common for African-Caribbean and Indian people. Over a third of Bangladeshi and African-Caribbean men lived in households headed by a person from social class III (manual), while the percentage living in households with heads from social class IV (partly skilled manual) was highest for South Asian men. Around a tenth of people lived in households with an unskilled (social class V) household head, and around a quarter of Pakistani and Bangladeshi women lived in households where the head was not allocated to a social class. There was little variation by age group, except for the relatively high percentage of African-Caribbean people aged 30–49 whose household head was from social class II.

There was a marked difference between Indian and Pakistani people and the other two ethnic groups in housing tenure (Table 3.19). Around a half of African-Caribbean people owned their own home, with a further third renting from a local authority, the remainder mainly renting from housing associations. About half of Bangladeshis lived in a dwelling rented from a local authority, with a further third living in owner-occupied accommodation and most rented accommodation being provided by the private sector. In contrast, well over 80% of Indian and Pakistani people lived in owner-occupied dwellings. There was very little variation in housing tenure by age group, except that the percentage of African-Caribbean people living in the social rented sector was highest among those aged 30–49 (Figure 3.10).

An important indicator of household deprivation is access to a motor vehicle (Table 3.20). Lack of a car can seriously restrict a household's activities and access to employment and social facilities, especially where public transport is deficient, and hence more affluent households generally tend to own more vehicles. The 1991 Census revealed that around a quarter of the population lived in households which did not own a car, with 24.6% of the white population and 34% of persons from minority ethnic groups living in such households.

The survey revealed marked contrasts between ethnic groups, the sexes and age groups in the degree of access to motor vehicles. In each ethnic group, a smaller percentage of women than men had access to a motor vehicle, while the percentage of both younger and older people with access to a car was smaller than the corresponding percentage of those aged 30–49 The percentage of men owning a car was twice as high in the 30–49 age group as for the 16–29 group. The level access to motor vehicles was greatest for the Indian ethnic group, in which over three-fifths of men owned a car and only a third did not. Car ownership was slightly greater in the Pakistani than in the African-Caribbean ethnic group, amongst whom more than half of men and nearly two-thirds of women did not have a car. Access to motor vehicles was least of all for the Bangladeshi ethnic group, with only a quarter of Bangladeshi men owning a car.

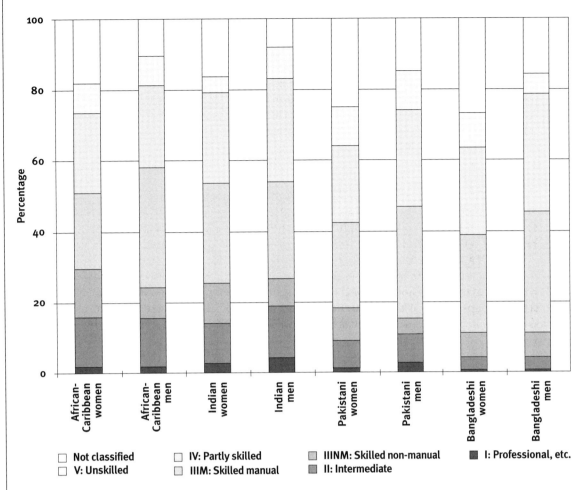

Figure 3.9: Percentage of residents by social class of household head, ethnic group and sex

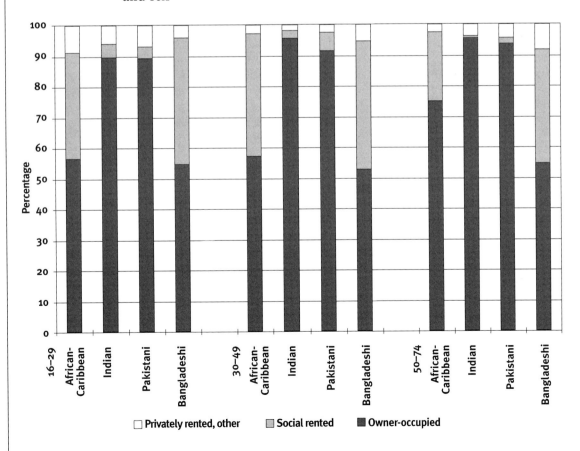

Figure 3.10: Housing tenure of respondents by ethnic group and age range

3.7 Country of birth, language ability and education

Country of birth

Just over half of African-Caribbean people covered by the survey had been born in the UK compared with around three-quarters of Indian and Pakistani people, but around 90% of Bangladeshi people had been born overseas (Table 3.21). On average, South Asian people had entered the UK as young adults (their average age at entry generally lay in the late teens or early twenties), while African-Caribbean people born outside the UK entered the country as children of older primary school age. Mean age at entry tended to increase with the age of the respondent; of African-Caribbeans born outside the UK, those aged 16–29 at time of the survey had been babies at their time of entry, while those aged over 50 at the time of the survey had, on average, been young adults when they entered the country. The larger percentage of young people from minority ethnic groups born in the UK was shown by the declining numbers of the overseas-born with declining age of respondent. The mean age at entry to the UK was greater for South Asians than for African-Caribbeans in each age group. Bangladeshi women aged 30–49 and 50–74 at the time of the survey were much older on average at the time they migrated to the UK than people from the other three ethnic groups, reflecting the relatively recent reunification of Bangladeshi families and perhaps a tendency for Bangladeshi families to bring older female relatives to live with them in the UK.

Language ability

The survey collected information on facility in the English language and in the language best understood from South Asian respondents. Table 3.22 shows that the ability to read and write English was greatest in the Indian ethnic group, while a smaller percentage of women than men were able to speak English. While nearly all Indian men and more than nine in ten Pakistani and Bangladeshi men could speak English, only three-quarters of Pakistani women and less than three-fifths of Bangladeshi women could speak English. For all three ethnic groups, and both men and women, the percentage able to read English was rather lower, but in each ethnic group, the percentage of men able to read English was higher than the corresponding percentage for women. Around half of South Asian women could read another language, compared with around two-thirds of Indian and Pakistani men, but just under half of Bangladeshi men.

Ability in the English language declined markedly with age, particularly for women. Almost all Indian and Pakistani men and women aged 16–30 could both speak and read English, but the level of ability of Bangladeshi women aged 16–29 in English was substantially less than that of other South Asian women. Of women aged 50–74, only just over half of Indian and Pakistani women could speak English, compared with only 17% of Bangladeshi women. Ability to read English declined with age for both sexes, but a substantially higher percentage of men than women could read English in all three South Asian ethnic groups. Among Indians and Pakistanis, the percentage able to read another language did not vary greatly with age, but this percentage also declined with age, most markedly for Bangladeshi women.

The survey probed further into the language ability of respondents who could speak or read English by asking them to report their own assessment of their ability to speak and read English (Tables 3.23, 3.24). Overall, more than three-fifths of Indian people reported that they could speak English very well, compared with half of Pakistani women, two-fifths of Pakistani men and Bangladeshi women and a third of Bangladeshi men, but a third of Bangladeshis and a quarter of Pakistanis could speak only a little English. The percentage who could speak only a little English was smallest for Indian men. Figure 3.11 combines the information in Tables 3.22 and 3.23 to demonstrate the contrast in ability in spoken English, showing that Indian men and Bangladeshi women lay at the extremes of ability. In each ethnic group, and for both men and women, a higher percentage of people aged 16–29 than older people were able to speak English very well; conversely, the percentage able to speak only a little English increased with age. Lack of ability to speak English was a particular problem for older Pakistani and Bangladeshi women, with three-quarters of Pakistani and all Bangladeshi women aged over 50 who could speak English able to speak only a little English.

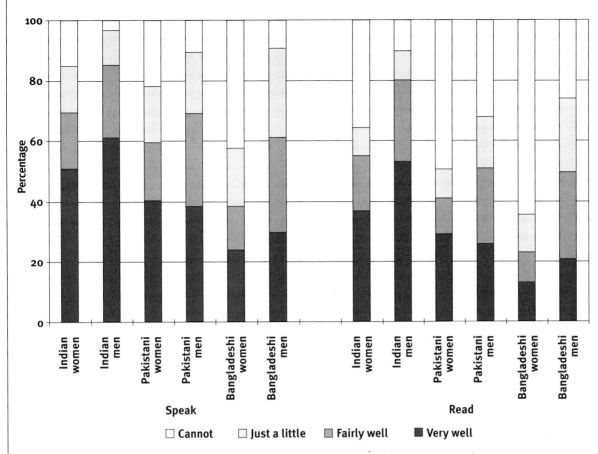

Figure 3.11: Ability of respondents in English by ethnic group and age range

A similar pattern by age sex and gender was evident in the percentage able to read English. Indian people displayed the best abilities in reading English, followed by Pakistani women and then Pakistani men and Bangladeshi people, less than a third of whom could read English very well. Conversely, a quarter of Pakistani men and a third of Bangladeshi people could only read a little English. Once again, ability in reading English was greatest in the youngest age group, declining with increasing age. Older Bangladeshi people exhibited very low levels of skill in reading English. Figure 3.11 demonstrates that, while the percentage of Bangladeshi and Pakistani men able to read English was higher than that for Bangladeshi women, a relatively large share of those able to read English had fairly limited ability in the language.

Table 3.25 presents the language best understood by respondents to the survey. While seven South Asian languages are listed with English in the table, people from most ethnic groups spoke a much more restricted range of languages. Indian people tended to speak Gujerati, Punjabi or English best, with nearly half of men and two-fifths of women speaking English best. Of South Asian languages, a higher percentage of both men and women could speak Gujerati than Punjabi. Half of Pakistani women spoke Punjabi best, followed by English, with under a fifth speaking Urdu best. In contrast, two-fifths of Pakistani men spoke Urdu best, a third spoke English best, and under a quarter spoke Punjabi best. Half of Bangladeshi women spoke Bengali best, with less than a third speaking Sylheti best, and a fifth speaking English best. Bangladeshi men were almost evenly split between Bengali and Sylheti in terms of the language they spoke best, with a sixth speaking English best. Younger South Asian people were much more likely than older people to speak English best, and had therefore lost some ability in South Asian languages. Nearly seven-eighths of Indian men and 70% of Indian women aged 16–29 spoke English best, with only 19% of women reporting that they spoke Gujerati best. Even among Bangladeshis, two-fifths of women aged 16–29 spoke English best. There was a marked contrast between the youngest age group and those aged 30–49, in which the percentage speaking English was only half as great. The percentage whose best language was South Asian increased with increasing age, being Gujerati for Indians, Punjabi for Pakistanis and Sylheti for Bangladeshis.

ducation

The majority of those born outside the UK attended school in their country of birth (Table 3.26). More than nine out of ten African-Caribbeans had done so, compared with around three-quarters of South Asians, with Pakistani women least likely to have been to school in their country of birth. Most African-Caribbean and Bangladeshi people had only obtained elementary education in their country of birth, while around a fifth of Pakistani people and a third of Indian people had finished secondary education in their countries of birth. A very small percentage of people born overseas had achieved post-school age qualifications before migrating to the UK. Relatively few people aged under 30 had been born overseas, and most of those born in India and Pakistan had received secondary education in their country of birth.

There were marked contrasts between ethnic groups in the highest educational qualification achieved (Table 3.27). Indians displayed the highest percentages with higher level qualifications, an eighth of men and a twelfth of women having degrees or their equivalent, while only 8% of Pakistani men, 5% of African-Caribbean women and 4% each of African-Caribbean men and Pakistani women had achieved such a high level of qualification. A higher percentage of African-Caribbean than Indian people held teaching qualifications or the equivalent of GCE A-level passes, while the most common qualification for all four ethnic groups was GCE O-level passes or their equivalent. The percentage of Bangladeshi people who had achieved this level of educational attainment was closer to the other ethnic groups than for higher level qualifications, with a very small percentage having obtained post-school age qualifications.

Two-thirds or more of Bangladeshi people held no educational qualifications, twice the rate for Indian men or African-Caribbean women, with around half of Pakistani people, African-Caribbean men and Indian women having no educational qualifications. This percentage was highest amongst people aged 50–74, with nearly all Bangladeshis in this age group having no educational qualifications. The highly qualified percentage (qualified to GCE A-level standard or better) was highest in the 30–49 age group, while the percentage with GCE O-level passes or their equivalent as their highest qualification was greatest in the youngest age group.

3.8 Religion

Table 3.28 presents the religious affiliation of respondents. These were more diverse for African-Caribbean people than South Asian people, but the largest single religion was Anglicanism, followed by Catholicism and Pentecostalism, etc. A number of less common faiths were mentioned, and a very small percentage mentioned Rastafarianism. Nearly all Pakistani and Bangladeshi people were Muslims, while Hinduism was the largest religion mentioned by Indian people, representing two-fifths of both men and women. Another third of Indian people were Sikhs, and a further fifth were Muslims. Around a quarter of African-Caribbean men and a tenth of African-Caribbean women had no religion, but almost no South Asian people professed to have no religion.

Amongst South Asians, there was little variation in religious affiliation by age, except that Muslims accounted for a much larger percentage of the 16–29 age group than of older people, with a correspondingly smaller percentage of Hindus in the youngest ethnic group. Amongst African-Caribbeans, the main variation with age was that around a third of men aged under 50 professed to have no religion, twice as high a percentage as for men aged over 50.

3.9 Conclusion

This chapter has set the scene for the remainder of the report, in summarising the characteristics of the survey population in terms of population and household structure, economic status, living conditions, migration, language use, education and religion. Most of the findings confirm the results of the 1991 Census of Population and surveys such as the 1994 Policy Studies Institute survey of ethnic minorities in Great Britain. While providing few surprises, this exercise does confirm that the survey of the health of black and minority ethnic groups in England succeeded in contacting a sample reasonably representative of the four minority ethnic groups.

Notes

1. The weighting procedure used Census of Population data for the three South Asian ethnic groups and the 'Black-Caribbean' census ethnic group.

2. D.W. Owen, 'Labour force participation rates, self-employment and unemployment', in V. Karn (ed.), *Ethnicity in the 1991 census: vol. 4, Employment, education and housing among the ethnic minority population of Great Britain* (HMSO, London, 1977).

3. A.E. Green, 'Patterns of ethnic minority employment in the context of industrial and occupational growth and decline', in V. Karn (ed.), *Ethnicity in the 1991 census: vol. 4, Employment, education and housing among the ethnic minority population of Great Britain* (HMSO, London, 1977).

4. D.W. Owen, *Ethnic minorities in Great Britain: housing and family characteristics* (NEMDA 1991 Census Statistical Paper 4, Centre for Research in Ethnic Relations, University of Warwick, Coventry, 1993).

4   General health status

Summary of the main findings

This chapter reviews the evidence from the HEA survey relating to the prevalence of certain key diseases, notably those associated with coronary heart disease and high blood pressure. It considers the rates at which people recalled that they had been advised of an unsatisfactory level of blood pressure, or that they had one of the selected conditions. Questions on these issues were asked at various points in the research interview: the relevant replies have been brought together in this chapter. Perceptions of health and the appropriate actions associated with these illnesses are also discussed.

- The prevalence of diabetes, in keeping with known clinical patterns, was reported to be very high, most notably among Bangladeshis.

- Despite well-established epidemiological evidence of excess mortality from coronary heart disease amongst minority ethnic groups, those interviewed generally reported levels of stroke and high blood pressure that were close to or less than national averages. African-Caribbean women were rather more likely to have been told that they had raised blood pressure.

- Lower levels of stroke, angina and heart attack among the survey population may be explained by their relative youth, while reports of raised blood pressure levels appear to be related to opportunistic screening during pregnancy.

- The survey shows that there is a considerable lack of understanding of the causes and implications of key ill-health conditions. Blood pressure levels are strongly believed to be most influenced by 'stress'.

- There are a number of areas where levels of knowledge vary between people in different age groups, although it is not always the case that younger people are better informed. Patterns also vary between the ethnic groups of the survey.

- 'Healthy Living' information has achieved a reasonable penetration, in that most of those surveyed were able to offer a selection of appropriate responses to questions on advice for a person with high blood pressure.

- People whose religion or culture discourages the use of alcohol or tobacco are less likely to suggest reductions in the use of these substances as a strategy to improve health.

- Overall, Bangladeshi men and women report strikingly worse levels of general health, including particularly high levels of stomach ulcer, heart disease and headache/migraine.

4.1   Blood pressure and related circulatory system disorders

It is well-established and widely accepted that people from the Indian subcontinent and Africa have a significantly higher rate of death from coronary heart disease and that levels of stroke in both these groups and people originating in the Caribbean Commonwealth are also seriously in excess of the national average.[1] Mortality from hypertensive disease is between four and seven times as high in the Caribbean-born UK population and raised in all minority ethnic groups. There are some gender differences: recent studies show that mortality from circulatory disease is significantly higher in migrant Bangladeshi men but not in women, and that Bangladeshi men also show a sixfold excess over white males in deaths from diabetes.[2]

A major focus of the HEA Health and Lifestyle Survey was to investigate various aspects of this question, including both a review of the numbers of people who said they had been diagnosed as suffering from high blood pressure,[3] and a series of questions testing the understanding of the condition in the ethnic minority populations.

Reported recall of prevalence of selected conditions

All respondents were asked whether they had ever been told by a doctor or nurse that they had one of a number of circulation-related disorders. Detailed analyses of these data are found in Table 4.1. As Figure 4.1 shows, there were considerable differences between ethnic groups in the HEA survey, and a notable difference overall between these minority groups and the level of diabetes reported in the HSE.

The data show that the rates of (reported) prevalence of stroke in the minority population were close to those for the national average. The number saying that they had been told they had high blood pressure was rather less than the national average. However, there appeared to be rather higher rates of angina/heart attack, and very much higher rates of diabetes in the four minority groups considered, compared to the national average. As expected (Table 4.1), prevalence rates increase with age, and diabetes, angina and heart attacks are very uncommon in those aged under 30, although an important exception is found among Bangladeshi women reporting diabetes (5%). Overall, men from the minority groups reported rates of diabetes two or three times as high as the national average, while for women the apparent relative risk was three or four times the expected level. Pakistani men were somewhat less likely to report having been told that they had had a stroke, while African-Caribbean men and women were very much more likely to have been told that they had raised blood pressure.

	African-Caribbean	Indian	Pakistani	Bangladeshi	England (HSE 94)
Female					
Diabetes	9.1	5.4	7.5	10.9	1.9
High blood pressure	29.1	15.0	11.6	10.8	18.3
Stroke	1.0	1.0	1.0	0.4	1.6
Angina	3.2	1.7	1.4	4.6	*
Heart attack	0.9	0.9	0.6	0.7	1.7
'Other'	2.5	0.6	1.6	3.1	na
Base n	*1043*	*1492*	*1729*	*1682*	
Male					
Diabetes	5.4	6.8	9.7	12.2	2.9
High blood pressure	16.5	12.3	9.4	11.1	15.3
Stroke	2.0	2.3	1.1	2.5	1.8
Angina	2.8	2.7	1.9	8.4	*
Heart attack	2.9	2.1	3.8	3.9	3.8
'Other'	3.9	0.8	2.8	6.6	na
Base n	*929*	*1497*	*1752*	*1859*	

*HSE reports heart attack and angina combined as ischaemic heart disease.

Figure 4.1:   Q15 Have you ever been told you suffer from (selected circulatory disorders) (percentage replying 'yes' to each condition)

It would appear that to a large extent the relatively low prevalence of stroke, angina and heart attack can be seen to relate to the relative youth of the minority ethnic population. Among the population aged 16–29, there were very few who report any condition other than diabetes or raised blood pressure. The highest rates of reported diabetes in this age group were found among the Bangladeshi females, who also reported a much greater prevalence at age 30–49, somewhat higher than for the men of this ethnic group. It would appear that health checks in pregnancy, a form of opportunistic screening, played a significant role in discovering diabetes (Table 4.2a). In the youngest age group, high blood pressure was most often reported by women, which may also be related to tests during pregnancy.

Among the middle-aged group, women continued to report higher rates of high blood pressure than men, and Pakistani and Bangladeshi people were very much more likely to report having been told that they had diabetes. (The rates for African-Caribbean men and women were rather less than the national average.) Bangladeshis were also somewhat more likely to report a diagnosis of angina or 'other' heart conditions.

Highest rates of disease were reported by the older age group, and for diabetes these considerably exceeded the levels reported by the majority (white) population. The highest rate of diabetes reported in the HSE was 6.4% among men aged 55–64: this is less than half that reported by all ethnic minority groups, male and female, and less than a quarter of the rate for African-Caribbean women (29%) and Pakistani men (26%). Men were more likely to have experienced a stroke or angina than women, and again the highest rates were reported by Bangladeshi men (and for heart attack, among Pakistani men).

It is possible that the higher rates of blood pressure noted among women are related to pregnancy. Around half of the women reporting that they had been told that they had high blood pressure said that they had been told this when they were pregnant (Table 4.2b). Indian women were least likely to have been pregnant when told that their blood pressure was high, while Bangladeshi women were much more likely (in two out of three cases) to report having been pregnant at the time. However, 40% of these women had also been told that they had high blood pressures when not pregnant, with Pakistani and African-Caribbean women being slightly more likely to have been given this advice. Only one in four of Indian women who had been told that their blood pressure was high while pregnant had also been told that they had high blood pressure when not pregnant.

It is probable that many of the women had their blood pressure checked as a routine measure when attending for contraception and ante- or postnatal care, and the proportions reporting being diagnosed when pregnant are very much greater among the youngest age group. Younger Pakistani women (and middle-aged Bangladeshi women) were somewhat more likely to have been found to have high blood pressure when not pregnant, but this these groups also have the highest fertility rates. The data do not allow us to know at what age the pregnancy or diagnosis occurred, so few further conclusions can be drawn from them.

Extent and recall of blood pressure screening

At a later point in the interview, all respondents were asked if their blood pressure had been checked by a doctor or nurse. The question was phrased rather differently to that reported in the previous section of this chapter. More than three-quarters of those asked this question replied that they had been tested, with females consistently more likely to have had their blood pressure checked. There were important differences between the ethnic groups. African-Caribbean men and women were most likely to have had their blood pressure checked. Bangladeshi people, particularly men, were considerably less likely to have had this done (Table 4.3). There were also age effects in the pattern of responses. Among the older age group, more than nine-tenths of the population had been checked, although Pakistani women were rather less likely to have had their blood pressure measured. Pakistani men were also less likely to know the outcome of the test. Young Bangladeshi men were rather less likely to know whether their blood level had been tested, and middle-aged men from all three Asian groups were consistently less likely to have had theirs checked. There appears to be a high level of recall of the result of the most recent test, among those who remembered having their blood pressure measured (Table 4.4).

Lower levels of having been tested were reported from the youngest age group, but even here more than two thirds reported having had a blood pressure test. Fewer than half of the Bangladeshi young men had been checked, and relatively low rates were also recorded among Pakistani and Indian young men, in comparison with female responses. Given that most of the younger South Asian women who had had their blood pressure checked had been pregnant at the time of the test, and that a similar pattern also appears for Bangladeshi women in the middle age group (Figure 4.2; Table 4.5), it is clear that opportunistic screening at antenatal consultations has played a significant role in raising these levels of coverage.

Age Group	African-Caribbean	Indian	Pakistani	Bangladeshi
16–29				
Yes	21	72	50	92
No	79	28	50	8
Base	*8*	*14*	*15*	*9*
30–49				
Yes	26	13	36	58
No	74	88	64	42
Base	*37*	*19*	*15*	*19*

Note: Only one African-Caribbean woman aged over 50 reported that she had been pregnant at the time of her last blood pressure check. Due to small base numbers, percentage in this table should be treated with caution.

Figure 4.2: Q69 (if blood pressure tested) Were you pregnant at the time of the test? (percentage saying 'yes')

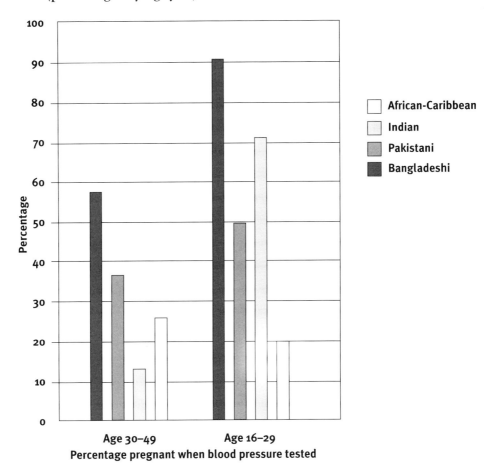

As shown in Table 4.4, the majority of those who reported that their blood pressure had been checked remembered that they had been advised of the result. There were a few exceptions, notably among younger Indian and (male) Bangladeshi respondents and older Pakistani men, in each of which groups one in ten did not remember or 'was not told' the result of the test. A small number of people recalled being told that their blood pressure was lower than normal, but no pattern arises from these responses, except that women were slightly more likely to have been told this. Highest rates of recall that the level was raised were found among African-Caribbean women, and to a lesser extent among Bangladeshi and Indian older men, consistent with the data shown for answers to Q15 (Have you ever been told that you had high blood pressure?). There are, however, certain anomalies, and the prevalence rates from the two different questions do not agree closely, since the data for one (Q15) refer to 'ever' having been told, and (Q68) data in Table 4.4 to 'the most recent occasion'.

Levels of understanding and knowledge

While the majority of the people in the survey reported that their blood pressure had been tested, and most of them were able to recall the outcome of that test, it is important to note that not everyone was clear what was meant by the term 'high blood pressure' (Figure 4.3; Table 4.6). Knowledge or understanding of this term was tested in a variety of ways, including a direct question (Q63 Do you know what is meant by the term 'high blood pressure'?). In particular, it can be seen that highest rates of understanding of this term were found among younger African-Caribbean men, and particularly low rates were reported by Bangladeshi women, with the oldest being the least likely to understand it, while middle-aged men of all three South Asian ethnic groups were the most likely age group to know about the condition. It is, of course, possible that some people gave 'socially acceptable' responses, feeling that they should not express ignorance of such a topic.

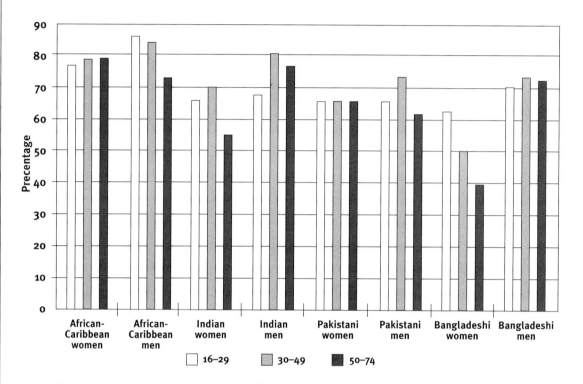

Figure 4.3 Proportion understanding 'high blood pressure'

Given the exposure to these conditions which is represented by the above-reported rates of disease, it is also of interest to explore the degree to which members of the communities concerned understand them and are aware of the risk factors associated with each. The HEA questionnaire approached the issue in several ways, asking both what the informants considered to be the *causes* of high blood pressure, but also what 'risks' were associated with having it. This may have led to some confusion, but the difference in questions produces illuminating findings.

The tables and figures show a clear pattern across all ethnic groups, and, in general, irrespective of gender. For all those surveyed, the most frequently mentioned cause of high blood pressure was given as 'stress', with nearly half the African-Caribbean women in the survey giving this response. While Bangladeshi women were half as likely to mention stress, this reflects rather a tendency to reply 'don't know' (nearly one in four) and to be markedly less likely to mention *any* cause than to have an alternative explanation.

The only group not placing stress as their primary cause were Pakistani males, slightly more of whom replied in terms of salt consumption. Salt was also mentioned by a very significant number of respondents in all groups, and it must be presumed that this reflects an awareness of the medical advice given to patients with hypertension to 'cut down' on salt intake, based on epidemiological evidence of raised levels of hypertension in societies where there is a high salt intake (including Japan). The other principal causes mentioned include obesity (around 15% of all respondents), alcohol (slightly more among men, and rarely by Bangladeshis), 'artery problems' and heredity. African-Caribbean women were particularly likely to mention the latter risk.

	African-Caribbean	Indian	Pakistani	Bangladeshi
Female				
Stress	47	36	33	18
Salt	23	18	25	11
Obesity	18	15	15	11
Alcohol	7	7	5	3
Heredity	7	2	2	3
Arteries	5	4	2	1
'Other'	33	18	21	7
Don't know	6	11	11	24
Base n	*820*	*982*	*1082*	*923*
Male				
Stress	42	39	29	23
Salt	19	22	29	11
Obesity	15	18	15	15
Alcohol	7	9	9	3
Heredity	2	2	5	2
Arteries	3	3	3	1
'Other'	24	21	16	14
Don't know	12	10	11	26
Base n	*748*	*1132*	*1197*	*1348*

Note: Interviewers were instructed not to prompt respondents, but to record as many causes as were mentioned: the question was only put to those replying 'yes' to Q63.

Figure 4.4: Q65 What are the causes of high blood pressure (percentage mentioning each)

As the full data (Table 4.7) show, there are few age-related differences, although older Pakistani women were particularly likely to refer to stress as a cause. Similarly, there may be a lifestyle element in the fact that older people were less likely to refer to salt as a risk factor, while younger respondents, male and female, were less likely to blame alcohol. Awareness of the role of family history is also a middle-aged and predominantly African-Caribbean characteristic in respect of heart disease. For many of the explanations proffered, there were more differences between middle-aged people and the old or young than were associated with an 'age gradient'. That is to say, middle-aged groups tended to differ from both older and younger people, and there was not a 'learning curve' from younger to older. This suggests a lifestyle and lifestage effect.

There are a number of major areas of risk associated with a diagnosis of hypertension, which include many of the issues identified by respondents to the HEA survey. In nearly all categories of the sample, the replies indicated an awareness of the danger of a 'heart attack' as being of highest priority, particularly among men. The exception was both genders of Bangladeshi people, who were considerably less likely to say this, and much more likely to reply 'don't know'. Men were also, in many cases, aware that there was an association with stroke, but the group with the highest awareness of this was African-Caribbean women. Men of this ethnic group were if anything slightly less likely to mention stroke despite the clear epidemiological evidence that exists, which has often been referred to in media oriented to this group. Asian women, by contrast were relatively less likely to mention strokes.

A few people in all groups also mentioned coronary heart disease. On the other hand, for most groups, 'headache' was the second or third mostly common response, and was mentioned particularly often by Bangladeshi men (and, slightly less often, by Bangladeshi women). Similarly, but perhaps more usefully, a small but significant group of people were aware of an association with diabetes. Although the two are not directly associated, hypertension is common in people with the form of diabetes (NIDDM) most commonly found in the minority ethnic population. This form can lead to complications, requiring more assertive treatment of the disease(s). Both, indeed, seem to have similar causes, notably an association with increasing age and obesity,[5] for which increased exercise is likely to be seen as a worthwhile preventive strategy. The link between hypertension and blindness or renal disease was not mentioned by enough respondents to be reported separately.

	African-Caribbean	Indian	Pakistani	Bangladeshi
Female				
Stroke	40	17	13	9
Heart attack	35	31	30	19
CHD	15	11	14	4
Obesity	6	8	10	6
Diabetes	7	6	7	6
Headache etc.	7	19	15	17
Other	24	17	13	7
'Don't know'	9	7	10	18
Base n	*820*	*982*	*1082*	*923*
Male				
Stroke	21	22	20	10
Heart attack	42	43	40	31
CHD	7	11	11	6
Obesity	7	9	10	5
Diabetes	5	8	6	3
Headache etc.	7	14	12	21
Other	23	18	16	14
'Don't know'	12	5	7	15
Base n	*748*	*1132*	*1197*	*1348*

Note: Interviewers were instructed not to prompt respondents, but to record as many causes as were mentioned: the question was only put to those replying 'yes' to Q63.

Figure 4.5: Q64 Perceived risks of having high blood pressure (percentage mentioning each)

	African-Caribbean	Indian	Pakistani	Bangladeshi
Female				
Heart trouble	43	30	28	18
High blood pressure	7	6	5	5
Stroke	1	6	4	2
No ill effects	2	3	4	4
Male				
Heart trouble	31	33	34	16
High blood pressure	4	7	8	4
Stroke	3	2	5	2
No ill effects	1	4	2	3
Base: all respondents				

Note: Interviewers were instructed not to prompt respondents, but to record as many causes as were mentioned.

Figure 4.6: Q8 Medical problems arising from lack of exercise (percentage mentioning each)

With very few exceptions, the three 'generations' represented in the survey gave very similar responses (Table 4.8). There was slightly less awareness of the risk of coronary heart disease among older people, but the proportions mentioning heart attacks were similar across the four ethnic groups and two genders. Awareness of stroke, on the other hand, increased with age, except among the Bangladeshi population. Older people too were more likely to mention headaches, except among the African-Caribbean sample. Older Pakistani women (from a small sample) were very much more likely to refer to obesity as a risk.

In order to approach the issue from a different direction, respondents to the survey were asked what medical problems they associated with a lack of exercise. This question was asked near the start of the interview, and without prompting, to obtain unbiased replies that were not 'informed' by subsequent more technical questions about personal health. While an association with 'heart disease' or 'heart trouble' was observed, relatively few people (with the possible exception of

Pakistani males and to a lesser extent, Indian men) made the link with blood pressure, and almost none mentioned the risk of a stroke.

It should however be noted that a (very) few people mentioned that lack of exercise could lead to 'poor circulation'. The most encouraging thing about responses to this question is the lack of people feeling that exercise was not beneficial, or, to be precise, that there were no ill effects from a lack of exercise. In this respect, there were no detectable 'ethnic' or gender differences – this seems to be 'common knowledge' and accepted wisdom. However, the table does also show some more significant differences, notably the particularly low level of awareness amongst Bangladeshi women and men that exercise could protect against heart disease. It is also strange, given that the African-Caribbean women were most likely to be aware of the connection, that males from this category were no more likely than Asian men to be aware of this fact.

Considerable insight may also be obtained by considering the kinds of advice that people felt that they would offer to a friend, relation or other acquaintance with high blood pressure. This undoubtedly reflects their perceptions of advice given both directly to their significant others and colleagues, and available (accurately or misleadingly) in the media and 'common knowledge'. Respondents were shown a card listing nine specific actions, and asked, 'If somebody you knew wanted to reduce their risk of having high blood pressure, which of these pieces of advice would you give them?' Avoiding (or combating) stress was not one of the options offered. In view of the 'popular belief' expressed earlier, this may have affected the answers given. Very few people, however, said there was nothing that could be suggested.

As with previous data, the full breakdown by age as well as sex and ethnic group is presented in Tables 4.9. The overall pattern, as represented in Figure 4.7, is apparent, but there are some age-related variations that may be relevant to health promotion work. In particular, older Pakistani, African-Caribbean and Bangladeshi men (and Bangladeshi women) seemed markedly less likely to suggest weight reduction as a strategy, while older Asians were much more likely to suggest reducing alcohol intakes. Salt reduction was also generally unpopular among older people, except for the African-Caribbean respondents, who were most likely to suggest this among the middle age group. It is a complex picture, which repays careful study.

	African-Caribbean	Indian	Pakistani	Bangladeshi
Female				
Get more exercise	45	31	29	15
Lose weight	50	38	37	28
Reduce fats	48	40	35	29
Reduce alcohol	46	28	28	17
Reduce salt	55	37	37	23
Stop smoking	39	25	29	20
Reduce sugar	32	24	19	17
Eat more starch	15	10	11	10
Eat more vegetables	49	30	32	21
'Don't know'	3	5	8	11
Base n	820	982	1082	923
Male				
More exercise	31	35	30	18
Lose weight	43	44	41	30
Reduce Fats	43	41	37	31
Reduce alcohol	36	40	34	18
Reduce salt	39	35	37	18
Stop smoking	27	33	30	24
Reduce sugar	27	25	22	17
Eat more starch	16	13	14	8
Eat more vegetables	38	37	33	23
'Don't know'	5	4	5	14
Base n	748	1132	1197	1348

Figure 4.7 Q66 What advice would you give to someone with high blood pressure? (percentage mentioning each item)

It is clear that many, indeed, nearly all, of those surveyed felt able to offer some advice, although again Bangladeshis (particularly the men, of whom 14% said 'don't know') were rather less likely to make specific recommendations. Among the women, African-Caribbeans were considerably more likely to offer each item of advice. Indian men, on the other hand, were at least as likely (and frequently more so) to offer particular suggestions, although African-Caribbean men were more free with their advice than Asian men in general. The data demonstrate a significant penetration of 'healthy living' advice in these populations, with the ranking of advice being similar to the priorities set out in HEA documentation relating to the Health of the Nation initiative. In particular, losing weight, reducing fats and salt in the diet and eating more vegetables were highlighted by more than a third of respondents and nearly half the African-Caribbean women. Taking more exercise was also a priority for this latter group while rather less frequently mentioned by men and Asian women. Men, on the other hand, were much more likely to suggest giving up smoking and reducing sugar intake. It is also interesting that a significant number of men (particularly African-Caribbean and Pakistanis) seemed to feel that a diet including more starchy foods (potatoes, rice, bread) would be an advantage. We cannot tell whether this reflected a feeling that high fibre foods were beneficial, or if this was a more general observation.

It should also be noted how Bangladeshis, who were less likely to be sure and mentioned many things less than others, were particularly less likely to suggest reduction of alcohol. Even so, a significant number did mention it. Pakistanis were not much less likely to mention alcohol than Indians, despite being much more like the Bangladeshis in the proportion being Muslim. Indian women, who are more likely to be Sikhs, did not mention smoking so frequently (it being against their religion) but Indian men by the same token were the most likely to urge this course of action. Very few people indeed said that they have no ideas on the subject, and most made recommendations that seem to be in line with accepted medical ideas.

4.2 Other conditions and long-standing illnesses

The 1991 Census for the first time included a health status question, asking everyone whether they had a 'long-standing illness or condition'. This was included because it had been found to be a reliable proxy for overall health status, but was difficult to interpret without any comparative data using the same measure of ethnic group. Prevalence of a long-term limiting condition was also found to be closely related to age. The HEA 1994 survey (Q12) asked a slightly more detailed question: 'Do you have any long-standing illness, disability or infirmity? By long-standing, I mean something that has troubled you over a period of time or that is likely to affect you over a period of time.' The phrasing of this question is significantly different from the census term (of a 'long-term limiting condition') and it is therefore not possible to make a direct comparison between the results of the two. However, the question as used in the HEA then went on to ask (if the answer had been a Yes), 'What is the matter with you?' and to probe for other conditions. The results, while not directly useful for epidemiology, provide an illuminating picture of perceptions of health, and give some guidance as to the key issues of chronic ill health affecting the various communities.

When broken down into categories corresponding to the International Classification of Diseases groups at the coding stage, using the judgement of the coders as to the appropriate definition of some of the replies given, a very large number of conditions were reported. These included a very small number of people with a cancer (neoplasm 0.2%), 'poor hearing' or deafness (0.5%), and other ailments that would probably not have been considered as 'disabling' by formal medical opinion, even if as personally distressing as piles/haemorrhoids (three people). Some of those replying to this question did mention the circulatory disorders already discussed, so that 0.6% of the men mentioned a stroke, largely among the Bangladeshi and African-Caribbean groups. Overall, it appears that the most commonly mentioned conditions (Figure 4.7) were in fact those covered by the more detailed inquiries reported above: diabetes (6% of men, 4% of women), high blood pressure or other heart conditions, asthma and various degenerative problems, such as arthritis and 'other joint problems'. It should also be noted that the levels of diabetes and other conditions mentioned in reply to this question were very much lower than those already reported. This may be a product of the use of the phrase 'troubled you'. It should be emphasised that this is not a report of the prevalence of diagnosed illness. The 'disorders of the blood and blood-forming organs' category which would include any reference to sickle cell disease or the other haemoglobinopathies, such as thallassaemia, was mentioned by only about 0.5% in all groups, but slightly more often (1.3%) by African-Caribbean women. A strikingly higher rate of mention of headache and migraine was reported by Bangladeshi women (4.2%) when compared to either African-Caribbean or Indian women (1.2% and 1.6% respectively).

	African-Caribbean	Indian	Pakistani	Bangladeshi
Female *Yes*	37	24	26	34
Heart attack/angina	1.0	–	0.6	–
Blood pressure	9.7	3.6	1.8	3.1
Other heart	1.4	1.9	3.4	6.6
Diabetes	6.1	2.6	2.7	5.2
Asthma	6.5	3.8	4.7	2.3
Stomach ulcer	0.9	0.9	1.0	4.7
Arthritis etc.	8.3	3.8	3.5	2.9
Male *Yes*	29	27	31	38
Heart attack/angina	1.5	1.6	1.3	4.0
Blood pressure	3.8	4.8	3.7	5.0
Other heart	0.6	–	2.9	6.9
Diabetes	3.8	3.8	5.2	9.5
Asthma	3.8	4.8	4.3	3.6
Stomach ulcer	1.2	1.5	2.0	7.8
Arthritis etc.	3.5	1.9	4.3	5.0

Base n: all respondents

Note: Only selected conditions reported in this table, that is, conditions affecting less than 5% of any (sub)group are excluded. Similarly, because of low prevalence, data here are reported to 1 decimal place: except that – = less than 0.5%

Figure 4.8 Q13: Reported prevalence of 'long-term' ill health (Q12) and specific conditions (percentage reporting each)

Overall, the replies to this question illustrate generally higher levels of ill health among the Bangladeshi population. In particular, much higher rates of heart attack and other heart disease were reported by Bangladeshi men; 'other heart diseases' were also very common among Bangladeshi women. We do not have any further information as to what these might be. High blood pressure was much more commonly reported by African-Caribbean women, but apparently rare among female Pakistanis. African-Caribbean women and Bangladeshi men were the most likely to report diabetes to this question. Bangladeshis of both genders were evidently subject to high levels of concern about the presence of stomach ulcers. Asthma, on the other hand, was relatively uncommon in Bangladeshis but raised among African-Caribbean women; the patterns appear to differ considerably between men and women of the four ethnic groups. Arthritis was most common among Bangladeshi men and African-Caribbean women. In none of the most frequently mentioned complaints were Indian or Pakistani people the most likely to report the condition, although Pakistani women had relatively high rates of asthma. When taken with the findings of the previous section, however, it would appear that the reporting of ill health conditions is not robust to variation in the way the question is asked. This point alone is of considerable significance to health promotion work.

Notes

1. R. Balarajan and V.S. Raleigh, *Ethnicity and health: a guide for the NHS* (Department of Health, London, 1993).

2. R. Balarajan and V.S. Raleigh, 'Patterns of mortality among Bangladeshis in England and Wales', *Ethnicity and Health* 2(1/2): 5–12.

3. In the absence of the possibility of conducting full blood pressure measurements, as was done for the HSE and ADNFS, a question on recall of a diagnosis was the best proxy that could be arranged.

4. It is not a simple matter to establish comparative rates between ethnic minorities and the national total population. There can be no direct comparison with the national HSE, since that depended on a slightly different basis of questioning, and age groups covered, but for certain conditions (diabetes, stroke, BP, IHD, i.e. heart attack and angina combined) some estimates may be obtained. In particular, we had expected the HSE to demonstrate higher prevalence rates for most conditions because it covered a significant number of respondents aged over 65, while these were only exceptionally included in the HEA survey.

5. NIDDM (non-insulin dependent diabetes mellitus,) the 'late onset' form of the disease, is normally treated by diet rather than self-injection. There is some evidence that the 'Asian form' of diabetes represents a development of insulin resistance and that other aspects of heart disease in Asians also represent a clinically different picture (P.M. McKeigue, G. Miller and M.G. Marmot, 'Coronary heart disease in South Asians overseas: a review', *Journal of Clinical Epidemiology* 42(7): 597–609; and A. Samanta, A.C. Burden and C. Jagger, 'A comparison of the clinical features and vascular complications of diabetes between migrant Asians and Caucasians in Leicester', *Diabetes Research Clinical Practice* 14(3): 205–13). A useful discussion about the risks of diabetes is found in H. Keen, *Blood pressure and diabetes: everyone's concern. Report of a working party* (RR Association for Zeneca Pharma, UK, Chineham, Hants, 1994).

5 Knowledge of health and health-promoting behaviour

Summary of the main findings

- When asked about their general health, the majority of people in each ethnic group rated their health as good (very good or fairly good) for their age (African-Caribbeans 86%, Indians 86%, Pakistanis 80%, Bangladeshis 73%) (Section 5.2).

- In each ethnic group, men and women aged 50–74 years were significantly more likely than younger men and women to rate their health as poor (very poor or fairly poor) for their age. The highest proportion was found among Bangladeshi people, among whom two-thirds (62%) of adults age 50–74 years assessed their health as poor for their age (Section 5.2).

- When asked about the link between behaviour and serious illnesses, the majority of people in each ethnic group reported an awareness that there are things people can do to reduce the risk of getting serious illnesses (African-Caribbeans 81%, Indians 76%, Pakistanis 72%, Bangladeshis 56%). However, in each ethnic group, the proportions reporting that people can do things to reduce the risk of getting serious illnesses were smaller than those reporting that people can do things to improve their health or help themselves to stay healthy (Section 5.3).

- When asked about the most important things people can do to improve their health, high proportions of those who had thought there are things that people can do to improve their health or to help themselves stay healthy identified healthy eating and taking regular exercise. Other health-promoting behaviours, including not smoking, were identified by very small proportions in each ethnic group (Section 5.4).

- Three-quarters of African-Caribbean people (75%), almost three-quarters of Indian people (71%), two-thirds of Pakistani people (66%) and half of Bangladeshi people (52%) reported that they did something on a regular basis to improve their health or to help themselves stay healthy (Section 5.5).

5.1 Introduction and background

The extent to which individuals engage in health-promoting behaviours and are prepared to modify risk behaviours, such as unhealthy eating and cigarette smoking, will depend, in part, on their own assessments of their health state, their awareness of the links between health behaviour and health/illness and their knowledge of what constitutes 'healthy behaviour'. This chapter reports, in the following four sections, on these aspects of respondents' health awareness and knowledge.

Section 5.2 reports on self-assessed health. It is widely accepted that people's own assessments of their health are an important component of health surveys. Respondents' own assessments of their health provide a general measure of their subjective feelings about their health and how they experience symptoms and biomedical conditions. Self-assessed health correlate well with objective measures of health, including eventual morbidity and mortality and has been found to be more closely associated with health service use than medical condition.[1]

While it is generally accepted that the causes of many illness are multi-factorial, it has been established that adopting certain health-promoting behaviours can modify people's risk of developing illnesses and diseases. Section 5.3 reports on respondents' awareness of this link between behaviour and health/illness. First, it examines whether respondents had an awareness that there are things people can do to maintain and promote good health. Second, it looks at whether respondents had any awareness that people can do things to reduce their risk of getting serious illnesses.

Sections 5.4 and 5.5 report on the subgroup of respondents in each ethnic group who believed that there are things people can do to improve their health or to help themselves stay in good health. Section 5.4 reports on respondents' knowledge of activities that promote and maintain health. Section 5.5 looks at the health-promoting activities that respondents report themselves to be involved in on a regular basis to improve their health or to help themselves stay healthy.

5.2 Self-assessed health

Health surveys of the UK population suggest that the majority of people rate their own health to be good.[2] Although the question format used in the current survey was slightly different to that used in other surveys, the findings are broadly in line with those reported for the adult population over age 16 years in the 1994 HSE. Large proportions in each ethnic group assessed their own health to be good for their age. The current survey utilised a single item measure from the 1991–2 Health and Lifestyles Survey of Black and Minority Ethnic Groups, thus allowing comparisons between the data from the two surveys.

Figure 5.1 shows respondents' perceptions of their own health. Respondents were asked to rate their health from 'very good' to 'very poor' for their age. Eight in ten African-Caribbean (86%), Indian (86%) and Pakistani (80%) people rated their health as good (fairly or very good). Among Bangladeshi people, this decreased to 7 in 10 respondents (73%), suggesting that a smaller proportion of Bangladeshis than other groups rate their own health as good for their age. These findings are very similar to those evident in the findings from the 1991–2 Health and Lifestyles Survey of Black and Minority Ethnic Groups.

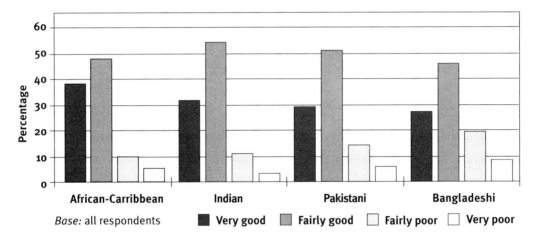

Figure 5.1: Self-assessed health by ethnic group

Health surveys of the general population suggest that there are some differences in self-assessed health between men and women.[3] Figure 5.2 describes differences in self-assessed health between men and women evident in the findings from the current survey. Although there were no significant differences between the proportions of men and women reporting good health (fairly good/very good health), there were some differences in the proportions of men and women reporting 'very good' health. Among African-Caribbean, Indian and Pakistani people, men were more likely than women to assess their health as 'very good' for their age. This finding is broadly in line with that reported in the HSE 1994[4] for the wider adult population in England. Among Bangladeshi people, although slightly more women than men reported 'very good' health, these apparent differences were not statistically significant.

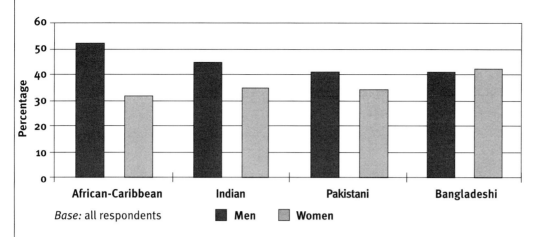

Base: all respondents   ■ Men   ■ Women

Figure 5.2: Proportions reporting very good health by sex

As might be expected, older men and women were more likely than younger men and women to assess their health as poor (fairly/very poor). Figure 5.3 examines this pattern for each ethnic group, illustrating some interesting differences between groups in the proportions of adults aged 50–74 years who reported poor health. Among African-Caribbean and Indian people aged 50–74 years, the proportions were relatively small, with a quarter of men and women rating their own health as poor. Among Pakistani people, the proportions assessing their health as poor increased to a third of women and almost a half of men. Among Bangladeshis aged 50–74, this figure increased to almost two-thirds for both men and women. Within all ethnic groups, for both men and women, there was a pronounced increase from the middle age band to the oldest age band in the proportions who assessed their health as poor. This pattern is similar to that found in the 1991–2 Health and Lifestyles Survey of Black and Minority Ethnic Groups (Figure 5.3).

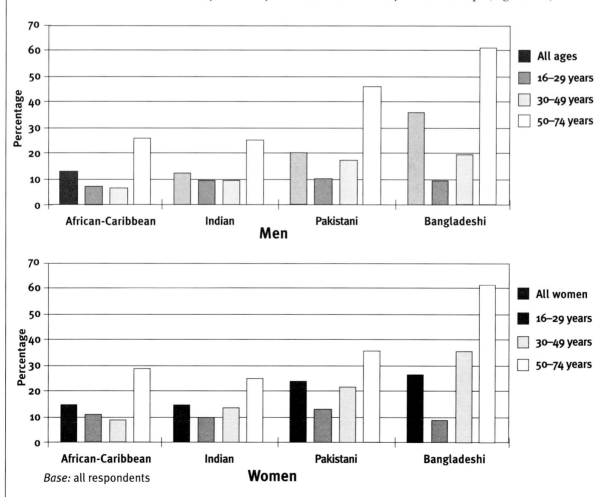

Base: all respondents

Figure 5.3: Proportions describing health as poor for their age by age group

5.3 Awareness of a link between behaviour and health/illness

The current survey attempted to provide some measure of people's awareness of the relationship between health behaviour and health state. The questionnaire explored this issue in two ways. First, respondents were asked, 'Is there anything people can do to improve their health, or to help themselves stay healthy?' Later, respondents were asked, 'Is there anything people can do to reduce their risk of getting serious illnesses or not?'

Large proportions in each ethnic group reported that they thought that people can do things to stay healthy or improve their health. The highest proportion, for both men and women in every age group, was found among African-Caribbean people, with 9 in 10 reporting that they thought there are things people can do to stay healthy or improve their health. The corresponding proportions for Indian and Pakistani people were also high (8 in 10 respondents), with the lowest proportion, 7 in 10, found among Bangladeshi people. In every age group, Bangladeshi men and women were less likely than other groups to report that they thought there are things people can do to improve their health or stay healthy (Figure 5.4; Table 5.2).

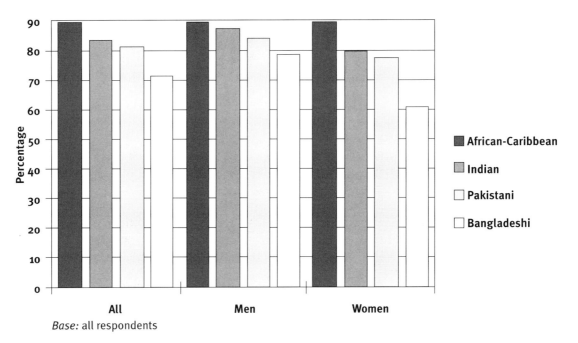

Base: all respondents

Figure 5.4: Proportions in each group by sex reporting that people can do things to improve their health

Among Indian, Pakistani and Bangladeshi people, men were more likely than women to report an awareness of the link between behaviour and health maintenance/improvement. This was most evident for Bangladeshi men and women, among whom 8 in 10 men but only 6 in 10 women stated that they thought that there are things people can do to improve their health or to keep themselves healthy. Among African-Caribbean women and men, there were no statistically significant differences (Figure 5.4).

Within each ethnic group, the proportions of adults reporting an awareness that people can do things to stay healthy or improve their health decreased as age increased: younger men and women within each ethnic group were more likely than older adults to state that healthy behaviour can promote and maintain good health. Even though smaller proportions of adults aged 50–74 years reported an awareness of the link between behaviour and health, the proportions of adults in the oldest age group who thought that people can do things to improve or maintain their health remained fairly high. The exception to this was Bangladeshi women, among whom only 40% aged 50–74 years reported that that they thought there are things people can do to improve health or stay healthy. This was half of the proportion found among African-Caribbean women in the same age group (Table 5.3).

Among Indian, Pakistani and African-Caribbean people, the proportions who reported that they 'don't know' if there are things people can do to improve their health or to help themselves stay healthy was small (less than 8%). The corresponding proportion for Bangladeshi respondents was more than double that for other groups, and can be largely accounted for by the relatively large minority of Bangladeshi women (26%) who stated that they did not know if there is anything people can do to maintain or improve their health. The proportion who said they did not know whether there is a link between health behaviour and promoting or maintaining health was highest among Bangladeshi women aged 50–74 (46%).

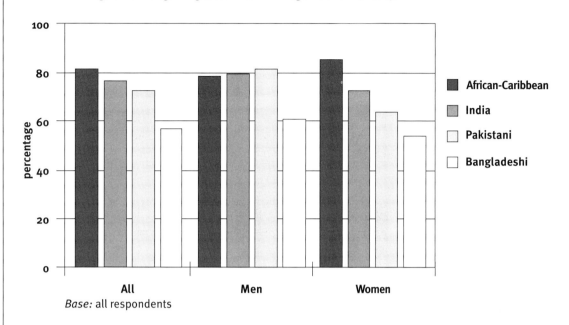

Base: all respondents

Figure 5.5: Proportions in each group by sex reporting that people can do things to reduce the risk of getting serious illnesses

Respondents were also asked whether there is anything people can do to reduce the risk of getting serious illnesses (Figure 5.5). Although a majority in each ethnic group identified a link between behaviour and getting serious illnesses, the proportions were smaller than those for the proportions of respondents who identified a link between behaviour and health improvement. African-Caribbean people were most likely, and Bangladeshi people least likely, to identify that people can do things to reduce the risk of serious illnesses. Among the South Asian groups who took part in the survey, in each age group men were more likely than women to report that people can do things to reduce the risk of serious illnesses. Among African-Caribbean people, this picture was reversed, with women in each age group more likely than men to state a link between behaviour and preventing serious illness. Across the groups, the general pattern was that young adults aged 16–29 were more likely than older adults aged 50–74 years to say that there are things people can do reduce the risk of serious illnesses (Table 5.4).

5.4 Knowledge about health-promoting activities

Respondents who answered 'yes' to the question 'Is there anything people can do to improve their health, or to help themselves stay in good health, or not?' were asked to identify the most important things which people can do to improve their health or to help themselves stay healthy. Figure 5.6 shows the health-promoting activities most commonly identified by this subgroup of respondents. The data suggest that, with the exception of eating a healthy diet and taking regular exercise, other behaviours generally accepted by health professionals as health-promoting (not smoking, not getting overweight, avoiding fatty foods, moderate alcohol consumption) were identified as health-promoting by only small proportions of respondents in each group. There were some significant differences between groups for some of the main health behaviours identified. Bangladeshi people were less likely to identify eating a healthy diet, taking regular exercise and not smoking as health-promoting than the other South Asian groups that took part or African-Caribbean people. The following subsections report on the patterns for the three health behaviours most commonly identified by respondents: healthy eating, regular exercise and not smoking.

As Figure 5.6 shows, eating a healthy diet was the health-promoting activity most commonly identified. It was most commonly identified by men and women of all ages, in each ethnic group. It was identified as health-promoting by 82% of African-Caribbean people, 81% of Indian and

Pakistani people and 74% of Bangladeshi people. Among African-Caribbean people, a slightly higher proportion of women than men identified healthy eating as a health-promoting behaviour but no clear pattern by age was evident, with high proportions of adults in each age group identifying healthy eating as health-promoting. A similar gender pattern to that found among African-Caribbean people emerged for Indian and Pakistani men and women, with greater proportions of women in each group identifying healthy eating. However, among Indian and Pakistani men and women there were some clear age differences. The data identify that in both groups, older adults were significantly less likely to identify healthy eating as an important health-promoting activity, suggesting that they may have less knowledge about the link between healthy eating and good health than younger adults. There were no significant gender or age differences in the proportions of Bangladeshi men and women identifying healthy eating as health-promoting.

The second most commonly identified health-promoting behaviour was taking regular exercise. The findings suggest that Indian, Pakistani and Bangladeshi men were more likely to identify taking regular exercise as health enhancing than their female counterparts. Differences between African-Caribbean men and women were not statistically significant. When age was examined, a similar pattern to that observed for healthy eating was evident, with older adults in each ethnic group least likely to identify taking regular exercise as an important health-promoting activity. The proportions of older Bangladeshi adults identifying taking regular exercise as health-promoting was particularly small (only 3 in 10 adults aged 50–74 years).

As Figure 5.6 illustrates, only small proportions (less than 1 in 5) in each ethnic group identified not smoking as an important health-promoting activity. Differences between men and women were not significant among African-Caribbean and Indian people, but among Pakistani people, a slightly larger but significant proportion of men identified not smoking as health-promoting. Within the Bangladeshi group, where smoking rates among men were particularly high, it was women rather than men who were more likely to identify not smoking as health-promoting. With the exception of the Bangladeshi group, where no age differences were apparent, adults over 50 in all other groups were less likely than younger counterparts to identify not smoking as health-promoting.

Health behaviour	African-Caribbean %	Indian %	Pakistani %	Bangladeshi %
Healthy eating	82	81	81	74
Taking regular exercise	77	74	70	60
Not smoking	19	15	17	18
Not drinking too much	14	12	12	9
Not worrying too much	3	7	12	6
Getting a good night's sleep	7	6	7	15
Avoid getting overweight	2	6	10	8
Avoid fatty food	5	10	11	13
Psycho-social factors	9	8	7	6
Don't take drugs	3	4	6	8

Base: Those who perceived there are things people can do to improve their health or stay healthy.

Figure 5.6: Most commonly identified health-promoting behaviours

5.5 Involvement in health-promoting activities

The current survey included a measure of the extent to which respondents perceived themselves to be involved in activities that promote health. It should be noted that questions about involvement in health-promoting behaviour were only asked of the subgroup of respondents who perceive that there are activities that people can do to stay healthy or to improve their health. The proportions of respondents in the current survey who felt that they were doing something on a regular basis for their health appear higher than the proportions reported in the earlier 1991–2 survey. This is due to differences in the bases used to calculate the proportions of respondents (the 1991–2 survey report calculated the proportions of respondents who perceived themselves to be involved in health-promoting activities as a proportion of all respondents in each group).

Half to three-quarters of respondents who were asked, reported that they participated in a health-promoting activity/activities on a regular basis to improve their health or to help themselves stay healthy (Figure 5.7). As a group, African-Caribbean people were most likely and Bangladeshi people least likely to report regular participation in a health-promoting activity. African-Caribbean and Indian men aged 16–29 years had the highest rates of participation and Bangladeshi men and women aged over 30 years the lowest rates of participation. Among Indian and Pakistani people, men were significantly more likely than women to be participating in health-enhancing activities. Among Bangladeshi and African-Caribbean men and women, there were no statistically significant differences in the proportions of each sex who reported regular involvement in health-promoting activities.

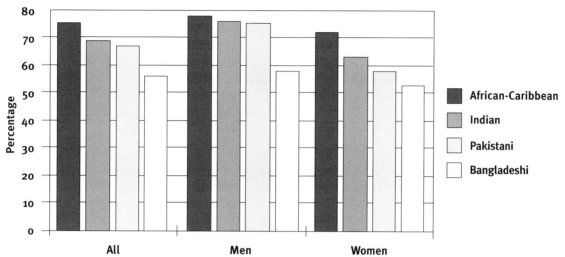

Base: Those who perceived there are things people can do to improve their health or stay healthy

Figure 5.7: Proportions participating in health-promoting activities on a regular basis

Figure 5.8 shows the main health-promoting activities respondents said they were engaged in on a regular basis. Only two activities were reported by large proportions of respondents in each group. The most commonly reported activity was taking regular exercise, mentioned by two-thirds to three-quarters of respondents. Healthy eating was the second most commonly reported activity, with half of respondents in each group saying that they ate a healthy diet regularly. However, as data reported in Chapter 8 suggests that respondents' knowledge of healthy foods varied widely, it is not clear to what extent the diet-related health-promoting behaviours reported here by respondents can be classed as meeting the guidelines laid down in the Committee on Medical Aspects of Food Policy report.[4]

Other behaviours widely held by health professionals as 'health promoting', such as not smoking, not drinking too much alcohol and avoiding getting overweight were mentioned by very low proportions of respondents in each ethnic group. It is not clear, however, to what extent this could be explained by respondents' failure to report activities they were involved in but which they were not aware would be regarded as health-promoting or were not consciously doing to promote good health.

Health Behaviour	African-Caribbean %	Indian %	Pakistani %	Bangladeshi %
Taking regular exercise	74	71	63	65
Eating a healthy diet	50	53	56	50
Not smoking	10	8	8	16
Avoiding fatty foods	7	12	15	15
Not getting overweight	3	6	6	8
Not drinking too much alcohol	8	8	8	11
Not worrying	3	4	6	4
Getting a good night's sleep	4	5	7	10

Figure 5.8: Most frequently reported health-promoting activities engaged in by those who felt that they were involved in a health-promoting activity on a regular basis

Figure 5.9 looks at the number of health-promoting activities respondents reported that they were involved in. The findings were similar across the groups, with just under half in each group reporting that they were involved in one health-promoting activity and just over half reporting involvement in two or more activities. Among African-Caribbean, Indian and Bangladeshi people, slightly larger proportions of women than men reported involvement in two or more activities. Differences between age groups were apparent only within the African-Caribbean and Indian groups, among whom a slightly higher proportion of adults over 50 than younger adults reported involvement in two or more activities.

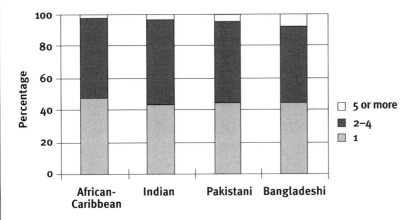

Figure 5.9: Number of activities engaged in

5.6   Conclusions

People's assessments of their own health provide an important measure of health. The data reported here suggest that large majorities in each group assessed their own health as good. The proportions who rated their health as good decreased with increasing age. As might be expected, older adults in each group were less likely than younger adults to report good health. It was notable that Bangladeshi men and women in each age group were more likely to report poor health than other groups. The proportion of Bangladeshi men and women over 50 who reported poor health was particularly high.

The extent to which African-Caribbean, Indian, Pakistani and Bangladeshi people are likely to adopt health behaviours and modify risk behaviours linked with cardiovascular and other diseases will depend, in part, on whether they believe that there are things that they can do to maintain or improve their health and reduce the risk of serious illnesses. The data described in this chapter suggest that across the groups, large proportions believed that there are things people can do to promote their health and reduce their risk of serious illnesses. Although large proportions of respondents identified healthy eating and regular exercise as health-promoting behaviours, the proportions identifying other behaviours linked to cardiovascular and other common causes of disease and premature death were small.

While large proportions of those who perceived that people can do things to improve their health or stay healthy reported that they were involved in health-promoting activities, few reported involvement in health-promoting activies other than healthy eating and regular exercise. It was notable that Bangladeshi people were significantly less likely than people in other groups to perceive a link between behaviour and health and illness or to report a perception of being involved in health-promoting activities.

Notes

1. A. Bowling, *Measuring health: a review of quality of life measurement scales* (Open University Press, Buckingham, 1991).

2. M. Blaxter, *Health and lifestyles* (Routledge, London, 1990); D. Cox, F. Huppert and M. Whichelow, *The Health and Lifestyles Survey: seven years on* (Dartmouth Publishing , Aldershot, 1993); Joint Health Surveys Unit, *Health survey for England, 1994* (London, 1994).

3. Joint Health Surveys Unit, *Health survey*; Blaxter, *Health and lifestyles.*

4. Joint Health Surveys Unit, *Health survey*; Blaxter, *Health and lifestyles.*

5. Department of Health, *Committee of Medical Aspects of Food Policy Report* (HMSO, London, 1994).

Cigarette smoking and the use of chewing tobacco products

mary of the main findings

- In general, smoking rates among African-Caribbean, Indian, Pakistani and Bangladeshi people were the same as or lower than those found among the wider population of England. However, smoking rates varied widely within and between ethnic groups (Section 6.2).

- Cigarette smoking appeared to be a significant risk behaviour among all groups and 49% of Bangladeshi men, 29% of African-Caribbean men, 24% of Pakistani men and 15% of Indian men reported that they currently smoked cigarettes. Particularly high smoking rates were found among Bangladeshi men aged 30–49 (54%) and 50–74 (70%) (Section 6.2).

- Rates of current cigarette smoking were very low in general among Indian women (2%), Pakistani women (1%) and Bangladeshi women (6%). A notable exception was the rate of current smoking found among Bangladeshi women in the oldest aged group (50–74), among whom 14% reported currently smoking cigarettes. Cigarette smoking was more prevalent among African-Caribbean women, with 21% reporting that they currently smoked cigarettes (Section 6.2).

- In general, African-Caribbean, Indian, Pakistani and Bangladeshi men and women, on average, smoked fewer cigarettes per day than men and women in the wider population of England. An exception was found among Bangladeshi men, whose average (mean) daily consumption of cigarettes was similar to that for men in the wider population (Section 6.3).

- In all groups, half to three-quarters of current smokers had attempted to stop smoking on one or more occasion. Stopping smoking appeared to be a more recent phenomenon among African-Caribbean, Indian, Pakistani and Bangladeshi men and women than among the wider population of England (Section 6.4).

- Knowledge levels about the main diseases linked to smoking were low among men and women in all groups. In each ethnic groups, the serious illness most likely to be linked to cigarette smoking was lung cancer. Knowledge levels about the links between smoking and other respiratory diseases, heart disease and throat and mouth cancers were very low (Section 6.5).

- Chewing tobacco continues to be a widespread habit among Bangladeshi people but very limited among Indian and Pakistani people. Chewing tobacco is particularly high among Bangladeshi women over 30, among whom 8 in 10 report chewing of tobacco. Half (52%) of Bangladeshi women and a third (33%) of Bangladeshi men who smoked cigarettes also consumed tobacco through chewing.

6.1 Introduction and background

This chapter examines smoking patterns and the use of chewing tobacco. Cigarette smoking is a significant cause of disease and premature death in Britain, with smokers at greater risk than non-smokers of developing coronary heart disease, lung cancer and other respiratory diseases and cancer of the throat and mouth. Cigarette smoking has become a prominent target for health behaviour change. There are considerable variations within and between ethnic groups in patterns of smoking-related diseases[1] and smoking behaviour.[2] It has been suggested that black and minority ethnic groups in general appear to be at greater risk than white groups of developing coronary heart disease and some cancers.[3] Data on the cigarette smoking consumption and cessation patterns of African-Caribbean and South Asian people is then central, not only to increasing our understanding of smoking as a risk factor for coronary heart disease, strokes, lung cancer and respiratory diseases among these groups, but also to the design and implementation of health promotion programmes that seek to improve their health.

The HEA surveys of the health and lifestyles of black and minority ethnic groups in England are the main source of information on cigarette smoking among black and minority ethnic groups.[4] This chapter reports on cigarette smoking prevalence (Section 6.2) cigarette consumption (Section 6.3), smoking cessation (Section 6.4) and looks at knowledge levels about the health effects of smoking (Section 6.5) in the four groups included in this survey. In addition the use of chewing tobacco products among Indian, Pakistani and Bangladeshi pe 6.6). Data from the survey are compared, where it is possible and appropriate, wi the HSE 1994[5] to provide some measurement of how smoking consumption patterns among African-Caribbean, Indian, Pakistani and Bangladeshi people those for the whole population in England.

6.2 Smoking prevalence

Smoking prevalences were measured using the same question format used in other major surveys (General Household Survey, Health Survey for England, Health in England Survey) and in the previous 1991–2 survey of black and minority ethnic groups. Figure 6.1 shows the proportions of current smokers ('smoke cigarettes at all nowadays') in each ethnic group and compares them with those reported in the HSE 1994 for the adult population in England. Smoking prevalences for African-Caribbean, Indian, Pakistani and Bangladeshi people were generally the same as or lower than those recorded for the wider population in England.

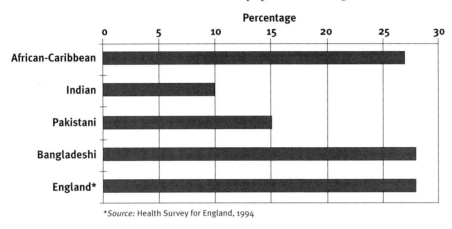

Source: Health Survey for England, 1994

Figure 6.1: Rates of current smoking

Rates of current smoking varied widely between and within the groups. Taking the groups as a whole first, high smoking prevalences were found among Bangladeshi (28%) and African-Caribbean people (27%), with lower rates among Pakistani (15%) and Indian people (10%). Figure 6.1 disguises notable differences in smoking rates between men and women within each group. While sex differences in cigarette smoking in the population in England as a whole have almost disappeared, sex differences among African-Caribbean, Indian, Pakistani and Bangladeshi people remain considerable. In every group, men had higher smoking rates than women. The current survey findings confirm those from the 1991–2 survey, suggesting that cigarette smoking is likely to be a significant risk behaviour for South Asian and African-Caribbean men. Very high smoking rates were found among Bangladeshi men (49%), particularly for those aged 30–49 years (54%) and aged 50–74 years (70%). The smoking rate for African-Caribbean men was lower (34%). The corresponding proportion for Pakistani men was 28% and for Indian men 18%.

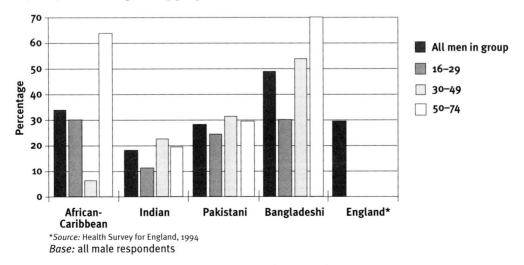

Source: Health Survey for England, 1994
Base: all male respondents

Figure 6.2: Current smokers: men in each group by age

In every group and at every age, women had lower smoking rates than their male counterparts (Figure 6.3). The highest smoking rate was found among African-Caribbean women (21%). Although smoking prevalences for African-Caribbean women were lower, at every age, than those recorded for women in the wider population in England, a similar pattern was evident with smoking prevalences declining with age, but at a faster rate than for the wider female population in England. African-Caribbean women aged 50–74 years had a very low smoking rate (4%). Among South Asian women, smoking rates were very low (Indian women 3%; Pakistani women 2%; Bangladeshi women 6%), continuing the pattern observed in the 1991–2 survey. A notable exception was the higher smoking rate found among Bangladeshi women aged 50–74 years, among whom 14% reported being current smokers.

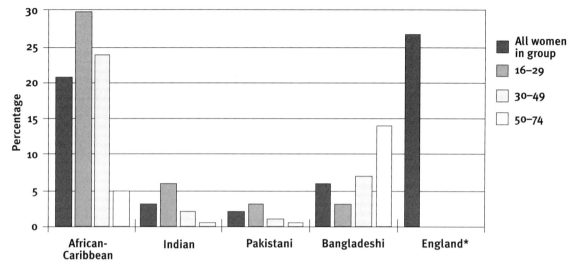

Source: Health Survey for England, 1994

Figure 6.3: Current smokers: women in each group by age

High majorities of current cigarette smokers in each ethnic group smoked on a regular basis. Figure 6.4 examines the smoking prevalences for current regular smokers (smokes one or more cigarettes a day) and compares them to those reported in the 1991–2 health and lifestyles survey of black and minority ethnic groups. As the data reported here is only the second survey of the health and lifestyles of black and minority ethnic groups in England, it necessary to report on trends in smoking rates with some caution, noting that any changes in smoking rates over time may be attributable to sample differences and not indicative of any general trend. Noting this caveat, data from the current survey suggest that the proportion of women in each group who smoke regularly remains largely unchanged. Among men, the pattern is more complex. The proportion of African-Caribbean men who reported that they were current regular smokers appears not to have changed since the 1991–2 survey. Among Indian and Pakistani men, there appears to have been a slight decrease in rate of current regular smoking and among Bangladeshi men, a slight increase in the proportion who reported currently smoking regularly.

	African-Caribbean		Indian		Pakistani		Bangladeshi	
	1991–2	1994	1991–2	1994	1991–2	1994	1991–2	1994
All	22	23	10	9	16	13	22	27
Men	29	29	20	15	30	24	42	46
Women	17	18	1	2	2	1	5	6

Figure 6.4: Proportions of current regular smokers in each group, 1991–2 and 1994 (percentage of all in ethnic group)

Figure 6.5 examines the respondents' self-reported cigarette smoking status: whether they were current smokers ('smoke at all nowadays'), ex-regular smokers or never regular smokers (never smoked or had never smoked regularly[6]). It shows that African-Caribbean, Indian, Pakistani and Bangladeshi women were more likely than the population of England to have never smoked

cigarettes regularly. Among Indian, Pakistani and Bangladeshi women the proportio͏
that they had never been regular smokers were very high (over 90%). Just under
of African-Caribbean women reported they had never smoked regularly. The pro͏
in each group who reported that they had never been regular smokers were muc͏.
those found among women. Among Indian, Pakistani and African-Caribbean ͏.
proportions who reported that they had never smoked were larger that the proportion fou͏.
the wider male population in England, with Bangladeshi men having a similar proportion of neve͏
regular smokers to that found in the wider male population of England.

Cigarette smoking status	African-Caribbean %	Indian %	Pakistani %	Bangladeshi %	Population in England* %
All					
Current smokers	27	10	15	28	28
Ex-regular smokers	10	6	5	6	26
Never/occasional smokers	63	84	79	66	46
Women					
Current smokers	21	3	2	6	27
Ex-regular smokers	7	2	8	2	21
Never/occasional smokers	72	96	96	92	52
Men					
Current smokers	34	18	28	49	29
Ex-regular smokers	14	9	9	10	31
Never/occasional smokers	52	73	63	42	40

*Source: Health Survey for England, 1994
Base: all respondents

Figure 6.5: Self-reported cigarette smoking status

6.3 Cigarette consumption

Daily cigarette consumption is reported in two ways: as the daily average (mean) quantity consumed per smoker per day and as the proportions smoking fewer or more than 20 cigarettes per day. Figure 6.6 shows the average daily consumption of cigarettes for men and women and how they compare to that found among the wider population in England. With the exception of Bangladeshi men, the general pattern is that South Asian men and women had a notably lower average daily consumption of cigarettes than men and women in the wider population in England. In England, the average daily cigarette consumption for men in 1995 was 15.6 cigarettes per day, and for women 13.3 cigarettes per day. Among men who took part in the survey, Indians and Pakistanis (11.6 cigarettes) had the lowest average daily consumptions. African-Caribbean men's average daily consumption of cigarettes was slightly higher (12.1 cigarettes). Bangladeshi men had the highest average daily consumption (15.6 cigarettes), which was just below that for the male population in England.

African-Caribbean, Indian, Pakistani and Bangladeshi women had lower average daily cigarette consumptions than the wider female population in England. The lowest average consumptions were found among African-Caribbean women (10.3 cigarettes) and Bangladeshi women (9.8 cigarettes), with slightly higher average daily consumption rates for Indian women (11.6 cigarettes) and Pakistani women (11.3 cigarettes).

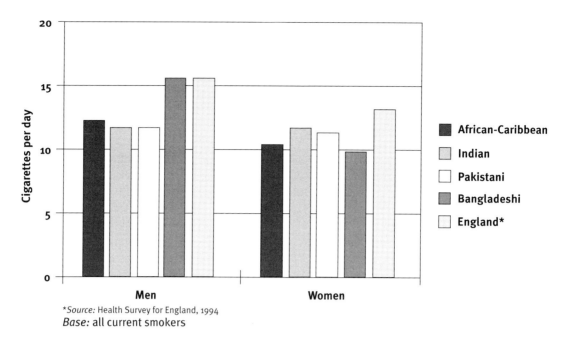

*Source: Health Survey for England, 1994
Base: all current smokers

**Figure 6.6: Current smokers: average (mean) daily cigarette consumption
(self-reported)**

Turning to the proportions smoking fewer than or more than 20 cigarettes per day, there were fewer heavy smokers (smoking 20 or more cigarettes a day) among African-Caribbean and South Asian respondents than among the population as a whole. Among male respondents, 8 in 10 African-Caribbeans (82%), Indians (80%) and Pakistanis (81%) and 7 in 10 Bangladeshis (69%) were light smokers (fewer than 20 cigarettes per day). The highest proportion of heavy smokers was found among Bangladeshi men (30%) and the lowest proportions among Indian men (19%). Among women, the majority in every group were light smokers, with 8 in 10 or more smokers in each group reporting that they smoked fewer than 20 cigarettes a day. Figure 6.7 shows the proportions of heavy and light smokers for men and women by ethnic group. Although the table suggests minor sex differences in the proportions of men and women who were heavy smokers, these were only statistically significant for Bangladeshi men and women. Among this group, a third more men than women were heavy smokers.

No. smoked daily	African-Caribbean %	Indian %	Pakistani %	Bangladeshi %	Population in England* %
Women					
0–19	86	88	82	80	74
20 or more	14	12	18	20	27
Men					
0–19	82	80	81	69	63
20 or more	18	20	19	31	37

*Source: Health Survey for England, 1994
Base: all current smokers

**Figure 6.7: Proportions of current smokers who reported smoking 19 or less
and 20 or more cigarettes per day**

Data for the whole population in England suggest that the percentage of smokers who are heavy smokers increases until it peaks at 45–54, after which it falls steeply with increasing age. For the groups reported here, no such pattern was evident, nor did any clear pattern by age emerge across the groups. However, notably high rates of heavy smoking were observed for Indian men aged 50–74 (42%), Pakistani women aged 30–49 (50%) and Bangladeshi men aged 30–49 (37%).

6.4 Smoking cessation

Current regular smokers and ex-regular smokers were asked about giving up smoking. African-Caribbeans and the South Asian groups reported on here were less likely to have given up smoking than those in the wider population of England. A third of Indian people (35%), a quarter of African-Caribbean people (28%) and Pakistani people (26%) and less than a quarter of Bangladeshi people (17%) who had ever smoked were now ex-regular smokers. This compares to just under half (46%) of the whole population in England. In 1994 among the population as a whole, fewer women than men who have ever smoked smokers were now ex-smokers. A similar pattern was evident among African-Caribbean men and women, but this pattern was reversed among Indian, Pakistani and Bangladeshi men and women (Figure 6.8).

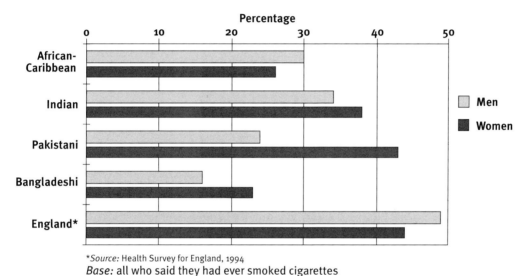

Source: Health Survey for England, 1994
Base: all who said they had ever smoked cigarettes

Figure 6.8: Proportions of ever smokers who reported that they were currently ex-regular smokers

Examining smoking cessation attempts among current smokers suggests that half to three-quarters of current smokers had attempted to give up smoking on at least one occasion (African-Caribbeans 63%, Indians 65%, Pakistanis 55%, Bangladeshis 71%) (Figure 6.9). High proportions of African-Caribbean (68%), Indian (89%), Bangladeshi (79%) and Pakistani women (59%) who were current smokers had attempted to give up smoking on at least one occasion. Among men, the ethnic group with the highest smoking rate, Bangladeshi men, also had the highest proportion of current smokers who had attempted to quit (71%). This suggests that a large proportion of Bangladeshi men have attempted to quit smoking but have been unsuccessful. Over half of Pakistani men (55%), African Caribbean men (59%) and Indian men (61%) who were current smokers had attempted to quit smoking. Within the groups, sex differences were only apparent among Indian people, with a greater proportion of female current smokers (89%) reporting that they had attempted to give up than male current smokers (61%). No clear pattern by age was evident.

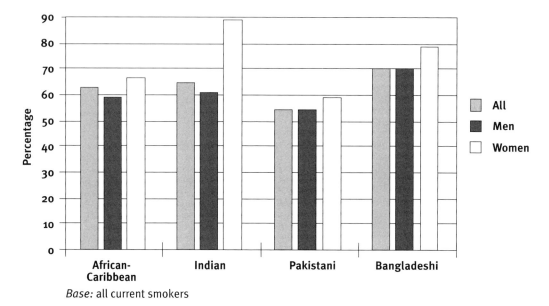

Base: all current smokers

Figure 6.9: Current smokers who have attempted to quit

Questions about stopping smoking were also asked of ex-regular smokers. The current survey confirmed the finding from the 1991–2 survey of black and minority ethnic groups that stopping smoking is a more recent phenomenon among African-Caribbean, Indian, Pakistani and Bangladeshi people than it is for the population in England as a whole. Whereas only 23% of ex-regular smokers in the whole population gave up smoking in the previous five years, the corresponding proportions for the groups taking part in the current survey were substantially higher (African-Caribbeans 41%, Indians 39%, Pakistanis 56% and Bangladeshis 60%). Figure 6.10 identifies when ex-regular smokers in each group gave up smoking. Although the data reported here broadly replicated the findings from the 1991–2 Health and Lifestyles Survey of Black and Minority Ethnic Groups, direct comparisons of the data are not possible, owing to slight differences in the way the categories were constructed (to allow data from the current survey to be compared with data from the HSE 1994).

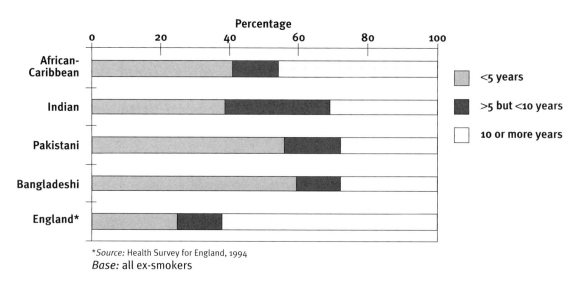

Source: Health Survey for England, 1994
Base: all ex-smokers

Figure 6.10: When ex-regular smokers gave up cigarette smoking

6.5 Knowledge about the links between cigarette smoking and disease

A key aim of the survey was to examine knowledge about the links between health behaviour and cardiovascular and respiratory diseases, so the survey attempted to measure respondents' knowledge of the links between cigarette smoking and specific diseases. Figure 6.11 shows the proportions in each group who perceived smoking to be linked to specific diseases. The data illustrate that for the main diseases linked to cigarette smoking (heart disease, stroke, lung cancer, respiratory disease and throat and mouth cancer), knowledge about the link between cigarette smoking and disease was relatively poor.

Beginning with heart disease, approximately a quarter of African-Caribbeans and South Asians perceived there to be a link between cigarette smoking and heart disease (African-Caribbeans 27%, Indians 23%, Pakistanis 27%, Bangladeshis 27%). In each ethnic group, women, as a group, appeared to have more awareness that cigarette smoking was linked to heart disease than men. When age was examined, the patterns were more complex. Among South Asian women, the knowledge that smoking can cause heart disease decreased with increasing age. Age differences among African-Caribbean women were not statistically significant. Among Indian and African Caribbean men, respondents aged 30–49 were more likely to report that smoking was linked to heart disease than men in other age groups. A slightly different picture emerged among Bangladeshis, with men aged 50–74 reporting less knowledge of the link between smoking and heart disease than men in other-age groups.

The serious disease most likely to be linked with cigarette smoking by each ethnic group was lung cancer. Half of African-Caribbean (52%) and Indian (52%) people and less than half Pakistani (47%) and Bangladeshi (41%) people identified a link between smoking and lung cancer. Among Indian, Pakistani and Bangladeshi people, men were more likely than women to report that lung cancer was linked with cigarette smoking. Among African-Caribbean people, a larger proportion of women than men identified a link between lung cancer and smoking. These differences between African-Caribbean men and women were small but statistically significant. For men and women in each ethnic group, knowledge of a link between lung cancer and smoking decreased with age.

Knowledge of a link between smoking and other respiratory diseases was poor. Less than 1 in 5 respondents in each ethnic group reported a link between smoking and respiratory diseases other than lung cancer (African-Caribbeans 16%, Indians 11%, Pakistanis 15%, Bangladeshis 12%). Differences between men and women followed a similar pattern to those for lung cancer with Indian, Pakistani and Bangladeshi men and African-Caribbean women more likely to report a link than their counterparts. No clear pattern by age was apparent.

Throat and mouth cancer, another serious illness and cause of death linked to smoking, was identified by less than 1% in each ethnic group, suggesting that information needs about the link between throat and mouth cancers and smoking are high.

Disease mentioned as linked to smoking	African-Caribbean %	Indian %	Pakistani %	Bangladeshi %
Heart disease				
All	27	23	27	27
Women	29	25	30	31
Men	24	21	25	24
Lung cancer	52	52	47	41
All				
Women	54	46	37	36
Men	50	59	56	45
Respiratory diseases				
All	16	11	15	12
Women	19	9	13	7
Men	13	12	17	15
Throat/mouth cancer				
All	<0.5	<0.5	<0.5	<0.5
Women	<1.0	<0.5	<0.5	<1.0
Men	<0.5	<0.5	<0.0	<0.5
Don't know of any disease linked to smoking				
All	7	10	14	18
Women	5	13	21	27
Men	9	7	7	8

Base: all respondents

Figure 6.11: Proportions mentioning selected diseases as linked to cigarette smoking

6.6 Chewing tobacco products

Tobacco can be consumed through chewing as well as through smoking. Chewing tobacco products is thought to be linked to an increased risk of mouth and throat cancers among users.[7] Tobacco is usually chewed on its own or mixed with betel nut or sopari (areca nut) or paan. Chewing tobacco products is a habit prevalent among some South Asian groups. The current survey asked Indian, Pakistani and Bangladeshi respondents about tobacco chewing on its own or with other products (paan, betel nut/sopari). Tobacco chewing (on its own or with other products) appeared to be widespread among Bangladeshi people but very limited among Indian and Pakistani people. Figure 6.12 shows the proportions in each groups who reported recent (within the last four weeks) chewing of tobacco on it own or with another substances (paan, betel nut/sopari). Among Bangladeshi people, a third (32%) of respondents reported recent chewing of tobacco. Among Bangladeshi women, the use of chewing tobacco was high among women aged over 30, with 8 in 10 (78%) women aged 30–49 and 9 in 10 (92%) women aged 50–74 reporting that they had chewed tobacco recently. Among Bangladeshi men, chewing tobacco was less common, but was used by over a third of men aged 30 or over. As only very small minorities of Indians (2%) and Pakistanis (1%) reported recent chewing of tobacco with or without other substances, the rest of this subsection will examine, in more detail, chewing tobacco use among Bangladeshi people only.

Chewing tobacco on its own was rare among Bangladeshi people. More commonly, it had been recently chewed with betel nut/sopari (by 29% of Bangladeshis). Chewing betel nut/sopari with tobacco increased with age among in both men and women. Among Bangladeshi women, this increase was much sharper than among men. Among women aged 50 or over, 8 in 10 reported recent chewing of tobacco with betel nut/sopari (83%). This compares to 3 in 10 men aged 50 or over. Tobacco was also chewed with paan by a quarter (23%) of Bangladeshis. A high proportion of Bangladeshi women (71%) and a smaller proportion of men (27%) aged 50–74 reported its use. These findings show a broadly similar pattern of chewing tobacco use to that found in the previous (1991–2) survey.

Smaller proportions of Bangladeshis (3% of women and 17% of men) were consuming tobacco through both chewing and smoking. Half of Bangladeshi women (52%) and a third of Bangladeshi men (33%) who said they were current smokers reported that they chewed a tobacco product. Among non-smokers, the proportions reporting that they chewed a tobacco product were smaller, with a third of women (36%) and a fifth of men (21%) reporting that they chewed a tobacco product.

The survey also asked about recent chewing of substances (betel nut/sopari or paan) without tobacco. Although there is sufficient evidence to show that the regular chewing of tobacco on its own or with other substances can increase the risk of developing throat or mouth cancer, there is not sufficient evidence to demonstrate a link between chewing of non-tobacco products and throat or mouth cancer. Chewing betel nut/sopari or paan without tobacco was also more widespread among Bangladeshi people than among Indian or Pakistani people. Among younger Bangladeshi women and Bangladeshi men of all ages, it was more commonly chewed than betel nut/sopari or paan with tobacco.

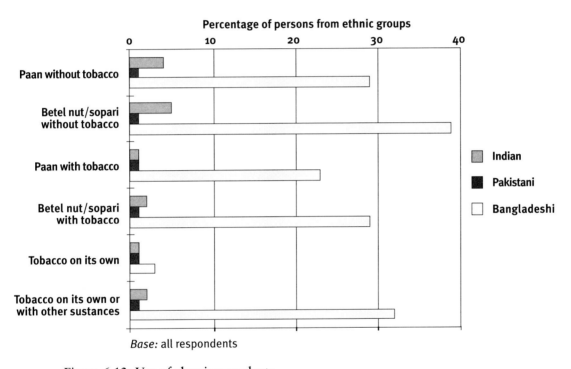

Base: all respondents

Figure 6.12: Use of chewing products

6.7 Conclusions

Patterns of cigarette smoking varied widely between and within the groups who took part in the survey. Cigarette smoking rates for each group taken as a whole in general appeared to be lower than those for the population in England as a whole. However, for some subgroups within the African-Caribbean community and the South Asian communities, smoking rates are particularly high. With the exception of Indian men, cigarette smoking appears to constitute a significant risk behaviour for African-Caribbean, Pakistani and Bangladeshi men. The smoking prevalence of Bangladeshi men was notably high. Among these groups of men, current smoking rates are higher than the target laid down in the Health of the Nation strategy and will need to fall substantially if the cigarette smoking target of no more than 20% is to be obtained by the year 2000. Cigarette smoking rates are lower among African-Caribbean women than among women in the population of England as a whole. Among Indian, Pakistani and Bangladeshi women, smoking rates are very low.

African-Caribbean, Indian, Pakistani and Bangladeshi men and women appear to consume fewer cigarettes per day than the English population taken as whole, and the groups surveyed contain fewer heavy smokers.

The data suggest that knowledge levels about the link between cigarette smoking and specific cardiovascular and respiratory disease appear to be low and could be improved significantly through sensitively targeted programmes that meet the information needs of individual groups. Further research into the most effective methods of helping each group to gain information about smoking-related disease would be a valuable prelude to the development of health promotion programmes.

The use of chewing products remains widespread among some Bangladeshi men and women. An important finding from this survey is that measures of tobacco consumption need to take into account that some people consume tobacco through smoking and chewing. Measures that only take account of tobacco consumed through smoking may underestimate tobacco intake, particularly among Bangladeshi people. In this survey, half of Bangladeshi women and a third of Bangladeshi men who said they were current smokers also said they chewed tobacco products. This survey did not seek to establish the extent of people's knowledge about the link between chewing tobacco products and disease. Currently, little is known about the extent of people's knowledge about the link between chewing tobacco products and disease, and research on the issue would be valuable.

Notes

1. K. Calman, *On the state of the public health: the Annual Report of the Chief Medical Officer of the Department of Health for the Year 1991* (HMSO, London, 1992).

2. K. Rudat, *Health and lifestyles: black and minority ethnic groups in England.* (Health Education Authority, London, 1994).

3. R. Balarajan and V.S. Raleigh, *Ethnicity and health: a guide for the NHS* (Department of Health, London, 1993).

4. Although black and minority ethnic respondents are included in the General Household Survey and HSE samples, the achieved samples sizes of black and minority ethnic groups are too small to permit separate annual analyses by ethnic group (aggregation of GHS data on minority ethnic groups across several years is available).

5. Joint Health Surveys Unit, *Health survey for England 1994*, (HMSO, London, 1996).

6. The category 'never regular smokers' consists of those who have never smoked cigarettes and occasional smokers who do not smoke cigarettes regularly (i.e. one or more cigarettes each day).

7. R. Bedi, 'Betel-quid and tobacco chewing among the United Kingdom Bangladeshi community', *British Journal of Cancer*, 74, suppl. XXIX (1996): S73–S77.

7   Activity and physical fitness

Summary of the main findings

- There was a clear consensus, unprompted, among all ethnic groups that taking exercise was one of the most important things that people could do to maintain their health. Rather fewer people reported following this advice.

- Bangladeshi people and Pakistani women were the least likely to be personally 'taking active exercise' for the sake of their health.

- Overweight (which was seen to be bad in itself) and heart disease were the health problems most likely to be said to be linked to (lack of) exercise: otherwise, there was a rather low level of awareness or knowledge about this issue.

- A variety of reasons were given for not participating in (energetic) leisure activity, some of which did vary between ethnic groups. White people (in a national sample) gave more excuses and were more likely to say that they were 'not sporty types'. Indian women were most likely 'not to have time', while Bangladeshi men were least likely to say this.

- There are certain reasons for not participating that appear to be specific to ethnic minority groups, notably modesty or avoidance of mixed sex activity and fear of going out alone, but language and culture were otherwise rarely mentioned as perceived barriers. Religion is important but modesty or avoidance of mixed sex settings or nudity is not confined to Muslims.

- A variety of 'good advice' relating to healthy living was proffered by respondents. This most commonly referred to not smoking, the need for a good night's sleep, avoiding overweight and not worrying. There were some variations between minority groups.

- Despite considerable variations in reported activity levels, perceptions of self-activity showed little relation to these.

- There was little difference in the aggregate amount of time spent on heavy housework and DIY or gardening between men and women or ethnic groups.

- There were considerable variations between gender, age and ethnic groups in the degree to which their (other) activities of daily living gave them opportunities for physical exercise. In particular this can be seen in relation to stair-walking, although very few people used stairs enough to obtain much benefit from this form of exercise.

- Walking is a common form of exercise among all people from minority ethnic groups.

- Significant numbers of people from all minority ethnic groups were active in caring for others (children and people with disabilities) which provided them with physical activity.

- African-Caribbean men and women were much more likely to engage in leisure sports, while Asian women were very much less likely to do so. Some sports or leisure activities are very much less likely to be engaged in by people from black and minority ethnic groups, but Bangladeshi men showed high levels of commitment to football, and African-Caribbean people to aerobics and body-building.

- Low levels of knowledge about the actual levels of effective physical activity were reported across the sample, and this may be a barrier to participation.

- Unemployment and patterns of employment among those in paid work have significant effects on levels of physical activity.

- Gender is a critical issue in both giving and taking advice related to exercise and healthy living, but it is difficult to isolate any specifically 'ethnic' factors which affect people's understanding of the issues.

7.1 Introduction

There is now a clear understanding that underpins much of the work of health promotion that an active lifestyle, that is, involvement in physical activity, is beneficial for health. Physical fitness, which need not necessarily relate to competitive levels of sporting prowess, is achievable at some level for all parts of society, and present recommendations are that everyone should attempt some 'moderate exercise' at least five times a week. At the time of the survey, a slightly different definition of desirable levels of activity was in use, that people should engage in 'moderate to vigorous exercise' on average at least three times weekly. Given the difficulties in assessing the true energy costs of any activity, and differences in perception of (or indeed, real variations in the challenge presented by) various activities, it is perhaps of more value here to concentrate on actual levels of reported behaviour and ideas about activity and physical fitness as they may differ between ethnic groups.

The analysis in this chapter, since the questions asked around this issue were located at a variety of points in the research interview, does not precisely reflect the sequence in which the data were collected. We have started by examining the data relating to perceptions and health beliefs before moving on to contrast these with the reported behaviour of respondents. In this, we feel that we reflect the process described in the 'health belief model', whereby expectations and values precede and affect actions.

7.2 Perceptions of exercise and health

At an early stage in the interview, all respondents to the HEA survey were asked the open (unprompted) question, 'What are the most important things which people can do to improve their health or to help themselves stay in good health?' A wide variety of answers were recorded, but there was a clear consensus that taking exercise was one of the most important of these. There was nevertheless some ethnic and gender variation in the pattern of replies. Similar but distinctive differences were also marked in the pattern of replies to a following question: 'What do you do to improve your health or to help yourself to stay healthy?'

	African-Caribbean %	Indian %	Pakistani %	Bangladeshi %
Females				
Q3: Most important	68	54	52	36
Q5: Done personally	47	32	25	18
Males:				
Q3: Most important	64	67	63	44
Q5: Done personally	49	48	44	29

Q3: To all those who replied 'yes' to the question, 'As far as you know, is there anything people can do to improve their health or help themselves stay in good health?' respondents were asked to list the 'most important' actions people could take. More than one (unprompted) answer could be recorded.

Q5: To all those who replied 'yes' to the question, 'And do you do anything yourself on a regular basis to improve your health or help yourself stay in good health?' respondents were asked to list what they did (unprompted). Take (regular) exercise was one answer. More than one could be recorded.

Figure 7.1: Proportion saying 'take regular exercise' as a health-maintaining or improving activity (Q3, Q5)

It is very clear that the majority of those questioned regarded 'taking exercise' as being very important, at least in the abstract. Men in general were somewhat more inclined to state this, ahead of other activities, but African-Caribbean women were in fact the most certain that exercise was a healthy activity. Bangladeshi women and men were least likely to state this, as they were also very clearly the least likely to be taking (or 'doing') exercise for their own health's sake. However, far fewer people in all groups appeared to be taking their own advice. Specifically, fewer than half the proportion of Pakistani women saying that exercise was important also said that they did some exercise for health reasons. A similar pattern was found among African-Caribbean and Indian men, only about three-quarters of whom appeared to follow their beliefs in action. A more detailed analysis of the replies to this question is given in Tables 5.3 and 5.5, where it can be seen that the proportions mentioning exercise decline sharply in older age groups, particularly in the Pakistani and Bangladeshi communities. Older Asian men (but not those in the youngest age range) were rather more likely than women to say that they considered exercise of value, while older African-Caribbean women seemed to be more likely to take exercise 'to maintain health' than their male peers.

It is hard to attribute these variations to any essential 'ethnic' factor. While Indian and Pakistani replies on the abstract, theoretical prioritisation of exercise were similar, they differed much more in their probability of actually reporting that they were taking exercise. As has been remarked, Bangladeshi patterns of reply rarely resembled those of the other 'Asian' groups. Gender clearly is an important issue to consider in giving (or in the taking) of advice for healthy living, probably connected as much with opportunities and alternative commitments as with attitude. It may also be considered that issues of 'body image' (discussed in Chapter 9) and awareness of diseases, some of which affect men and women differently, may also affect attitudes and active participation in voluntary exercise.

Respondents were asked which (if any) diseases they felt were caused by a lack of exercise. A wide variety of possible answers was allowed for, and a number of others were volunteered by respondents and recorded by interviewers. The most significant are recorded in Figure 7.2. This can be seen to show both gender and ethnic differences in knowledge or at least, in beliefs expressed in reply to the question. One might, for example, highlight the fact that men saw lethargy as a consequence of inactivity much more than did women.

	African-Caribbean %	Indian %	Pakistani %	Bangladeshi %
Female				
Overweight	37	43	41	40
Heart	43	30	28	18
Blood pressure	7	6	5	5
Stroke etc.	1	6	4	2
Diabetes	–	3	3	2
Joint problems	11	15	9	12
Respiratory	3	2	1	1
Lethargy	2	3	1	3
Cancer(s)[a]	1	2	1	0
'Other'[b]	12	12	8	5
None	2	3	4	4
Don't know	18	19	28	39
Male				
Overweight	34	42	51	40
Heart	33	34	33	16
Blood pressure	4	7	8	4
Stroke etc.	3	2	5	2
Diabetes	1	3	6	4
Joint problems	12	10	9	14
Respiratory	2	3	2	1
Lethargy	4	6	7	10
Cancer(s)[a]	0	1	2	1
'Other'[b]	16	17	14	9
None	1	4	2	3
Don't know	20	15	17	26

[a]Several cancers were mentioned, including bowel, lung and breast: replies here combine these.

[b]'Other', excluding replies coded to added categories devised during coding, such as constipation and some cancers and others mentioned in text below.

Figure 7.2: Q8 What serious illnesses or health problems, if any, are linked to not taking enough exercise?

It is also instructive to compare these findings with those revealed later in the survey, when people were asked, 'What health effects are likely if a person does not take enough exercise or do enough physical activity?' – a rather different way of asking the same question (Q75: see 'Perceptions of activity levels', p. 89; Figure 7.19 on exercise beliefs).

It is obvious that overall the ethnic minority population were aware of the connection between exercise and health, at least in very general terms. Virtually no one was willing to say that there were no diseases or health problems linked to lack of exercise. On the other hand, a significant proportion could not state for certain what those illnesses were, as many as two in five Bangladeshi women making this reply. Men in general were either better informed or less willing to admit ignorance, since only among the African-Caribbean group did the proportion saying 'don't know' exceed that of women from the same ethnic category. Even so, it is a matter for concern that around a quarter of women (and one in five men) would admit or claim not to know any health problems associated with a lack of exercise, while stating throughout the interview (in collective terms) that they were clearly aware of the benefits or value of exercise for health.

Obesity (or overweight) was the single most commonly mentioned issue, reflecting both an awareness of the link with exercise and that this was indeed a health problem. Perhaps surprisingly, and certainly worthy of comment in the light of the data on body mass (BMI), was the finding that the group least likely to connect overweight or obesity with lack of exercise was the African-Caribbean population, both male and female. Pakistani males were in fact the most likely to make this connection, although not noticeably the most likely to take exercise themselves. On the other hand, African-Caribbean women were much the most likely to associate lack of exercise and heart disease, which was mentioned by nearly a third of men (but half as many Bangladeshi males). Unusually, Bangladeshi women were more likely than men to say this, although less so than other Asian women (and in only a very small number of cases). The replies of Asian men and women in respect of heart disease were very little different. Other circulatory disorders were hardly mentioned, although a very few mentioned the need for exercise to protect against diabetes (which it will do, in an indirect fashion). A small number of people also mentioned stroke, which is also linked to blood pressure problems. It may be a matter for concern that awareness of the link between exercise and (protection from) stroke and diabetes was so low, particularly amongst the African-Caribbean population.

A significant number of other conditions were 'volunteered' by respondents, and the most commonly mentioned were added to the coding frame when questionnaires were being analysed. Perhaps the most interesting from the point of view of health promotion work was the substantial number of mentions of joint problems, arthritis and rheumatism. A very few people also mentioned 'back problems'. Clinical interest is growing in the maintenance of mobility (and prevention of osteoporosis), particularly amongst the older population, and it may be that, with the increasing onset of age amongst what has until very recently been a relatively young population of 'migrant/settler' origin, this is an area on which future campaigns could be built. Evidently there is an awareness of the potential for loss of mobility ('use it or lose it'), and one may assume a concern to maintain independence through personal mobility in these populations. This might also include reference to the problem of 'lethargy', volunteered by a small number of women and a rather larger number of men. It is tempting to relate this to the experience of retirement (whether on age grounds or involuntary). This last category of ill health might also be linked to the (small) number of references to 'mental illness'. It may be that some spirit of 'healthy mind, healthy body' continues to inform public opinion in these communities. In terms of issues other than these, however, a lack of exercise may not be seen as a major disadvantage, but there is some scope to build upon fears for heart health, incipient joint problems and obesity. Further, such campaigns could apparently be aimed at all ethnic groups, targeting most particularly the Bangladeshi, irrespective of gender, since this was a concern shared by all groups in the survey. It will, however, be necessary to explain more clearly the connection between the benefits of exercise and protection from other forms of harm, such as diabetes, perhaps by reference to obesity but probably building on existing positive images as well.

7.3   Perceptions of barriers to exercise

While it is generally agreed by respondents to surveys that exercise is a 'good thing', it is also clear that many are not taking what they would regard as 'desirable' levels of exercise themselves. A number of reasons are given for this, some of which may be regarded as self-justifying excuses and others clearly major structural barriers. The evaluation of these is not the role of this study, but it is important to observe the differing patterns of reasons given by men and women if these barriers are to be overcome through educational or promotional campaigns. Further, if it appears that the reasons given for not participating in 'additional' or voluntary, leisure-based exercise cannot be easily overcome, this places additional stress on the need (and value) for exercise to be obtained in the routine activities of daily life. It is also instructive to compare the differences between the ADNFS national study of the majority population (which included a small proportion of minority origin respondents, whose replies were not analysed separately) and the findings of the latest HEA Health and Lifestyles survey. The ADNFS recorded reasons for non-exercising in various ways, and grouped them into five major groups: 'physical' barriers (age, previous injury, etc.); access and availability (no clothes or equipment, cost, etc.); time constraints, 'emotional' reasons (fear of injury, shyness, etc.), or 'motivation'. Some interesting patterns emerge.

When given a list of reasons 'commonly said' to stop people from getting enough exercise, marked ethnic differences emerged, both between groups within the BMEG populations and between those subgroups and the national picture reported by the ADNFS. One of the most commonly selected reasons for not exercising according to the ADNFS survey – a perception critical to health promotion – is that people said they were 'not sporty'. While we should be cautious of creating or supporting 'ethnic stereotypes', this does seem to have been an essentially white perspective, since only about half as many members of the BMEG sample gave this response. Whatever the reasons underlying this, it does make it easier to promote an 'activities of daily life' approach to exercise if the notion of exercise is not inseparable from that of 'sport'. Ethnic minority respondents were also very unlikely to blame a prior injury (although other research does suggest that members of the ethnic minority population are in fact more likely to have suffered injury through domestic or work-related accidents[1]).

Lowest rates of reported injury (or at least lowest rates of those blaming injury for non-participation) were expressed by Bengali women, although rather higher rates were suggested by African-Caribbean women, who were still less likely than the national sample to say this. Ethnic minority respondents rarely replied that they were 'too fat', although, perhaps surprisingly, Bangladeshi men were somewhat more likely than most to say that they were 'too old'. In general, however, there was a markedly lower rates of attribution of blame for non-participation to what the ADNFS characterised as 'physical' reasons.

A slightly different pattern emerges when the question of 'available time' is considered. Not having enough time, while consistently a major reason given by ethnic minority people, was again about half as likely to be mentioned compared with the white population, and there was remarkably little difference between the minority groups. On the other hand, Pakistani and Bangladeshi women were very much more likely to plead child care responsibilities. Perhaps less surprisingly, relatively few men from any ethnic minority group claimed this. A small number of Asian women also reported that they were also caring for older relatives.

In terms of psychological or personal feelings also, there was less explicit mention of these as reasons for non-participation. Shyness was slightly less common across all groups, and fear of injury was markedly lower in all of the ethnic groups, with the exception of Bangladeshi women. Another aspect of this component (as defined by the ADNFS) was personal motivation, and this too was rather less often cited. Very few indeed claimed not to enjoy sport, although we cannot confirm whether in fact they had ever tried any. Significantly, it was women who (unlike those in the majority population) were most likely to claim that they needed their rest, and (like the majority women) were twice as likely as men to say they lacked energy. However, while we might have expected cost and/or equipment and clothing to have proved more of a barrier, this was not so except for African-Caribbean women, who evidently saw themselves as financially restrained. It is clear that the majority did feel that they could get access to necessary facilities and a partner to 'do it with', in this case rather less than half the proportion of whites who gave absence of a 'partner' as a reason.

	African-Caribbean	Indian	Pakistani	Bangladeshi	ADNFS
Female					
None	25	19	26	20	27
Physical					
'Not sporty'	13	17	14	17	38
Age ('too old')	3	5	4	4	7
Prior injury	12	5	4	1	15
Poor health	10	8	8	10	7
Too fat	6	3	5	2	14
Time					
'Have no time'	21	34	27	25	43
Young children	17	21	30	28	18
Work	12	18	10	9	21
Emotional					
Shyness	8	8	11	9	12
Fear of injury	2	3	1	6	5
Access					
No 'partner'	15	10	8	6	22
No facilities	7	7	10	9	12
Clothes/equipment	4	3	5	5	7
Cost	16	5	5	3	14
Motivation					
I need to rest	14	14	12	10	26
I'd not keep up	14	9	8	7	19
No energy	12	9	8	13	21
Don't enjoy it	5	3	5	7	13
Male					
None	38	36	36	30	37
Physical					
'Not sporty'	6	11	13	13	24
Age ('too old')	5	3	7	13	7
Prior injury	9	7	8	8	18
Poor health	8	8	8	10	11
Too fat	1	2	3	1	7
Time					
'Have no time'	20	25	20	15	41
Young children	4	6	6	4	10
Work	13	19	16	10	34
Emotional					
Shyness	1	2	3	5	4
Fear of injury	2	2	3	2	7
Access					
No 'partner'	7	6	5	6	14
No facilities	6	7	10	9	8
Clothes/equipment	3	2	3	6	5
Cost	7	5	5	4	9
Motivation					
I need to rest	8	9	10	7	25
I'd not keep up	9	5	7	7	12
No energy	5	4	4	6	13
Don't enjoy it	2	3	5	4	9

Note: Respondents were shown (or read) a list of items, after being told, 'I'm going to show you a list of things that people say stop them getting more exercise, and I'd like you to tell me which, if any, apply to you.' They were encouraged to offer more ('What others?'). Then they were shown a second list: 'And do any of the following stop you from getting more exercise?' (answers reported in Figure 7.4). Totals will sum to more than 100%.

NB: *Group headings* relate to groups used in the ADNFS analysis.

Figure 7.3: Q113 Reasons for not taking part in leisure activities (percentages selecting each item from a list)

These data, which consistently show lower numbers agreeing with or adopting the various excuses or reasons for not participating that were offered (on a 'show card'), can be interpreted in two ways. Given that we have observed that few said 'none' of the reasons fitted their case, it may be that black (African-Caribbean and Asian) respondents were less likely to select more than one or two reasons, while the white general population clearly gave several reasons. Secondly, we must consider the possibility that ethnic minorities, who may be able to draw upon different cultural resources, may also have had other reasons for not taking part in activities. Alternatively, it may be suggested that responses reflected a lack of experience in the sports. Those who have not tried to take part in a sport, such as golf or squash, may not know how expensive the equipment or fees can be.

The HEA, in addition to asking about and recording the same answers to this question as that used in the ADNFS, asked about a series of other potential barriers to participation in exercise activities outside the home, which we have termed 'ethnic' reasons in Figure 7.4 below. It is known that certain cultures and/or religions place restrictions on dress, modesty and relationships between the sexes, but it is not clear to what extent these are 'ideals' and how far people may see or cite them as barriers to their own activities. This survey provides an opportunity to test this, and again generates some remarkable findings. In particular, it should be noted that while (as might be predicted) men found themselves much less likely to be constrained by such pressures, there was a significant group of men, notably in the Bangladeshi community, who were so limited. Secondly, at least half of the 'Asian ' female population (again, perhaps excluding the Bangladeshi, for whom one-third would still agree) did not feel that any of the reasons put to them were real problems for their participation.

All respondents were offered or read a second show card, listing reasons for non-participation which might be deemed more likely to accord with previous research into ethnic minority lifestyles. In particular, these covered such issues as community pressures, 'modesty' and cultural distance (including language). There was some support for the suggestion of an 'ethnic/cultural barrier', particularly from the distribution of replies among the Bangladeshi population and to a lesser degree those of the other Asian female groups. On the other hand, most men and a clear majority (three-quarters) of the African-Caribbean women gave replies which would reject this suggestion, saying that none of the ideas listed applied to them. However, there were certainly some features and factors which it would be important to consider in planning facilities and promotion campaigns targeting minority groups and particularly Asian women,[2] as has been already noted by the Sports Council.

Modesty, whether a dislike of being in a mixed sex setting, or simply being in a place where other people bare their bodies, was a very clear disincentive amongst all Asian groups, irrespective of gender. Women, especially those whose religion was expected to be Muslim because of their Pakistan and Bangladesh origins, were particularly opposed to mixed sex facilities, but it is worth noting the number of men who also expressed some degree of embarrassment. Other predicted barriers, such as partner's and family disapproval, were identified, especially among Pakistani and Bangladeshi women, but not at particularly high levels. Much more significant was a fear by any women of going out alone, which contrasts with the earlier replies to the problem of having a partner for activity. It would seem that this reply reflected more than a lack of someone to play with, and may represent a fear of going out of the home and risking racial abuse or harassment. This, rather than any 'cultural' or 'ethnic' criterion, would seem to be the main deterrent, although the increased levels of harassment faced by members of black communities does however render this an 'ethnic' need.[3]

	African-Caribbean %	Indian %	Pakistani %	Bangladeshi %
Female				
My (marriage partner) would disapprove	–	4	10	9
Other members of my family would disapprove	1	4	10	9
I don't want to go to 'mixed sex' places	5	9	21	20
I don't like to go to places where I can't speak my language	1	5	8	10
I don't want to go to places where people show parts of their bodies	3	9	18	20
I have older relatives to look after	1	5	3	4
I don't like to go out alone	17	18	12	21
I would not know what to do	3	4	5	6
I never see anyone from my culture doing these things	1	6	7	9
None of these	74	59	48	37
Male				
My (marriage partner) would disapprove	1	2	2	1
Other members of my family would disapprove	1	–	2	2
I don't want to go to 'mixed sex' places	1	3	6	12
I don't like to go to places where I can't speak my language	1	4	3	5
I don't want to go to places where people show parts of their bodies	1	5	7	11
I have older relatives to look after	–	1	1	2
I don't like to go out alone	5	5	6	6
I would not know what to do	–	3	2	7
I never see anyone from my culture doing these things	–	2	2	6
None of these	90	82	77	63

**Figure 7.4a: Q114 HEA survey 'ethnic' reasons for not taking exercise
(proportion selecting each response, as Figure 7.3)**

In order to establish the degree to which certain explanations might be associated with a religious rather than a national culture, a further analysis was conducted (Figure 7.4b) which tests this issue explicitly. It can be seen that there are certain patterns, reflecting the anticipated association between Islam and 'modesty', but that other religious groups also have their own sensitivities. It would also seem that some Muslims, and Hindu women, might put forward a variety of alternative explanations or excuses for not participating.

	Christian %	Muslim %	Sikh %	Hindu %	'No religion' %
Female					
I'm not the sporty type	14	15	12	21	13
I need to rest and relax	13	11	14	16	18
I don't have time because of my work	14	10	20	20	20
I might get injured or damage my health	2	4	–	5	–
I haven't got the time	22	27	39	36	26
I have got young children to look after	16	25	22	17	18
I'm too shy or embarrassed	8	11	6	8	6
There's no one to do it with	15	6	15	8	10
None (of the 'common' list)	24	25	21	16	27
My (marriage partner) would disapprove	1	9	5	5	2
Other members of my family would disapprove	1	10	3	4	2
I don't want to go to 'mixed sex' places	4	20	10	7	8
I don't like to go to places where I can't speak my language	1	8	5	7	4
I don't want to go to places where people show parts of their bodies	3	19	5	8	6
I have older relatives to look after	1	3	6	5	5
I don't like to go out alone	18	16	18	18	17
I would not know what to do	3	6	3	4	3
I never see anyone from my culture doing these things	1	9	6	5	1
None of these (ethnic reasons)	73	43	59	60	74
Male					
I'm not the sporty type	7	14	3	13	6
I need to rest and relax	8	9	4	12	15
I don't have time because of my work	14	14	19	22	16
I might get injured or damage my health	1	2	6	2	4
I haven't got the time	22	19	22	25	23
I've young children to look after	5	6	5	6	5
I'm too shy or embarrassed	8	11	6	8	6
There's no one to do it with	4	6	7	11	9
None (of the 'common' list)	40	33	42	38	41
My (marriage partner) would disapprove	–	1	2	2	2
Other members of my family would disapprove	–	2	1	1	2
I don't want to go to 'mixed sex' places	2	9	2	2	–
I don't like to go to places where I can't speak my language	2	4	3	3	1
I don't want to go to places where people show parts of their bodies	2	9	1	5	0
I have older relatives to look after	–	2	0	1	1
I don't like to go out alone	4	6	3	5	5
I would not know what to do	0	5	2	3	1
I never see anyone from my culture doing these things	–	4	0	4	–
None of these (ethnic reasons)	91	70	83	83	87

Left margin labels: Allied Dunbar Health & Fitness Survey results; HEA's additional 'ethnic' reasons (repeated for Female and Male sections)

Figure 7.4b: Q114 An analysis of reasons for not taking exercise, by religion (percentage selecting each response, as Figures 7.3, 7.4)

75

It can be seen that there are certain reasons given that relate more closely to gender than to ethnicity. Not wishing to go out alone is common to women across all the religious groups, while other reasons appear to be more closely tied to a particular religion, or to females within a religious group. That said, it is also clear that religious belief can act as a constraint on the actions of men as well as women.

Certain other perceptions appear to be associated with religion. In particular, we note that Muslim men and women were considerably more likely to say, 'I'm not the sporty type,' but Hindu women were otherwise least likely to feel that any of the 'common' (i.e. reasons also reported in the general white population of the ADFNS survey) reasons covered their case. Generally, about 40% of all men, but only a third of Muslims, said that none of those reasons fitted their case. Equally, the majority of men from all religions other than Islam felt that none of the 'ethnic' reasons for non-participation applied to them, while Muslim women, and to a lesser extent women from the other major Asian religions, were more likely to feel that these fitted them. Not all of the reasons, however, were directly related to religious prohibitions. Hindu and Sikh males, and non-Muslim women, were more likely than many others to mention the problems of work, while it remains true that fewer Muslim women are found in employment. Sikh and Hindu women also more generally felt that they had no spare time, but there is no differentiation between the religions in the propensity of women to mention child care responsibilities. Embarrassment or shyness was slightly more often mentioned by Muslims, but was a factor for other religions, while Muslim women were most likely to anticipate disapproval from their husband or family. Muslims of both sexes were most likely to avoid mixed sex facilities, but this was also a factor affecting all Asian religions and a substantial number of Christians. Muslims and Hindus were both likely to be offended by nudity.

Virtually none of the respondents indicated that they were totally ignorant of sports and other means of getting exercise, or that a lack of 'role models' from their own cultural background was an issue. There may be some scope for developing promotional campaign materials around the existence of suitable role models, which would include the incorporation of 'ordinary' people of minority origin into materials. It is, for example, noticeable that African-Caribbean women were by a long way the least likely to think that there were no physically active people from their background, although it must be admitted that the super-fit black athlete is almost a stereotype of present-day British sport. At the same time, perhaps one in twelve Asian women did feel that they might be 'unusual', and this is one area where intervention might be relatively simple, although unlikely to affect male participation.

7.4 Perceived priorities for a healthy life

The final section of the health beliefs and actions element of the survey, before collecting the necessary basic factual data about the informants' age and household, was a question seeking the priority accorded in respect of eight 'commonly given' bits of advice on healthy living. Interviewers were instructed to read a list of factors, after the following introduction:

(Q117) I'm going to read out advice that people often give to those who want to be healthy. I'd like you to tell me how important you think each one is, for a person of your age who wants to be healthy.

Very few people indeed said that the advice (any of it) was totally irrelevant or even 'not very important', but there were some differences in replies which may have practical application.

In respect of those pieces of advice not seen as important, the data suggest that for African-Caribbean people generally less than 5% of any of the items of advice were seen as unimportant. The least likely to be seen as important was the value of not drinking too much alcohol, mentioned (as unimportant) by 6% females and 8% males. This does not mean that this group is more likely to run into difficulties with alcohol abuse, but nor does it mean that there is no problem there, as is being increasingly noted by specialist advice centres. A similar pattern was also found among Asians. Up to 11% of male Indians and Bangladeshis, but only 6% Pakistanis, felt alcohol was a low priority, while as many as 10% of Bangladeshi women did not see it as important, compared to under 5% of the other two groups. Interpretation of Likert score-type data, particularly when there appears to be a substantial consensus, is problematic, but these deviations from the overall picture appear to highlight some areas of potential interest to health promotion practitioners.

	African-Caribbean	Indian	Pakistani	Bangladeshi
Female				
Get out and about	67	63	66	65
Get good sleep	80	76	76	88
Avoid overweight	72	68	66	67
Avoid worry	71	64	64	71
Don't smoke	80	86	77	78
Get exercise	60	58	51	52
(Reduce) alcohol	62	76	75	79
Avoid fatty food	73	69	64	67
Male				
Get out and about	61	58	68	55
Get good sleep	73	72	69	72
Avoid overweight	71	64	70	61
Avoid worry	68	53	61	56
Don't smoke	68	70	76	67
Get exercise	56	56	64	52
(Reduce) alcohol	54	51	76	68
Avoid fatty food	63	51	70	64

Note: The question was offered in the form of a 'Likert Scale', respondents being asked if they thought each item was 'very important', fairly important', 'not very important' or 'not at all important'. Most replies fell in the first two categories.

Figure 7.5: Q117 Advice often given to keep healthy (percentages saying 'very important')

As has been repeated many times in the media and by those responsible for public health, smoking is the 'number one preventable behaviour', and this was consistently mentioned by women as being very important advice. Men, except those of Pakistani origin (where it would appear that smoking rates are actually very high), gave it a somewhat lower priority. Indeed, Pakistani men generally seemed to have a rather distinctive approach to the priority given to various bits of advice, ranking alcohol avoidance highly (as did the women) and seeing 'worry' ('avoid worrying too much') as the least of their priorities. This finding may accord with those of Currer,[4] who was investigating the applicability of the standardised questions of anxiety used to establish mental health. She noted that Pushtu speakers (Pakistani) in Bradford felt it was actually normal not to be in control of their lives, because, as they assumed everyone knew, it was better for God (Allah) to be in control. This would not, however, explain why Indian men were the least likely to see 'not worrying' as the most important advice to give.

Much greater concordance of opinion was found in relation to the question of getting a 'good night's sleep', where greatest agreement (after smoking, in the case of women) was found across all ethnic groups. Exercise was generally regarded as being a relatively low priority area for advice, especially among Asian women, although two-thirds of them (and of most men, with the significant exception of Bangladeshi men) felt that 'getting out and about' (which we take to refer to being active and perhaps getting a little basic exercise) was very important. It remains clear, however, that the priorities of 'ordinary men and women', whether of the majority population or of black and minority ethnic groups, differ in important ways from those of health professionals, at least in respect of the salience placed on 'getting exercise'. These data provide some indications which can be used to focus and accentuate advice in appropriate ways and to stress benefits or work on existing concerns, to ensure that messages are felt to be appropriate and welcome, thereby reinforcing existing health behaviour and facilitating within communities an atmosphere of positive reinforcement or support for health promotion workers. While they do show that there may be subtle and important differences between ethnic minority groups, they also show a remarkable degree of commonality, and some important similarities and differences from the perceptions of the majority population.

7.5 Self-perceptions of activity levels

In order to encourage uptake, as well as an understanding of the salience of an activity (in this case, the importance of taking exercise), it is important to have some understanding of the individuals' belief in their current personal level of participation. Questions in the survey therefore asked people how active and fit they thought they were, and how vigorous their work (if employed) was.

Perceptions of activity levels

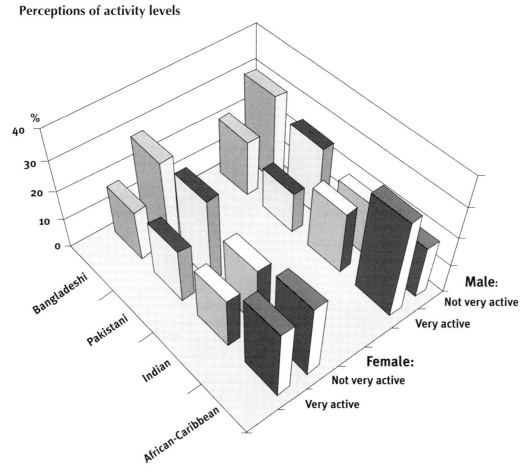

	African-Caribbean %	Indian %	Pakistani %	Bangladeshi %
Female				
Very active	24	17	18	17
Not very active	25	21	29	28
Male				
Very active	33	21	14	19
Not very active	18	18	24	29

Figure 7.6: Compared with other people of your age, how active would you say you were?

Given the variation in levels of exercise expressed above (e.g. in Figure 7.1), and in attitudes towards exercise, we might have expected to find rather more difference between groups in response to this question. It would appear that people have no great knowledge of the actual amounts of exercise obtained by others. If this is the case, then naturally they will have difficulty in assessing whether or not their own level of activity is appropriate or inadequate (or, more rarely, excessive). If the reported levels of activity are accepted, African-Caribbean men and women may have been justified in being more likely to see themselves as rather more active than their 'peers', but a substantial proportion of women in this category also saw themselves as relatively inactive. There was also among the African-Caribbean sample, a slight age effect (see Appendix, Table 7.2), in that those aged 30–49 were the most likely to see themselves as very active, while the older group were aware that their activity had declined. These differences were too small to be significant in any real sense. It is, however, possibly significant that Pakistani and Bangladeshi women, and men of the latter group, were most likely to be aware that they are relatively inactive. Pakistani men were certainly least likely to see themselves as 'very active'. An awareness of such self-referencing may assist in building on group self-image in developing demand for, and uptake of, recreational activity. Not perhaps surprisingly, about half the population in all groups saw itself as being around the average in its level of physical activity. It is, however, almost impossible to link these perceptions to actual practice.

Self-reported perceptions of fitness

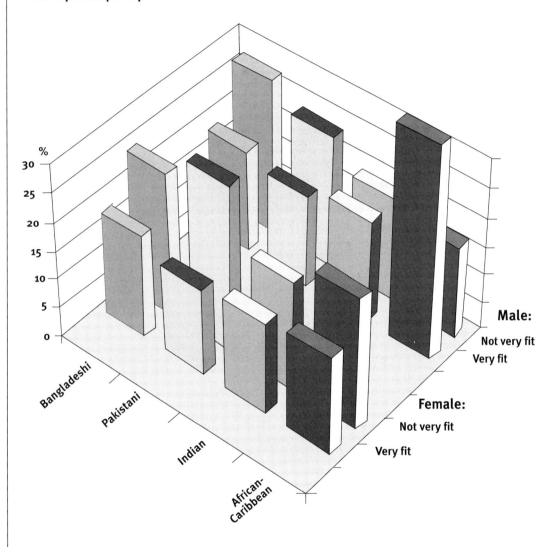

	African-Caribbean %	Indian %	Pakistani %	Bangladeshi %
Female				
Very fit	17	16	15	18
Not very fit	23	19	29	25
Male				
Very fit	30	18	16	18
Not very fit	16	18	23	27

Figure 7.7: Compared with other people of your age, how fit would you say you were? (Q110)

In general, but with the clear exception of African-Caribbean women, self-assessed fitness and self-assessed activity seemed to resemble each other very closely. The two concepts were clearly related in people's minds, and again, most people saw themselves as being in the majority. There were, however, a few striking differences. While the patterns of perceived relative fitness shown in Figure 7.7 and activity levels (Figure 7.6) were almost identical among the Asian respondents and African-Caribbean men, African-Caribbean women were considerably less likely to see themselves as 'very fit', despite being relatively 'active'. This was accentuated when considering the age groups, since the older people in this group were most likely to see themselves as having become less fit, while those aged 30–49 again were the most likely to see themselves as more fit than the average (see Appendix, Table 7.3).

	African-Caribbean %	Indian %	Pakistani %	Bangladeshi %
Female				
Self	52	63	59	41
Others	24	47	51	71
Male				
Self	61	65	59	46
Others	16	27	30	50

Figure 7.8: Do you think you/'most people' get enough exercise at present to keep fit? (proportion saying 'yes') (Q111, Q112)

It is interesting to note that the majority of people questioned felt that they at least, while not necessarily more active or fit than others, were getting 'enough' exercise, and that they were critical of 'most other' people as not getting enough. This represents a considerable challenge to health promotion, if people are satisfied with their own current levels of fitness. The exception to this seems to be found among the Bangladeshi communities, where less than half of both men and women felt that they were getting enough exercise, and a majority felt that others were doing better than them. Asian women as a whole were less critical of others, despite (with the exception noted, of Bangladeshis) being the most likely to feel that they personally were getting enough exercise. Such levels of personal complacency require sensitive challenging. There are here too some slight age effects. Younger African-Caribbean people were less likely to see themselves as getting enough, while the older group were most likely, and also to see others as getting enough. Young people were very unlikely to see enough exercise being got by others (only 15% of females, 11% of males) (see Appendix, Table 7.4).

In all of the above discussions, we are conscious that there is a question of reference groups. We have assumed that 'most people' or 'other people' is a general and appropriate term. However, it is clear that patterns of socialisation and experience will vary between groups, both in terms of age, gender, ethnicity and location as well as 'social class' and other issues affecting group lifestyle. If (for example) South Asian women's lives are largely spent in the company of other South Asian women, they may make their comparisons with that group, or with a perception of the majority society's lifestyle gained from television or gossip. Similarly, we are unable to be certain about the reference groups of young African-Caribbean people, and so on. For the sake of the analysis, we have necessarily assumed that each individual has related to 'people like us', based on their broad age and ethnic group (and gender) following the categories we have used in our analysis. This clearly may be an assumption too far.

	African-Caribbean %	Indian %	Pakistani %	Bangladeshi %
Female				
Yes – three or more	22	17	17	12
Yes – once	23	16	18	7
Yes to either	40	30	31	17
Male				
Yes – three or more	32	35	30	29
Yes – once	20	20	17	12
Yes to either	45	47	41	37

Figure 7.9: Q115, Q116 Do you do ... vigorous exercise three times a week or more (or at least once a week) for at least 20 minutes per occasion?

Despite the answers to previous questions, when asked a definite question about the probability of doing 'vigorous exercise' (defined as 'something which makes you out of breath or sweaty') for at least 20 minutes, rather fewer than half the informants could reply in the affirmative – and particularly small numbers of women from the Bangladeshi group did so. Overall, less than one in five women, and under a third of men, felt that they were as energetic as this on three or more occasions. It is possible that the recall of respondents was not so accurate, given the numbers claiming to take part in a variety of energetic activities on a fairly regular basis. Another feature of this table is that the apparent difference between African-Caribbean and Asian people seems to be somewhat lessened in their replies to this question. It is unclear to what extent this represents a 'real' difference, and to what extent the replies to this question are impressionistic and designed to respond to the perceived interest of the interviewer rather than a clear recall of activities that met the criteria. In fact, when asked more specific questions about the things people had done, rather more energy expenditure was elicited, so that it may be that people are underestimating their exercise levels, probably by omitting common tasks which are not regarded as being 'leisure' or 'work' and are thus 'taken for granted'. At the same time, since there are apparently obstacles to engaging in leisure or taking unproductive exercise and to setting aside time for healthy recreation, it is apparent that the more these 'taken for granted' actions can be encouraged, and an awareness of their beneficial aspects promoted, the greater will be the benefit to the community's health. It is therefore important to pay closer attention to those 'activities of daily life' which can provide 'free' exercise, which is the basis of current health promotion policy.

7.6   Actual levels of activity recorded in the HEA survey

Activities of daily life: cleaning, gardening and DIY

Despite the introduction of electric vacuum cleaners and other equipment, housework can still provide considerable opportunities (or challenges) in terms of physical exercise. The ADNFS and HSE recognise not only digging, chopping wood and mixing concrete, but also walking with heavy shopping for more than five minutes, scrubbing floors, cleaning windows and 'spring cleaning' as being of 'moderate intensity', while car washing, pruning or weeding and decorating (painting and wallpapering) are regarded as of 'light intensity'. These and other examples were shown to respondents to help them assess their replies to questions on 'activity at home'.

	African-Caribbean	Indian	Pakistani	Bangladeshi
Female				
Heavy housework (N)	*444*	*364*	*305*	*368*
Days/month	9.3	8.6	9.4	11.1
Duration[a]	121	123	121	88
Heavy DIY/Gardening (N)	*130*	*81*	*56*	*18*
Days/month	3.2	2.9	2.7	4.2
Duration[a]	142	152	118	135
Male				
Heavy housework (N)	*231*	*178*	*167*	*200*
Days/month	6.8	7.0	7.7	6.1
Duration[a]	84	118	109	76
Heavy DIY/Gardening (N)	*111*	*145*	*146*	*49*
Days/month	5.6	4.7	3.7	4.4
Duration[a]	161	164	171	118

Notes: Questions 78–85: the results are an amalgamation of the answers to this series of questions, and we cannot express data as a proportion of the total because of the complexities of the filtering in the way questions were asked.

Other surveys of such activity have found that data may be heavily skewed, with a small number participating in long periods of exercise: these averages relate only to those who said that they did *some* heavy work of that type.

[a]How long in total was spent on the activity on the most recent occasion – in minutes.

Figure 7.10 Numbers reporting participation in energetic 'activities of daily living'

It is perhaps not surprising that women in general were likely to spend more time, more often, on 'heavy housework'. In general, it would appear that most had spent about two hours in such activity on the previous occasion, and did so slightly more than twice a week. Bangladeshi women reported spending rather less time (even if more often) on 'heavy housework' and rather more in other 'DIY' activity and gardening, and women in all ethnic groups said that they did these latter about three times a month. In total, all women were averaging about 25 hours per month on the two forms of activity. Men, who were somewhat less likely to report doing housework, nevertheless spent appreciable amounts of time in these tasks as well as on 'heavy DIY' and gardening, so that they also accumulated a similar amount of time in energetic activity. Asian men, particularly from the Indian and Pakistani communities, reported spending almost as long on housework as the women, while men of African-Caribbean origin were more likely to spend their time in DIY and gardening. Bangladeshi men, despite saying that they did this at least once a week, spent rather less time on it, and gained least benefit overall from these 'activities of daily life'. Overall, there was a very close comparison between both men and women and between ethnic groups in the total amount of time dedicated to these activities.

Stairs

The HEA study asked both whether people went up and down stairs at home, and if so how often in a day and how many steps this involved; and also how frequently (times per day, days per week, number of steps) they climbed stairs at work or elsewhere other than their home. Indian and Pakistani people were most likely to use stairs in their homes, and Bangladeshis were considerably less likely to do so. Around one in ten respondents did not use stairs at home. For most other people stair use represented a significant number of steps, the modal value being 13 steps, which would be transited normally between about six and ten times daily. Reportage of these data was somewhat problematic, possibly partly because of uncertainty about the numbers of steps or recall of the normal number of times they were used. Overall, they suggest that most Asian respondents would go up (or down) stairs at home about five times a day. African-Caribbean respondents supplied slightly higher levels of use. Rather fewer used stairs away from home, probably using lifts or escalators in shops and offices: less than half (41%) gave data from which to make an estimate of this activity. An average for these of just under 120 steps/day (116 Asian; 125 African-Caribbean) was noted.

With other measures of reported physical activity, there are clear gender variations as well as differences in age groups, but in respect of stair walking females had virtually identical rates to men at home. Thus the data show that Asian women and men reported an average 'stair-mileage' of 139 compared to African-Caribbean women and men, who averaged 143 stairs daily. There are slight 'ethnic' variations in these values. According to the reported data, those of Indian origin climbed the most stairs in a day (women 151, men 140), while people of Bangladeshi origin got the least benefit from this potential source of exercise, men and women in this group averaging about 138 stairs/day at home. Away from the home, however, Asian men averaged 136 stairs/day compared to women's 89, and again the Indian group reported the highest rates and Bangladeshis the lowest. A similar but less marked gender imbalance was reported by African-Caribbean people, where women averaged a further 116 steps daily 'away from home', while men reported an average of 136.

There was a clear age effect among the Asian community, since those aged 50 or over were about three times as likely as others to report that they did not go up and down stairs at home – at all. It would also appear that one in four Bangladeshi women in the survey did not use stairs at home, probably because of living in flats, while slightly fewer men reported this, possibly because they were more likely to use stairs in the flats or outside their homes. Among Asian people, the most active appear to be those aged 30–49 but African-Caribbean men and women in this age group stepped up and down the lowest average number of stairs, while those younger and older were very similar.

	African-Caribbean	Indian	Pakistani	Bangladeshi
Female				
% using stairs at home	90	98	100	77
Average daily use at home	143	151	149	138
Average daily use away from home	116	135	82	53
Male				
% using stairs at home	88	95	99	81
Average daily use at home	160	141	139	138
Average daily use away from home	136	170	141	105

Note: The data reported here are calculated from the answers to questions 96–101.

Figure 7.11: reported stair usage (number of stairs climbed/descended per day)

The ADNFS survey suggested that a minimum level of 500 stairs/day should be reached to obtain a significant health and fitness benefit. Amongst the minority ethnic population, it can be seen that negligible proportions of people in the survey were reaching the levels of use suggested. Less than three in a hundred did as much at home, irrespective of gender or ethnic group. Equally few did much stair walking at work, where there may well be the maximum potential to 'take the stairs rather than the lift' and benefit thereby. The maximum usage 'away from home' appears to be among those African-Caribbean men who used stairs outside the home: just over 5% said they walked up and down more than 500 steps on a (typical) day.

Walking

The most common form of exercise taken – and probably the cheapest – is the simple act of walking, not just up and down stairs, but from place to place, whether as a means of getting somewhere (instrumental) or with no particular aim in view (recreation). Recreational walking, in this definition, need not be defined solely as that undertaken for pleasure or in 'pleasant' (rural or park) surroundings: it is possible to walk in urban settings, 'window shopping' or 'parading', or indeed, just for the exercise. One way or another, the majority, but certainly not all, of the population walk significant amounts. The survey, however, demonstrated that there were some gender and ethnic variations in levels of this activity, and that, while car ownership had some relevance, this made very slight difference to levels of walking overall (Figure 7.12).

	African-Caribbean %	Indian %	Pakistani %	Bangladeshi %
Female				
With use of car				
Short walks	78	77	80	76
(of these)				
Longer walks	69	70	74	56
Without car				
Short walks	89	82	84	84
(of these)				
Longer walks	69	79	67	62
Male				
With use of car				
Short walks	73	75	73	80
(of these)				
Longer walks	79	77	77	74
Without car				
Short walks	84	86	80	90
(of these)				
Longer walks	82	83	84	81

Note: Respondents to the survey were first asked (Q86), 'Have you done any walks of a quarter of a mile (5–10 minutes) or more in the past 4 weeks?' Those saying they had were asked (Q86) if they had walked for a mile or more (continuous walking for at least 20 minutes).

Figure 7.12: Proportions taking walks in previous 4 weeks (Q86–90)

Four out of five of all ethnic minority respondents in the survey reported going for at least short walks in the previous month. There was no 'ethnic' or gender variation in this figure, nor any reason to believe that this is 'minority specific' behaviour. Indeed, the ADNFS notes only that 'over 50%' of the general public walked regularly (their question was phrased slightly differently). Of those who had been for a walk in the last month, most had been for reasonably substantial walks of a mile (20 minutes) or more, the majority doing so regularly more than once a week. Indeed, about one in three women, and as many as two-fifths of men did so. Contrary to the earlier picture of Bangladeshi men's apparent relative inactivity, it is this group who were most likely to walk. The survey did not ask where and how this was done, but it can be seen (Figure 7.12) that those without cars were most likely to walk. In general, however, while those without cars were slightly more likely to walk than those who either owned or 'had the use' of a vehicle, these differences were slight. Possession of a car also seemed to make very little difference to the likelihood of having taken a longer walk. Women were rather less likely to have gone for longer walks, and Bangladeshi women were the least likely to have done so, while Indian women without cars were slightly more so.

Longer walks, defined as two miles or more, and taken by less than one in five of the general public, were also surprisingly common in all groups of ethnic minority men, although about 60% of women said that they never walked this far, with the notable exception of Pakistani women. Only one in five of women who did go for more than short walks would walk as far as two miles more than once a month, while twice as many men said they did so.

A significant factor in the exercise benefit of walking is of course the speed of walking. A long dawdle does not generally raise the heart rate or provide significant benefit to health (apart from possibly burning off a few calories) compared to a brisk stroll. However, exceptionally few people said that they walked at a fast pace (that is, more than four miles per hour), and, with the possible exception of African-Caribbean people, most walked at a less challenging pace. Interestingly, rather more women than men reported walking briskly, but even here they were in a clear minority, and while one in three Bangladeshi women said they did so at a brisk pace, considerably more of this group than of others said that they walked quite slowly. Very few Pakistani or Bangladeshi men walked briskly.

	African-Caribbean %	Indian %	Pakistani %	Bangladeshi %
Females				
A slow pace	11	11	13	17
A steady average	45	60	63	53
Fairly brisk or fast	44	30	24	30
Males				
A slow pace	9	16	13	15
A steady average	49	53	62	62
Fairly brisk or fast	42	31	26	23

Figure 7.13: Q90 Which of the following best describes your usual walking pace?

If any greater benefit to health is to be obtained from this form of exercise, it would appear that the maximum benefit will be obtained by encouraging people to walk more briskly, and perhaps a bit further, rather than merely encouraging more pedestrian activity in general. Those who presently never walk anywhere – a substantial minority – may have good reason and are unlikely to be persuaded to change.

'Caring'

It is clear from the replies given to the HEA survey that significant numbers of people were getting considerable health benefit from exercise undertaken in fulfilling the role of carer. This is an aspect of caring that has been little considered in the literature relating to carers, whether of the majority or ethnic minority population. Indeed, it may be problematic and certainly impacts on the overall patterns of daily living and amount of time available for other forms of exercise, as was remarked by many informants (see 'Reasons for not exercising' p. 72). It is also true that for many elderly (or older) carers, the effort of lifting and assisting a partner can be a health hazard. Another factor worthy of attention is the gendered nature of caring, although there are some distinctive 'ethnic' patterns that may run counter to stereotype.

From the table it can be seen that caring has a very significant impact on the population. One in ten ethnic minority women would expect to carry a child on at least some day(s) in the week, and nearly twice as many did so on most days. That is to say, between a quarter and a third of them spent some time in a week carrying a child. Of those surveyed, Pakistani women seemed to be the most likely to do so. Bangladeshi and Indian women spent rather less time carrying a child but were quite likely to push one in a pram or pushchair. The image of passive parenting amongst Asian families propounded by some child developmental studies is belied by the number of both male and females (one in five women, and about a quarter of the men) who played actively with a child at least some time in each week. When taken with those who played regularly on most days, this represents between a third and two-fifths of the women and a third of all minority ethnic males.

However, caring for an adult can be every bit as physically demanding, and one in eight women (somewhat more amongst the older groups) and one in twelve men were providing regular support for a person with disabilities. For at least half, and up to two-thirds of this group, this involved assistance with walking ('giving walking support'). One in three ethnic minority women (and nearly two-thirds of Bangladeshi women) had to lift or carry an adult on a regular basis, as did one in three African-Caribbean, about one in five Indian and Pakistani men, and about half of the Bangladeshi male community. Male carers were more likely, in general, to be pushers of wheelchairs, but about half the African-Caribbean women carers did so at some point in a typical week. This level of support is both physically demanding and tends to restrict personal opportunities to engage in other forms of recreation, giving particular force to the needs of minority carers to obtain 'respite' and other support services, which at the same time might enable them to take more advantage of opportunities for 'healthy recreation' in their leisure time.

	African-Caribbean %	Indian %	Pakistani %	Bangladeshi %
Female				
Child care				
Carry on some days[a]	9	10	13	13
Carry on most days[a]	20	16	29	14
Pram pushing	18	17	25	21
Play games 1–5 times weekly[b]	19	17	25	20
Play more often[b]	20	14	17	14
Help care for a disabled person	13	15	11	7
Of whom (N)	78	83	66	39
Lifting adult	34	36	38	63
Help adult walk	64	64	54	37
Push wheelchair	51	18	12	18
Males				
Child care				
Carry on some days[a]	11	12	12	22
Carry on most days[a]	11	14	15	9
Pram pushing	8	7	7	9
Play games 1–5 times weekly[b]	23	25	20	25
Play more often[b]	13	11	12	8
Help care for a disabled person	5	10	9	8
Of whom (N)	23	40	45	37
Lifting adult	33	21	23	53
Help adult walk	46	56	67	44
Push wheelchair	37	15	30	28

[a]Q102 'In an average week on how many days, if any, do you carry a child around?' Answers regrouped to 'none/1–5 days/most days'.

[b]Q104 'And in an average week, on how many days if any do you play games with a young child that involve you in physical effort?'

Figure 7.14: Proportions getting exercise through caring activity

Leisure activities and exercise

The natural instinct when discussing exercise and physical activity is to consider the various forms of leisure pursuit in which people engage. The HEA survey, like the ADNFS, presented respondents with a comprehensive list of leisure activities which might involve some degree of physical exertion. There were, however, a number of differences between the ADNFS study and that of the HEA. The HEA list was generally much shorter than the selection of activities covered by the ADNFS study. This part of the enquiry (unlike the section dealing with 'reasons for non-participation) did not include such ethnic-specific sports as kabaddi (a rapidly growing competitive sport from the Indian subcontinent akin to the old game of 'British bulldog'[5]), Equally, however, it did not include such traditional British 'sports' as snooker and darts, which might be classed as relatively physically inactive. Other sports covered by the ADNFS might be pursued by ethnic minority people, such as fishing and rambling, but were not included. Since most reports of 'countryside' activities draw attention to the absence of ethnic minorities, this is unlikely to affect significantly the overall conclusions of the study. The urban bias of the HEA sample, reflecting the facts of ethnic minority population distribution (see Chapters 2 and 3) also makes it unlikely that many people would have been found engaged in such activity.

	African-Caribbean	Indian	Pakistani	Bangladeshi	ADNFS
Female					
None of the following	47	66	69	82	na
One activity	27	18	17	11	
Two or more	26	16	14	7	
Bike/exercise bike	10	8	4	2	12
Squash	–	0	1	–	1
'Exercises'	23	13	16	8	18
Aerobics	25	11	9	3	12[a]
'Other' dance	16	7	2	3	18
Weight training	7	2	2	1	2
Swimming	10	10	4	2	19
Run/jogging	11	6	6	2	2
Football etc.	1	1	1	1	1
Tennis/badminton	2	5	6	3	5[b]
Other	3	3	4	2	na
Male					
None of the following	47	50	61	60	na
One activity	20	24	16	18	
Two or more	33	26	23	22	
Bike/exercise bike	15	11	9	9	16
Squash	–	2	1	1	4
'Exercises'	30	22	17	14	18
Aerobics	10	3	2	2	3[a]
'Other' dance	11	2	1	1	12
Weight training	16	16	13	11	8
Swimming	9	9	5	7	17
Run/jogging	15	12	10	11	9
Football etc.	16	19	15	24	10
Tennis/badminton	4	9	9	13	6[b]
'Other'	9	8	9	5	

NB: 'None' and 'other' cannot be compared as the ADNFS included questions on bowls, snooker, darts, fishing, rambling, golf, ten-pin bowling and table tennis. They also recorded that 3% men (ten in the past year) had played cricket. HEA did not ask about this sport. HEA did, however, accept 'exercise bike' as cycling.

[a] Aerobics: ADNFS asked about keep-fit and aerobics separately. HEA combined these.

[b] Tennis and badminton: ADNFS recorded each of these separately (combined here).

Figure 7.15: Participation in leisure activities

The most striking fact, initially, is that two-thirds of Asian women (four out of five Bangladeshis) and over half the Asian men, had not participated in any of those activities listed, while half of both African-Caribbean men and women took part in at least one. Even fewer claimed to have performed two or more in the previous four weeks ('the maximum limit of reliable recall' [ADNFS]). Certain sports were notably absent from the ethnic minority catalogue of replies, especially squash. This is played by 4% – a small but significant minority – of the national male population, but, despite the game's origins in India, very few Asian males (and virtually no African-Caribbeans) played it. Less surprisingly, no Asian women reported playing football or rugby, while this 'national sport' (of many countries) was enjoyed by a very significant proportion of ethnic minority men and up to 20% of Bangladeshi males. This is particularly interesting in the light of the virtual absence of 'cultural role models' in this sport, recent press reports suggesting that there is only one 'commercial' professional football player of Asian origin currently in Britain. However, other press coverage has discussed racialised exclusion from the organised sport, and the existence of informal Asian leagues in many towns.

The practice of jogging is also performed at near to national levels, indeed, at rather higher levels among African-Caribbean women. The levels of jogging among Asian (especially Indian and Pakistani) women are perhaps surprising in the light of relatively low levels of walking and other activity away from the home. This might repay further qualitative investigation, since they may have a different understanding of the question. Overall, however, the picture is of generally lower than national participation in any of the activities, including bicycling, in which the HEA included the use of static 'exercise' bikes. This is true also of social dancing, although it is not clear whether that term was understood to include either religious and classical Indian dance, or indeed the popular bhangra. This is an energetic Punjabi dance style, which in some forms has elements of Morris dancing, and at other extremes is a popular Asian 'disco-dance' style much performed at weddings. The figures for swimming repeat or confirm previous reports, despite the increasing provision of women-only sessions in most urban leisure centres.

These differences are often related to gender, in that men and women show different patterns both nationally and in the ethnic minority groups. There are also points at which the 'ethnic' patterns show greater significance. In particular, African-Caribbean people are much more likely, and Bangladeshis much less, to take part in exercises ('keep fit' etc.) irrespective of gender. A similar pattern is found in weight training, which is perhaps the only major sport other than (male) football in which black and minority ethnic groups consistently and significantly exceed national levels of participative activity. It remains possible that there was some form of bias operating in the sample, which might render such comparisons inaccurate. Certainly the minority ethnic population is considerably younger on average than the white majority, but these patterns do appear to be consistent when taking age into account.

Overall, it can be seen that African-Caribbean people are generally the most involved in sporting activities, and that the three Asian groups have some similarities, but not consistently so. At times the populations of Indian and Pakistani origin are more similar, and at others, Bangladeshi and Pakistani patterns are distinct from those of Indian origin. In so far as these relate to 'national' origins, such differences are likely to erode fairly rapidly as the British-born Asian population reaches maturity. One area where African-Caribbean sporting levels are well below those of the Asian population is in 'tennis and badminton'. As these two were combined for the HEA survey, we cannot be sure how far this might be related to more 'indoor' facility provision. While some better-equipped modern centres offer 'indoor' tennis, these are relatively rare. Opportunities may perform a partial role in dictating patterns of activity, as in walking or rambling, and provision of weight training clubs (which do seem to predominate in inner city areas and modern sports centres). Qualitative research will be required to explore why particular areas of provision (or activity – not all of these require large capital investment) are under-utilised. The area of greatest concern perhaps is the great under-participation in swimming, both male and female, since there are few areas of black and minority ethnic group settlement which do not have at least a network of Victorian public baths, and normally also more modern facilities.[6]

Perceptions of activity levels

One possible barrier to exercising may be a perception that there is a threshold below which no benefit will be obtained. If this were to be the case, then participation which is not driven by other benefits, such as enjoyment (or necessity, in the case of walking up stairs, perhaps) will be minimised and deterred by the slightest obstacle. There is now an increasing realisation among health exercise promotion professionals that motivation and 'reward' plays a key role in exercise

	African-Caribbean %	Indian %	Pakistani %	Bangladeshi %
Females				
Is there a minimum: % saying yes?	88	73	72	66
If yes, how often is necessary?				
1–2 times weekly	38	28	20	17
Most days or more often	18	38	35	50
Males				
Is there a minimum: % saying yes	80	84	82	80
If yes, how often?				
1–2 times weekly	29	25	21	21
Most days or more often	14	32	34	36

Q70: 'If a person is taking any of these kinds of exercise or doing other physical activities in order to keep fit, do they need to do it a certain number of times each week ... or not?

Figure 7.16: Q70, Q71 Perceived minimum frequency of exercise required for fitness

behaviour. The survey therefore asked a number of questions about perceived limitations to benefiting from exercise.

Clear support was expressed for the belief that exercise needs to be regular to be beneficial, in line with most current medical opinion. Over three-quarters of those surveyed agreed that there is a minimum frequency required. Among men of all ethnic minority groups, 80% agreed with the statement; among women Bangladeshis were less likely to agree (and more uncertain), while nearly 90% of African-Caribbean women felt a basic minimum was essential. That said, the African-Caribbean women, and to a lesser extent the men of this group, who saw a threshold set the minimum lower, at once or twice a week, while over half the Bangladeshi women and a third of all Asian men (irrespective of national or ethnic origin) placed the minimum frequency as being 'on most days' or even higher. It is uncertain from the data whether a fear of commitment or the need to do something so often is off-putting, on the lines of, 'If I cannot do it every day, there is no value in doing it at all.' On the other hand, it is strange that the group most likely (on other evidence) to be taking regular exercise is that which sets the lowest threshold.

Table 7.17: Perceived minimum length of exercise required for fitness (Q72–73)

	African-Caribbean %	Indian %	Pakistani %	Bangladeshi %
Female (N)	597	505	419	439
Yes	84	84	87	89
Under 15 mins	14	24	26	21
Over 30 mins	44	25	29	25
Don't know	4	4	4	9
Male (N)	397	430	589	483
Yes	80	85	82	90
Under 15 mins	10	18	12	11
Over 30 mins	51	36	45	49
Don't know	6	3	3	3

Q72: 'Does a person have to take exercise or do physical activities for at least a certain length of time on each occasion for it to help them keep physically fit, or not?'

Note: A relatively large proportion of the sample were not asked this question: the data may therefore be less reliable.

As well as frequency, that is, having the ability to find time on most days in a week, there is also the question of duration. Nearly everyone in the survey, and particularly in this case the Bangladeshis (male and female), felt that, if exercise was undertaken for the sake of health and fitness, it should last for a certain length of time. Surprisingly, few people felt unable to specify a limit to this, but the data also show that a very large proportion of respondents (8% African-Caribbean, 12% Indian and Pakistani, 21% of the Bangladeshi group) were not asked the first question and were excluded from the table above. This may suggest that they had indicated at the previous question that they did not wish to pursue this line of discussion further. On the basis of the data available, it does seem that there was a degree of difference between the African-Caribbean and Asian women, the former feeling that any bout of beneficial exercise should be over 30 minutes long, while the majority of Asian women opted for 15–30 minutes, interestingly more in line with current recommendations. Among men of all groups a more 'macho' line was presented, with half of all African-Caribbean and Bangladeshi men (but only one in three Indians) feeling that to do good exercise should be for more than half an hour. It is nevertheless significant that the majority of black and minority ethnic groups do recognise that too short a time spent in exercising has no benefit, and that for a large number the current advice (20 minutes 5 times a week) is close to their own perception of the optimum. There is no cultural barrier to the acceptance of this advice, and it provides a baseline of agreement on which healthy living campaigns can be developed.

	African-Caribbean %	Indian %	Pakistani %	Bangladeshi %
Female				
Feeling exhausted	3	6	8	12
Sweating/breathless	15	24	26	40
Raised heartbeat	60	44	38	24
Should not make any difference to heart	19	15	12	5
Don't know	4	10	16	19
Male				
Feeling exhausted	9	7	9	10
Sweating/breathless	20	28	27	41
Raised heartbeat	51	45	37	33
Should not make any difference to heart	12	16	21	7
Don't know	9	4	6	10

Q74: 'If a person is taking exercise or doing other physical activities in order to keep physically fit, which of the following statements best describes how much effort they need to put into it? It should leave you feeling exhausted; it should leave you feeling out of breath and sweaty; it should make your heart beat a bit faster than normal and make you feel slightly warmer; or it should *not* make your heart beat any faster than normal.'

Figure 7.18 Perceived minimum intensity of exercise required for fitness (Q74)

It is worth noting that a significant proportion of Asian women, notably the Pakistani and Bangladeshi, said that they did not know how energetic exercise should be. A surprisingly large proportion of Bangladeshi women (one in seven) felt that it should leave them feeling exhausted, a perception likely to turn people against participation. Male and female Bangladeshis, and to a slightly lesser extent the other Asian groups, were also most likely to feel that the minimum level of effort required for beneficial exercise was to become sweaty and breathless, which may also be a disincentive to those who are not accustomed to exercise or see no other (social) benefit from it.

African-Caribbean women, and men to a lesser extent, were most likely to provide an answer close to the advice offered by many GPs, that it should challenge the body system sufficiently to raise the heartbeat. A few people in all groups (not much differentiated) felt that healthy exercise should not make any difference to the heart rate. It is evident that this aspect of 'healthy exercise' will require considerably more attention in future promotional activities.

We have referred earlier to perceptions of the health effects of not getting enough exercise. The question was repeated in less precise terms towards the end of the interview, and certain interesting points emerge. The modification of the phrasing to omit reference to 'serious health problems' led to a slightly different emphasis.

A clear majority associated (lack of) exercise and physical activity with weight problems. Two-thirds of Indian and Pakistani men and women felt that lack of exercise led to obesity, and around a further one in three saw it (or perhaps the resultant obesity) as being linked with heart problems. Perhaps surprisingly, or perhaps because, as noted earlier, some were doing exercise for body-building purposes, rather fewer African-Caribbean and Bangladeshi people made the link between (in)activity and excess body mass. In the case of Bangladeshi women, who were most likely to say 'don't know', only one-third saw a connection with obesity. This group, on the other hand, were most likely to be concerned with mobility, problems of joint stiffness and the like. Overall, around one in five of all those in the survey, with few gender or ethnic differences, saw a need to exercise to keep joints supple. This is an important factor and increasingly being recognised by geriatricians. It would be useful to build upon an existing perception of this priority, particularly in these communities.

	African-Caribbean %	Indian %	Pakistani %	Bangladeshi %
Females				
Overweight	51	65	65	68
Diabetes	1	3	7	6
Heart disease	30	30	31	28
Stroke	3	3	4	4
Joints	17	24	15	26
Backache	4	6	8	7
Breathlessness	15	19	15	20
Inability to cope	5	6	4	4
Minor ailments	3	5	5	1
Tiredness	12	4	7	3
Blood pressure	2	2	4	3
Become lazy	5	2	3	1
Don't know	11	10	13	19
Males				
Overweight	49	62	68	60
Diabetes	–	6	6	4
Heart disease	30	34	39	22
Stroke	3	5	5	2
Joints	16	19	19	15
Backache	2	4	5	2
Breathlessness	12	14	11	7
Inability to cope	5	5	4	4
Minor ailments	2	4	5	3
Tiredness	9	6	3	9
Blood pressure	2	6	6	2
Become lazy	5	7	8	8
Don't know	11	8	6	15

Note: Responses elicited in survey and not pre-coded following pilot testing of original frame.

Figure 7.19: Health effects of insufficient exercise (Q75; cf. Q8 above)

The second most commonly mentioned ill effect was heart disease but since this had been the focus of much of the interview, this was perhaps not surprising. On the other hand, breathlessness was mentioned by nearly as many people as referred to joint problems This seems to be a major concern, notably among the Asian women (but, surprisingly, not in the same ratios amongst the male ethnic minority groups). It may be that there is a link to concerns about childhood asthma. A significant number of other minor illnesses were also mentioned, including 'tiredness' and a few mentions of blood pressure, but 'inability to cope' (rather similar to 'tiredness') was more commonly mentioned than the more clinically significant connection to stroke and (indirectly at least) diabetes. Interestingly, diabetes was virtually only ever mentioned by Asian people. It is, however, important to note in health promotion work that there is this concern and connection with the role that exercise can play in combating an unhealthy psychological (or psychosomatic) state. No one said that there were no ill effects, and one or two suggested that lack of physical challenge could lead to 'becoming lazy'.

7.7 'Objective' measures of activity and exertion

Previous studies of physical activity and health in the general public, such as the ADFNS study, and the recommendations of the Health of the Nation initiative[7] have posited recommended levels of activity which are based upon an aggregation of activities, not all of which need to be at the same level of exertion. Thus individuals might be advised to move 'up' a stage from taking no physical activity to 'at least one period of at least 30 minutes of moderate activity a week', and from this eventually to perhaps three periods of vigorous activity of 20 minutes duration. In this sense, 'moderate activity' is defined as having an energy cost of between 5.0 and 7.5 kcals/minute, while 'vigorous intensity' activities are expected to have an energy cost of 7.5 kcals/minute or more. Examples of the former would include brisk walking, heavy housework and gardening, or cycling if this did not make the person out of breath or sweaty. Running or physical activity that made the participant sweaty and breathlessness, including swimming and cycling, and certain occupations, would be classed as 'vigorous'. Using these categories and the more detailed information provided to the HEA survey, it is possible to classify respondents into the categories of two 'activity group' measures by using a complex algorithm. One measure identifies 'moderate' activity levels, and the other can be compared with the classifications of the HSE, which also identifies vigorous exercisers. The former (ALOV30J) groups people into one of four categories; the latter (OC20SUM) into a sixfold typology based on the previous month's activity levels. It should be noted that these two measure slightly different concepts, and it would be possible to be 'sedentary' on one measure and very active on the other. The notion of vigorous exercise largely refers to voluntary and additional (i.e. recreational and sporting) activity – a very few occupations will deliver this.

ALOV30J: Average weekly participation in at least moderate activity

	Activity level (per week, average)
Group 1	Less than one occasion of 30 minutes moderate activity
Group 2a	1–2 occasions of (at least) 30 minutes duration
Group 2b	3–4 occasions of (at least) 30 minutes duration
Group 3	5 or more occasions of at least 30 minutes moderate activity

---

OC20SUM: Frequency-intensity activity level (the categories used in the ADFNS)

	Number and intensity of activity events in previous 4 weeks
Level 0	No occasions of even moderate level activity
Level 1	1–4 occasions of at least moderate level activity
Level 2	5–11 occasions of at least moderate level activity
Level 3	12 or more occasions of (only) moderate level activity
Level 4	12 or more occasions of either (mixed) moderate and vigorous activity
Level 5	12 or more occasions of vigorous activity

These indicators are derived variables, and do not directly relate to any specific single question in the surveys. It should be noted that they will therefore reflect a complex mixture of answers to several questions, and may not always be entirely culture-free, since members of various groups may interpret questions about 'heavy housework', for example, differently, despite the use of show cards with examples of likely activity.

Figure 7.20: Categories of activity groups (ALOV30J and OC20SUM)

Overall, national data suggest that about one in three of the national population can be classed as 'sedentary' (i.e. Group 1), while a quarter of women and a third of men are 'regularly active' (Group 3). It can be seen from the data (Figure 7.21) relating to 'moderate activity' that among the BMEG population of this survey, about half of the Asian population was categorised as sedentary, with only Indian men and both sexes in the African-Caribbean population having levels of activity similar to the national average. Even more striking was the proportion of Pakistani and Bangladeshi men who reported themselves as being in the Level 0 group, never taking any more vigorous exercise. On the other hand, more men within the black and minority groups were likely to be 'committed exercisers', taking part in at least three sessions of 20 minutes' worth of vigorous activity weekly (Level 5), including 14% of Bangladeshi men and 11% of African-Caribbean men, compared to 10% in the national population.

	African-Caribbean %	Indian %	Pakistani %	Bangladeshi %
Males				
Sedentary (Group 1)	32	38	47	50
Medium (Group 2)	30	29	24	25
Regular active (Group 3)	38	33	29	26
Females				
Sedentary (Group 1)	31	47	50	53
Medium (Group 2)	44	36	26	29
Regular active (Group 3)	25	17	14	18

Figure 7.21: Activity levels – moderate medium-length exercise (ALOV30J)

Reference to the more detailed information in the tables (Table 7A) suggests that, not unexpectedly, there is an age differential. This is greatest among the Asian groups, where there is a very marked increase in the proportions 'sedentary' from the youngest to oldest group, and older Asian women demonstrate particularly low levels of physical activity. Among the African-Caribbean groups, however, it is the middle-aged group who demonstrate the highest levels of physical activity. It is also the case that there are fewer 'ethnic' differences and a less marked gender differential in the younger age group, since although there are slightly more sedentary Asian young women, the numbers taking more regular exercise are quite similar across ethnic groups. Pakistani and Bangladeshi women in the middle age group also show a considerable decrease in the proportion exercising regularly.

	African-Caribbean %	Indian %	Pakistani %	Bangladeshi %
Males				
Sedentary (Level 0)	21	28	37	39
Low–medium (Levels 1–2)	28	29	27	27
Moderate (Levels 3–4)	40	31	24	21
High (Level 5)	11	13	12	14
Females				
Sedentary (Level 0)	19	32	36	39
Low–medium (Levels 1–2)	34	36	38	34
Moderate (Levels 3–4)	39	27	22	25
High (Level 5)	8	5	4	2

Figure 7.22: Levels of shorter vigorous and moderate activity (OC20SUM)

When considering more vigorous or more complex patterns of exercise as measured by the OC20SUM variable (Figure 7.22, also Table 7B, p. 96) there are many similarities but certain key differences. Clearly the definition of a shorter period of activity (20 minutes rather than half an hour) affects the likelihood of participation. In particular, it can be seen that, among the 'committed vigorous exercisers' (i.e. those engaging in more than 12 occasions of vigorous activity in a month), there are very few differences between men of the four ethnic groups, while only the Bangladeshi women (2%) fall below the national average (and African-Caribbean women are twice as likely to be in that group). The real differences can be seen to lie in the middle of the table, where a distinct gradient develops in intermediate levels of commitment and activity, Pakistani and Bangladeshi men showing considerably lower levels of activity than either Indian or African-Caribbean males. The differentials among Asian women are less clear, except at the higher rates of activity. When age is brought into the equation (Table 7B) it can be seen that differences between groups are greatest among the youngest and oldest, while there is little difference between men and women's patterns in the 30–49 age group. Vigorous exercise, however, is very clearly a prerogative of the young, with few except African-Caribbean men (and women to a lesser extent) taking any vigorous exercise over the age of 29. However, in the youngest age group, Indian and Bangladeshi males appear to be the most committed to vigorous activity, in contrast to the pattern in other ages.

Very little of this physical exertion is obtained in work-place activity. Partly this may be related to the predominantly urban lifestyles of the black and minority ethnic population and the fact that nowadays only a limited number of occupations, particularly in 'primary' industries, such as farming and mining, can be classified as very physically demanding. Perhaps more significant (Table 7C) is the relatively low involvement in the labour market, through exclusion or choice, that can be seen also in the earlier analysis of the demographic data (Chapter 3). This is particularly marked among Asian women, among whom 91% of Bangladeshi women were not in employment. There are also very high levels of non-engagement in the labour market (i.e. being a student, carer or unemployed) among the younger people of all age groups. Most of the men and women in jobs were in occupations classified as 'inactive' or, at best, 'light activity'. This, it should be noted, is in stark contrast to the perceptions of respondents mentioned earlier (Q77, Section 7.5). Equally, it may be that their particular roles within an occupation or work-place were more demanding than the formal definition of their job would indicate. This would certainly be compatible with the earlier findings of Lee and Wrench.[8] Indeed, the highest level of physical exertion among the HEA survey respondents was marked among the (few) Bangladeshi women in employment, nearly half of whom were rated as in 'moderate active' work, while African-Caribbean men, particularly in the middle- and older-aged group were also more often in physically demanding jobs than any other group.

7.8 Conclusions

It is clear that an improvement in the levels of physical activity is required in all ethnic groups, whatever definition of target activity is adopted. It can also be demonstrated that there are both gender and ethnic differentials in participation. These do not arise from major ethnic differentials in perceptions of the value of exercise, and with some exceptions there is not a distinctive 'ethnic' pattern of 'excuses' or reasons for not taking more exercise. There is, however, a poor understanding among most groups of the precise health benefits of exercise, and of the connection between specific types of ill health and activity levels. Complex patterns of variation can be observed, and it may be necessary to consider the needs and potential to increase participation of each ethnic group (and, within those, the sexes), separately. Age also has its effects, generally, but not always, independently of the other issues: it is not always the younger people who are most physically active. The chapter overall demonstrates a number of areas where intervention might be most appropriately targeted. These conclusions may not, overall, be very different from those to be drawn for the majority ('white') population, but we have tried to illustrate just how and where they may differ, and the importance of taking some of the culturally specific issues into account.

Table 7A: Levels of participation in moderate intensity activity

Code	African-Caribbean		Indian		Pakistani		Bangladeshi	
	Female %	Male %	Female %	Male %	Female %	Male %	Female %	Male %
16–29								
Group 1	24	23	36	24	39	30	42	24
Group 2a	31	24	32	24	30	21	26	24
Group 2b	21	14	14	13	14	11	7	11
Group 3	23	39	19	40	17	38	24	39
Base number	*178*	*114*	*208*	*129*	*281*	*235*	*307*	*213*
30–49								
Group 1	22	23	45	36	57	48	59	54
Group 2a	26	17	22	20	22	20	22	15
Group 2b	22	17	13	7	6	5	6	6
Group 3	31	44	20	37	15	27	13	24
Base number	*270*	*140*	*283*	*227*	*186*	*268*	*233*	*183*
50–74								
Group 1	51	48	72	62	59	76	74	81
Group 2a	15	15	16	20	25	8	13	10
Group 2b	12	4	5	1	9	1	5	2
Group 3	21	33	7	17	6	15	8	7
Base number	*193*	*174*	*107*	*107*	*50*	*124*	*63*	*171*

Note: See explanation in text and Figure 7.19 for details of classification of groups.

Table 7B: Vigorous and moderate activity (over previous month)

Code	African-Caribbean Female %	African-Caribbean Male %	Indian Female %	Indian Male %	Pakistani Female %	Pakistani Male 5	Bangladeshi Female %	Bangladeshi Male %
16–29								
Level 0	11	10	20	11	23	18	30	17
Level 1	14	14	21	17	24	17	17	11
Level 2	27	20	21	16	19	16	19	20
Level 3	21	21	18	11	20	15	24	13
Level 4	18	17	11	15	5	11	6	9
Level 5	9	18	9	31	9	24	4	31
Base number	*178*	*114*	*208*	*129*	*281*	*235*	*307*	*213*
30–49								
Level 0	10	10	32	26	44	39	43	38
Level 1	13	16	16	11	17	11	17	17
Level 2	22	13	16	16	16	17	18	11
Level 3	35	33	28	33	21	24	21	24
Level 4	12	16	4	8	2	3	1	6
Level 5	8	13	3	6	–	5	–	3
Base number	*270*	*140*	*283*	*227*	*186*	*268*	*233*	*183*
50–74								
Level 0	42	39	56	56	53	68	61	69
Level 1	10	10	18	15	13	11	16	15
Level 2	15	11	13	10	19	4	9	6
Level 3	27	36	13	17	15	16	13	10
Level 4	2	1		1		–	–	
Level 5	5	3	1	2		–		
Base number	*193*	*174*	*107*	*107*	*50*	*124*	*63*	*171*

Table 7C: Reported levels of physical activity at work (WORKACTY)

Code	African-Caribbean Female %	African-Caribbean Male %	Indian Female %	Indian Male %	Pakistani Female %	Pakistani Male %	Bangladeshi Female %	Bangladeshi Male %
16–29								
Not applicable[a]	61	66	64	56	76	61	84	65
Inactive	26	19	31	24	27	18	8	14
Light	52	39	45	59	51	49	48	50
Moderate	22	42	24	18	22	33	44	37
Base number[b]	*178*	*114*	*208*	*129*	*281*	*235*	*307*	*213*
30–49								
Not applicable	43	33	51	25	89	45	97	52
Inactive	29	31	19	26	20	28	(9)	17
Light	29	18	51	37	67	41	(33)	48
Moderate	41	52	30	37	13	31	(58)	35
Base number[b]	*270*	*140*	*283*	*227*	*186*	*268*	*233*	*183*
50–74								
Not applicable	69	66	81	64	94	80	100	95
Inactive	2	9		18	(59)	21	#	(7)
Light	42	26	(88)	64		41	#	(78)
Moderate	56	65	(12)	17	(41)	38	#	(14)
Base number[b]	*193*	*174*	*107*	*107*	*50*	*124*	*63*	*171*

Base: Those whose replies to the question on occupation were sufficient to assign them to a level of physical exertion based on the normal activities of the occupational category.

[a] Not applicable: Those who were not working, for whatever reason, and could not answer the question.

This proportion is calculated from total base number: membership of activity groups recalculated from those remaining.

[b] Percentages based on very small numbers of eligible respondents in other age groups are indicated by brackets (*nn*). (When unweighted base for subgroup less than 20).

Empty cells are marked with this symbol.

Notes

1. This question has been researched by the Royal Society for the Prevention of Accidents and reported on in a so-far unpublished report: *An equal right to safety* by A. Parmar (1997).

2. Sports Council, *Black and ethnic minorities and sport* (Sports Council, London, 1994).

3. Racial harassment has been extensively researched and demonstrated to be a reality of everyday life. Figures from the British Crime Survey show that both men and women from African-Caribbean and Asian communities are much more likely than whites to suffer from 'contact crimes' and abuse: M. Fitzgerald and C. Hale, *Ethnic minorities: victimisation and racial harassment* (Home Office Research Study 154, Home Office, London, 1996).

4. C. Currer, 'Concepts of mental well- and ill-being: the case of Pathan mothers in Britain', in C. Currer and M. Stacey, *Concepts of health, illness and disease: a comparative perspective* (Berg, Leamington Spa, 1986).

5. The British Kabaddi Association is based in Dudley and produces leaflets and a newsletter to promote the sport. It may be contacted c/o Mrs P. K. Dhani, Dept. of Education and Community Services, Sandwell MBC, PO Box 41, West Bromwich B70 9LT.

6. A qualitative enquiry into perceptions of health and health facilities in Birmingham did find considerable unmet demand for leisure facility provision, and clear misperceptions of availability: M.R.D. Johnson and C. Verma, *It's our health too: Asian men's health perspectives* (Research Paper 26, Centre for Research in Ethnic Relations, University of Warwick, Coventry, 1998).

7. In particular, the consultation paper of the Physical Activity Task Force, *More people more active more often* (Department of Health, London, 1995). See also the tabulations and analysis of the *Allied Dunbar National Fitness Survey* (Health Education Authority and Sports Council, London, 1992), the *Health Survey for England* (N. Bennett, T. Dodd and J. Flatley *et al.*, Office of Population Censuses and Surveys, London, 1995) and *Health in England 1996* (Hansbro, Bridgwood, Morgan and Hickman, Office of National Statistics and Health Education Authority, London, 1997).

8. G.L. Lee and K.L. Wrench, 'Accident-prone immigrants: an assumption challenged', *Sociology* 14(4) (1980).

8   Diet and nutrition

Summary of the main findings

- About half in each ethnic group (African-Caribbeans 50%, Indians 47%, Pakistanis 53%, Bangladeshis 54%) perceived their own traditional diets to be healthier than Western diets (most foods eaten by people in this country) (Section 8.2).

- Only small minorities in each ethnic group (African-Caribbeans 13%, Indians 17%, Pakistanis 13%, Bangladeshis 10%) said that they preferred eating British- or European-style foods to their own traditional foods (Section 8.2).

- Traditional foods constituted a major component of the diets eaten at home by Indian, Pakistani and Bangladeshi people, with 8 in 10 Pakistani people (79%) and Bangladeshi people (83%) and 7 in 10 Indian people (71%) reporting that all or most of the foods they consumed at home in the last week consisted of traditional foods. Eating traditional foods at home was less common among African-Caribbean people, with only 1 in 3 respondents reporting that all or most of the meals eaten at home during the last week consisted of traditional foods of some kind. For both African-Caribbean people and the South Asian respondents who took part in the survey, eating traditional foods away from home was less common (Section 8.3).

- Dietary restrictions for cultural or religious reasons were uncommon among African-Caribbean people (22% reported restricting their diets) but widespread among Indian people (80%), Pakistani people (97%) and Bangladeshi people (97%) (Section 8.4).

- Perceived understanding of key terms used in healthy eating messages varied widely across groups and between terms. Large proportions (three-quarters or more) of African-Caribbean people reported understanding the terms 'starchy foods', 'dietary fibre' and 'fat', with a smaller proportion (about half) reporting an understanding of the term 'saturated fat'. Indian, Pakistani and Bangladeshi people reported lower rates of perceived understanding of each term (Section 8.5).

- Among those who said they understood individual dietary terms, knowledge of foods high in starch, dietary fibre, fat and saturated fat was patchy and often poor across all ethnic groups (Section 8.6).

- Knowledge of the links between diet and cardiovascular and other specific diseases was poor in general, particularly among Bangladeshi people (Section 8.8).

8.1   Introduction and background

A large body of evidence suggests eating habits are linked to a range of health problems, including circulatory diseases, cancers, diabetes and obesity. While it is generally accepted that many of these diseases are multi-factorial, diet is thought to be a modifiable risk factor that should be considered central to programmes of prevention.[1] Healthy eating messages are likely to have a central place in health promotion programmes to prevent and reduce the risk of cardiovascular disease and other health problems among black and minority ethnic groups. The current survey offered an opportunity to map people's understandings of diet as a risk factor for diseases among the Indian, Pakistani, Bangladeshi and African-Caribbean communities. The survey concentrated on four aspects of diet: perceptions about and use of traditional foods (Sections 8.2 – 8.4); knowledge and understanding of dietary terms commonly used in healthy eating messages (Sections 8.5, 8.6 and 8.7); knowledge of the links between diet and specific diseases and health problems (Section 8.8).

8.2   Perceptions of traditional foods

It has been suggested that, in general, the traditional diets of the African-Caribbean, Indian, Pakistani and Bangladeshi communities are closer to current dietary recommendations for dietary fat and fibre than those of the general UK population.[2] However, little is known about how African-Caribbean and South Asian groups view them and the extent to which they are a component of their diets. Through a series of questions about people's perceptions and use of traditional foods, the current survey provides some evaluation of the role that traditional foods play in the diets of respondents and maps some of the difficulties they encounter in trying to include traditional foods in their diets.

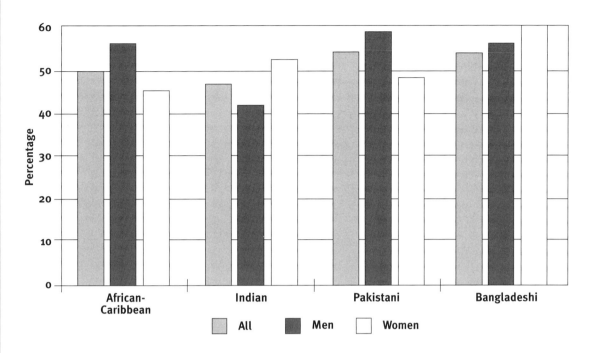

Figure 8.1: Proportions agreeing that their traditional foods are healthier than most foods eaten by people in this country

Figure 8.1 examines respondents' views about whether traditional foods are healthier than foods eaten by most people in this country. It suggests that about half of African-Caribbean (50%), Indian (47%), Pakistani (53%) and Bangladeshi (54%) people perceived their own traditional foods to be healthier. There were some significant differences within the South Asian groups between men and women. Among Indian and Bangladeshi people, women were more likely than men to identify traditional foods as healthy, whereas among Pakistani people this picture was reversed, with men more likely than women to report that traditional foods are healthier than foods eaten by most people in this country. There were also some significant age differences among South Asians. The perception that traditional foods are healthier than foods eaten by most people in this country in general appeared to increase with age for both men and women.

Among African-Caribbean people, differences between men and women were also apparent, with African-Caribbean men more likely than African-Caribbean women to perceive traditional foods as healthier than foods eaten by most people in this country. Age also appeared to shape beliefs among African-Caribbean people. Among men and women, respondents aged 50–74 were less likely than younger African-Caribbean people to report that traditional foods are healthier.

Only a small proportion of people in each group (African-Caribbeans 13%, Indians 17%, Pakistanis 13%, Bangladeshis 10%) reported that they preferred eating British- or European-style food rather than their own traditional food. Among African-Caribbean people, a preference for British or European food did not appear to be shaped by age or gender. Among Bangladeshi people, a higher proportion of women than men reported a preference for British or European food. For Indian men and Pakistani women only, preferences for British or European food decreased with increasing age.

8.3 Consumption of traditional foods

Figure 8.2 looks at the consumption of traditional meals eaten at home in the seven days prior to the survey. While traditional foods appeared to constitute the major component of the diet of South Asian respondents, they featured less often in the diets of African-Caribbean respondents. Among the South Asian groups, 8 in 10 Bangladeshi (83%) and Pakistani people (79%) and 7 in

10 Indian people (71%) reported that all or most of the meals they had eaten at home consisted of traditional foods. Among African-Caribbean people, this proportion fell to 1 in 3 people (33%). The general trend among all groups was that men were more likely than women, and adults aged 50 years or more were more likely than younger adults, to report that all or most of the foods they had eaten at home in the last week included traditional foods of some kind.

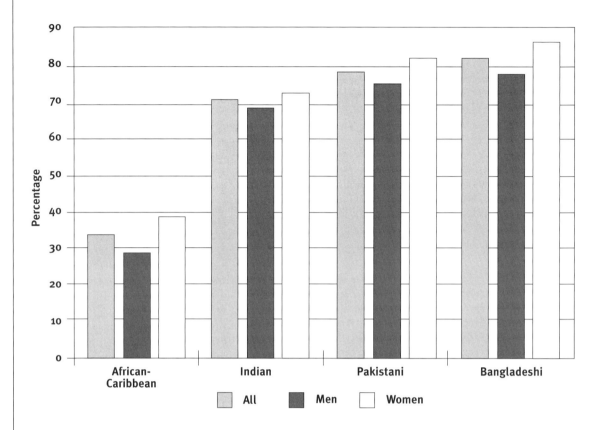

Figure 8.2: All/most meals eaten at home in last week included traditional foods of some kind

Traditional meals were less likely to form part of people's diets when eating away from home (Figure 8.3). Among African-Caribbean people who had eaten away from home in the last week, only a small minority (11%) reported that meals included traditional foods of some kind. Among South Asian people, the proportions were higher (Indians 32%, Pakistanis 44%, Bangladeshis 44%). Indian and Pakistani women were more likely than their male counterparts to have reported that all or most meals eaten away from home included traditional foods. Among Bangladeshi and African-Caribbean people, the pattern was reversed, with a higher proportion of men than women reporting that all or most meals eaten away from home in the last week included traditional foods. Within the South Asian communities only, the proportion reporting that all or most of the meals eaten away from home in the last week consisted of traditional foods increased with age. As no data was collected on where meals were eaten away from home (for example, in other people's houses, in the workplace, etc.), it is not clear to what extent these differences reflect the different places and circumstances under which people of different ages and sexes eat away from home.

Respondents were asked whether it could be difficult to get traditional foods when eating away from home. Just over a quarter of Indian (30%) and Pakistani people (27%) and just under half of Bangladeshi people (45%) agreed that they found it difficult to get traditional foods to eat when eating away from home. Some small but significant gender differences were apparent among Indian and Bangladeshi people, with more women than men in both groups reporting difficulties in getting traditional foods away from home. Among the South Asian groups who took part, the general trend was that younger people were significantly more likely than older adults in each group to report difficulties in getting traditional foods when eating away from home (although age differences were not significant for Bangladeshi women). Getting traditional foods when away from home was also an issue for African-Caribbean people, with half of men and women (53%) agreeing that it was difficult. Among African-Caribbean women, difficulties getting traditional foods away from home decreased with age (age differences among men were not significant). However, it is unclear, for all ethnic groups, to what extent gender and age differences may reflect differences in eating venues.

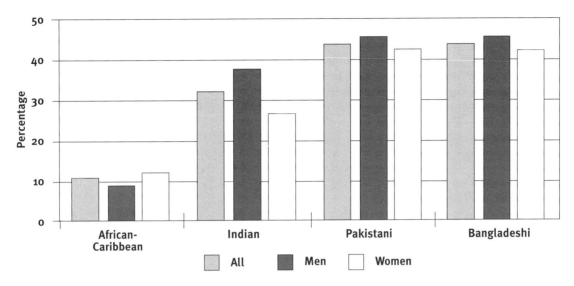

Figure 8.3: All/most meals eaten away from home in last week included traditional foods of some kind

8.4 Dietary restrictions

Eating patterns vary considerably within any population as a result of cultural and religious influences, and these factors are known to be key influences shaping the diets of South Asian and African-Caribbean people.[3] The survey provides some measure of the prevalence of dietary restrictions and the types of foods restricted among the populations surveyed.

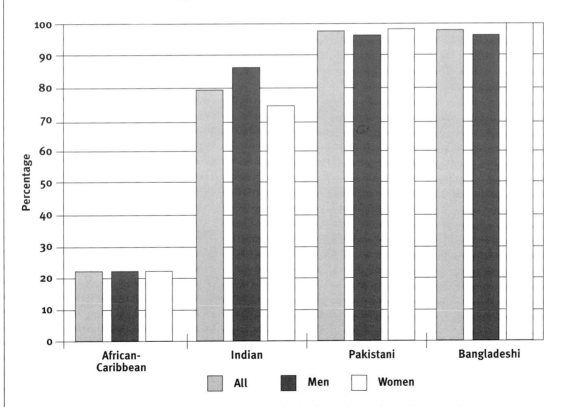

Figure 8.4: Proportions restricting their diets for cultural or religious reasons

Figure 8.4 shows the proportions in each groups who reported that they restricted their diets. It suggests that dietary restrictions were uncommon among African-Caribbeans. This is likely to reflect the fact that a high proportion of African-Caribbeans in the UK are Christians, whose diets are largely free from religious restrictions. A minority of African-Caribbeans (22%) stated that they did restrict their diet for religious or cultural reasons. Although there were no differences in the proportions of men and women who reported dietary restrictions, there were some significant age difference among men, with African-Caribbeans aged 50–74 less likely than younger adults to restrict their diets. It is unclear to what extent people who restricted their diets did so for religious or cultural reasons, or both. The most common food cited as restricted (Figure 8.5) was pork (including pork products), which was not eaten by 14% of African-Caribbeans from a range of religious groups, including Seventh Day Adventists, Rastafarians, Baptists and Church of England/Wales faiths. The proportions reporting that they restricted other foods were very small. As the total proportion of African-Caribbean respondents who reported that they restricted their diet was low, and the proportions reporting that they did not eat specific foods was very small, any further analysis by religion was not possible.

Food reported as restricted	African-Caribbean %	Indian %	Pakistani %	Bangladeshi %
Pork (including pork products)	14	30	82	86
Beef	3	43	15	9
Meat that isn't halal	<1	19	72	68
Meat of any kind	1	26	4	4
Animal fat of unknown origin	<1	10	26	32
Drinking alcohol	1	13	33	54

Base: all respondents

Figure 8.5: Proportions of respondents reporting that they do not eat specific foods for religious or cultural reasons

In contrast, dietary restrictions among Indian, Pakistani and Bangladeshi people were much more widespread, reflecting the strong influence of religion across the groups, and religious diversity between and within groups. Eighty per cent of Indian people, 97% of Pakistani people and 97% of Bangladeshi people reported that they restricted their diets for religious or cultural reasons. Whereas a higher proportion of men than women reported dietary restrictions among Indians, among Pakistani and Bangladeshi people, higher proportions of women reported dietary restrictions, although the differences between Pakistani men and women were very small.

Among Indian people, the food mostly commonly cited as not eaten for religious or cultural reasons was beef, with 43% reporting that they did not eat it. Non-beef eaters were predominantly Hindus and Sikhs, with half of each religious group reporting that they did not eat beef. Pork was not eaten by just under a third of Indian people (30%), three-quarters (73%) of whom were Muslims. A quarter (27%) of Indian respondents, predominantly Sikhs and Hindus, reported that they did not eat meat of any kind. A fifth (19%), the majority of whom were Muslims, reported that they only ate halal meat. Among Indian Muslims, a quarter (24%) reported not eating animal fat of unknown origin and a third (35%) reported not drinking alcohol.

A majority of Pakistani people (82%) and Bangladeshi people (86%) reported that they did not eat pork. As 9 in 10 Bangladeshi and Pakistani respondents were Muslims, this and other findings on dietary restrictions are likely to reflect the strong religious influence of Islam. Eating only halal meat was also reported by three-quarters of Bangladeshi (69%) and Pakistani Muslims (77%), and not eating animal fat of unknown origin was reported by a third of Bangladeshi (33%) and a quarter of Pakistani Muslims (37%). Not drinking alcohol was reported by a third (34%) of Pakistani and half (54%) of Bangladeshi Muslims.

8.5   Perceived understanding of dietary terms

This section examines people's understanding and knowledge relating to selected 'healthy eating' messages. People's ability to change their diets in response to healthy eating messages depends in part on whether they have been able to understand key terms within these messages and any information attached to them. The survey sought to establish people's understanding of four commonly used dietary terms: 'starchy food', 'dietary fibre', 'fat' and 'saturated fat'. Respondents were asked whether they themselves felt that they understood each term. The data suggest that

Dietary term	African-Caribbean %	Indian %	Pakistani %	Bangladeshi %
Starchy food				
All	91	64	46	26
Women	94	63	39	19
Men	87	57	42	23
Dietary fibre				
All	75	57	45	29
Women	79	58	39	21
Men	67	51	39	27
Fat				
All	95	91	84	91
Women	96	93	77	92
Men	94	89	87	89
Saturated fat				
All	54	46	35	20
Women	55	43	24	16
Men	50	43	36	17

Base: all respondents

Figure 8.6: Proportions reporting that they understood what was meant by the dietary terms

reported understandings of the terms varied widely across groups and between terms. Figure 8.6 presents these findings.

Starchy food

Respondents understanding of the term 'starchy food' varied widely across the groups surveyed. A very high proportion of African-Caribbean people reported that they understood the term (91%). A slightly higher proportion of African-Caribbean women (94%) than men (87%) reported an understanding of the term. Across all age groups, high proportions of African-Caribbean men and women reported that they understood the term starchy food, although those least likely to report an understanding were male and female respondents aged 16–29.

Among the South Asian groups, the proportions who reported an understanding of the term were significantly lower, with 3 in 5 (64%) Indian people, 2 in 5 (46%) Pakistani people and 1 in 5 (26%) Bangladeshi people reporting that they felt that they understood what was meant by the term 'starchy food'. Among Indian people and Pakistani people there were no significant differences between the proportions of men and women who reported an understanding of the term. Among Bangladeshi people, a slightly higher proportion of men than women reported that they understood the term 'starchy food'. Among South Asian people, the proportions who reported that they understood the term 'starchy food' appeared to decrease with age, with people in the younger age group (16–29) more likely than people in older age groups to report an understanding. Small proportions of Pakistani and Bangladeshi adults aged over 30 years reported that they understood the term.

Dietary fibre

A similar pattern emerged when respondents' understanding of the term 'dietary fibre' was examined. Three-quarters of African-Caribbeans (75%) reported that they understood the term, of which eight in ten were women and seven in ten were men. Moderately high proportions of African-Caribbeans reported understanding the term across the age groups. Although age appeared to be a factor related to men's understanding of the term dietary fibre, with men in the youngest age group most likely to report an understanding of the term, among women age did not appear to be related to their understanding of the term.

The proportions of South Asian groups who reported that they understood the term 'dietary fibre' were lower than that reported for African-Caribbean people, with Indian people reporting the highest rate (57%) of understanding and Pakistani people (45%) and Bangladeshi people (29%) lower rates. Higher proportions of Indian and Pakistani women than men reported that they understood the term 'dietary fibre'. This picture was reversed among Bangladeshi people, with more men reporting that they understood the term. Across all groups, the general pattern was that a reported understanding of the term 'dietary fibre' decreased with increasing age (the exception was among Indian men, among whom age differences were not significant). Only small proportions of Bangladeshi men and women aged 30 years or older reported that they understood what was meant by the term 'dietary fibre'.

Fat and saturated fat

A reported understanding of the term 'fat' was very high across the groups. Nine in ten African-Caribbean people (95%), Indian people (91%) and Bangladeshi people (91%) said they understood the term. The proportion fell to 8 in 10 among Pakistani people (84%). Among African-Caribbean people, although some differences were apparent, with more younger adults than older adults reporting that they understood the term, reported understanding of the term remained high across the age groups. Among South Asian people, Indian and Bangladeshi women were more likely than their male counterparts to report that they understood the term 'fat'. Among Pakistani people, men were more likely than women to report they understood the term. Among South Asian men and women, the proportions reporting that they understood the term 'fat' decreased with increasing age, but remained high generally across the age groups.

The term 'saturated fat' appeared to be generally less well understood than the term 'fat'. Among African-Caribbean people, half (54%) reported an understanding of the term. This proportion was lower than for any other dietary term. A slightly higher proportion of African-Caribbean women than men reported that they understood the term, and adults aged 50–74 were less likely than other adults to report an understanding. Among South Asian people, 46% of Indian people, 35% of Pakistani people and 20% of Bangladeshi people said that they understood the term 'saturated fat'. Although a higher proportion of Pakistani men than women reported an understanding of the term, differences between Indian and Bangladeshi men and women were not significant. Among Pakistani and Bangladeshi people, men and women aged 50 years or over were least likely to say they understood the meaning of the term (no age differences were apparent among Indian).

8.6 Knowledge about foods high in starch, fibre, fat and saturated fat

Respondents who reported that they understood what was meant by the key terms discussed above were asked to give some examples of foods which contained 'a lot of' starch, dietary fibre, fat and saturated fat. Figures 8.7, 8.8, 8.9 and 8.10 show the proportions of respondents in each group who identified the main sources of starchy foods, dietary fibre, fat and saturated fat in the diet. The subsections below look at knowledge of each food constituent in more detail.

Starchy foods

As Figure 8.7 illustrates, knowledge about foods high in starch was mixed. Rice and potatoes were most commonly identified as high in starch. However, bread (including nan, chapati, puri, roti and poppodum), a high starch food common to the diets of many African-Caribbean and South Asian groups, was not commonly cited. Yams/plantain/sweet potatoes were identified by less than half of African-Caribbean people as high in starch, even though they form part of the traditional African-Caribbean diet. Starchy foods that are particularly high in dietary fibre, such as wholemeal/brown bread or brown rice were mentioned by very few respondents in each group.

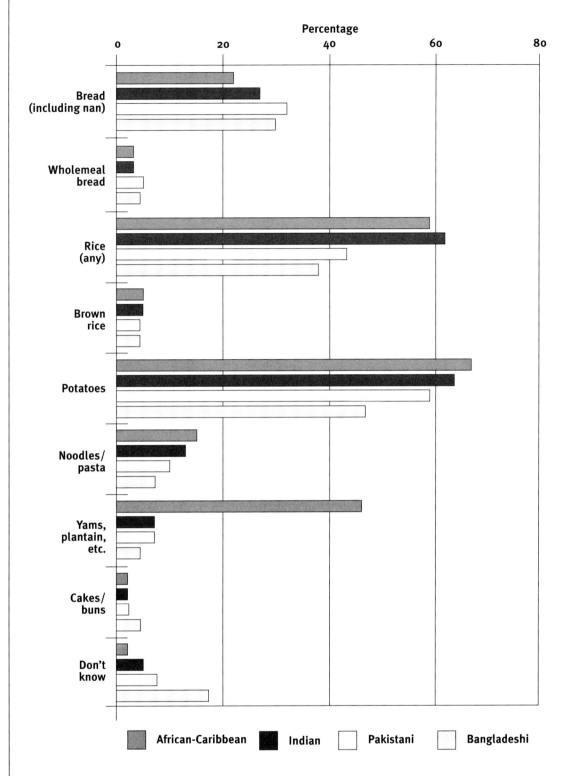

Figure 8.7: Proportions identifying specific foods as high in starch

Dietary fibre

Of those respondents who reported that they understood what was meant by the term dietary fibre, relatively small proportions were able to identify commonly used foods that contain dietary fibre. Wholemeal bread appeared to be the most commonly reported source of dietary fibre by each group. The proportions identifying vegetables and fruits as good sources of dietary fibre were extremely low in all groups. Figure 8.8 shows the proportions in each group identifying specific foods as high in dietary fibre.

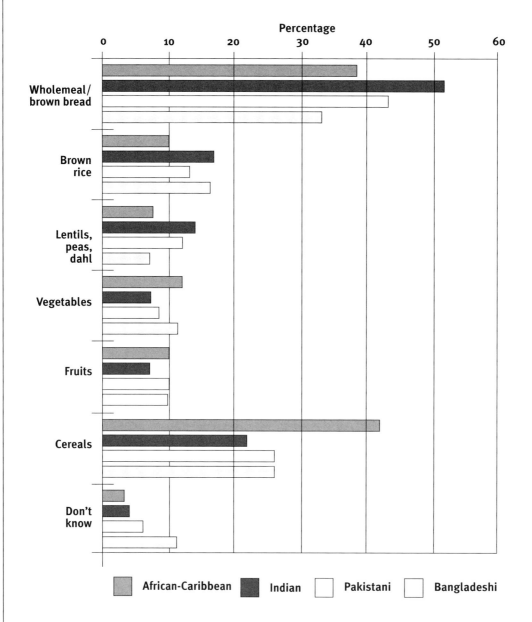

Percentage

Wholemeal/ brown bread

Brown rice

Lentils, peas, dahl

Vegetables

Fruits

Cereals

Don't know

■ African-Caribbean ■ Indian □ Pakistani □ Bangladeshi

Figure 8.8: Proportions identifying specific foods as high in dietary fibre

Fat and saturated fat

Knowledge of the common foods that are high in fat and high in saturated fat was relatively poor in all groups (Figures 8.9 and 8.10). Among African-Caribbean respondents who said they understood what was meant by the term 'fat', only half (51%) identified red meat and a third (32%) identified butter as foods high in fat. African-Caribbean people's knowledge of foods containing saturated fat appeared to be poorer than their knowledge of foods containing fat in general. Less than a fifth (18%) of African-Caribbean people identified red meat and just over a quarter (27%) identified butter as high in saturated fat. Two in five (19%) African-Caribbean people reported that they could not identify any foods which are high in saturated fat.

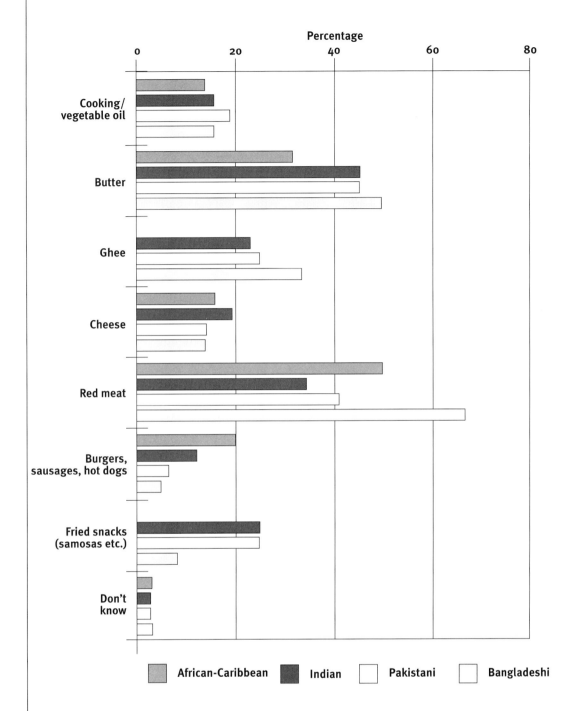

Figure 8.9: Proportions identifying specific foods as high in fat

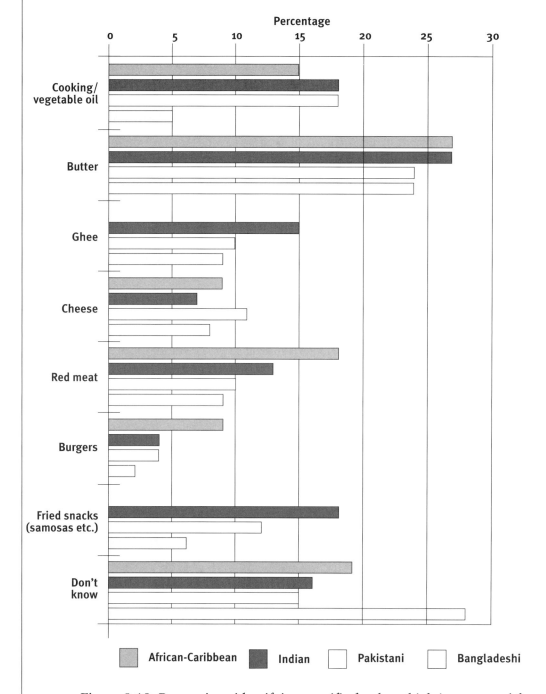

Percentage

African-Caribbean   Indian   Pakistani   Bangladeshi

Figure 8.10: Proportions identifying specific foods as high in saturated fat

Among the South Asians groups, where the consumption of red meat is relatively common (Pakistanis and Bangladeshis), moderate proportions identified red meat as source of fat. Approximately half of each South Asian group (Indians 46%, Pakistanis 46%, Bangladeshis 51%) identified butter as a high fat food, but significantly lower proportions identified it as a food high in saturated fat. Knowledge about ghee as a product high in fat or saturated fat was not widespread among any South Asian group.

8.7   Knowledge of ways to reduce dietary salt

In addition to examining knowledge about common food constituents, the survey also explored respondents' knowledge of ways to reduce salt in the diet. Figure 8.11 describes the responses in each ethnic group. Among African-Caribbeans, the most commonly reported method of reducing salt in the diet was cutting down or avoiding particular foods. Just over a third (37%) of African-Caribbean respondents said they just cut out or avoid particular foods, with a further 12% saying that they would use less salt in cooking or put less salt on food in addition to cutting out or avoiding particular foods. Just over a quarter (27%) said they would not cut out or avoid particular foods but would use less salt in cooking or put less salt on food. Among South Asian respondents, the most commonly reported method of reducing salt was using less salt in cooking or putting less salt on food (Indians 32%, Pakistanis 38%, Bangladeshis 34%). Smaller proportions said they would cut out/ avoid particular foods only or cut out/avoid particular foods and cut out or reduce salt in cooking and on food. As Figure 8.11 demonstrates, small but significant proportions of respondents said that they did not know of ways to reduce salt in the diet. Figure 8.12 describes the particular foods that those who reported that they would cut down or avoid particular foods to reduce salt in the diet listed. Crisps, salted peanuts and other salty snacks were most commonly cited by each groups as foods they would cut down on or avoid in order to reduce their intake of salt.

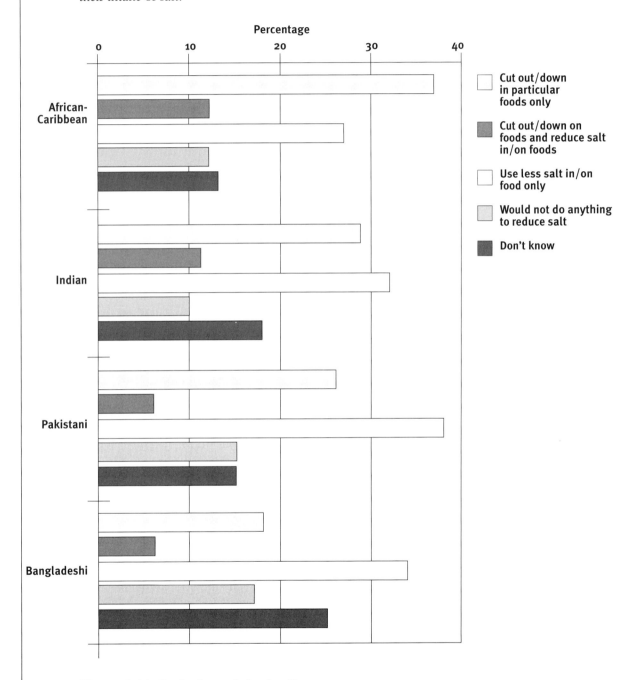

Figure 8.11: Reducing salt in the diet

Foods cut down or avoided	African-Caribbean %	Indian %	Pakistani %	Bangladeshi %
Processed food/tinned food	16	19	14	6
Ready-prepared meals	7	9	9	5
Salt cod/mackerel/beef	30	8	11	9
Bacon	22	16	3	4
Crisps, roasted peanuts, salty snacks, etc.	32	49	57	49
Other	35	33	35	42

Base: Respondents who said they would cut down or avoid particular foods to reduce their salt intake.

Figure 8.12: Foods respondents would cut down on or avoid in order to reduce salt intake

8.8 Knowledge of the links between diet and disease

The survey provided an opportunity to examine knowledge levels about the link between diet and diseases/health problems. Figure 8.13 illustrates that the proportions of respondents who were able to identify a link between diet and specific diseases varied widely between ethnic groups and across different diseases. In all groups, the proportions linking diet with specific diseases were generally low. Respondents were most commonly able to identify a link between heart disease and diet. Among African-Caribbean people, half (51%) said they thought that heart disease was linked to diet, with a third more women than men appearing knowledgeable about diet as a risk factor for coronary health disease. Among Indian people and Pakistani people, just under half of respondents (Indians 45%, Pakistanis 42%) reported that they thought there was a link between diet and heart disease. Among Bangladeshi people, the corresponding proportion fell to a quarter (25%). Among African-Caribbean and South Asian groups, knowledge of diet as a risk factor for heart disease decreased with age, with adults over 50 less likely than other adults to state a link between the two.

Knowledge about diet and strokes, a cardiovascular disease prevalent among African-Caribbean people, was poor among African-Caribbean and South Asian groups. Three per cent or less from each group identified diet as a risk factor for strokes. There appeared to be a greater awareness of a link between raised blood pressure and diet, although the proportions able to identify this link with diet were relatively small. Among African-Caribbean people, women were slightly more likely than men to report a link between both diet and strokes and diet and raised blood pressure. The links between diet and bowel cancer, cancer generally and 'stomach problems' were identified by very few respondents.

Disease health problem	African-Caribbean %	Indian %	Pakistani %	Bangladeshi %
Heart disease				
All	51	45	42	25
Women	60	45	42	23
Men	41	44	42	27
Raised blood pressure				
All	16	13	14	8
Women	21	14	13	8
Men	11	12	14	8
Strokes				
All	3	3	2	3
Women	4	3	3	2
Men	<1	3	4	2
Over weight/obesity				
All	19	19	18	15
Women	19	20	16	10
Men	19	18	20	19
Cancer in general				
All	7	4	3	2
Women	8	5	5	2
Men	5	4	1	2
Bowel cancer				
All	<1	<1	2	<1
Women	1	1	<1	<1
Men	<1	<1	3	1
Anaemia				
All	<1	<1	<1	<1
Women	<1	<1	<1	<1
Men	<1	<1	<1	<1
Don't know				
All	20	23	28	39
Women	14	25	30	45
Men	27	22	25	33

Base: all respondents

Figure 8.13: Diseases most frequently reported as linked with diet

8.9   Conclusions

A number of important findings emerge from the dietary data. Traditional foods were the main component of the meals eaten at home by Indian, Pakistani and Bangladeshi people, but are less commonly consumed at home by African-Caribbean people. Only small proportions in each group reported a preference for British- or European-style food rather than their own traditional food. It was evident that some respondents found it difficult to get traditional foods when eating away from home.

A substantial proportion of people in each group may not be aware that their traditional diets are, in general, closer to dietary recommendations for fibre and fat than Western diets. Only about half of people in each group perceived their own traditional food to be healthier than the foods consumed by most people in this country.

The survey sought to establish people's understanding of four key dietary terms commonly used in health education messages: 'starchy food', 'dietary fibre', 'fat' and 'saturated fat'. The data suggest understandings of the terms varied widely across groups and between terms. Across all the groups, high proportions reported an understanding of the term 'fat', lower proportions understood what was meant by 'saturated fat'. A high proportion of African-Caribbean people reported an understanding of the terms 'dietary fibre' and 'starchy foods', with lower proportions of South Asian groups reporting an understanding of these terms.

Respondents' perceptions that they understood key dietary terms was not necessarily confirmed by the data. Commonly used foods high in starch, dietary fibre, fat and saturated fat were often not identified by respondents as foods high in these dietary constituents. Knowledge about foods high in starch, dietary fibre, fat and saturated fat, can be best be described as patchy among all groups. In addition, knowledge of the links between diet and cardiovascular diseases and diseases more generally was poor, particularly among Bangladeshi respondents. Together, these findings suggest that key nutrition education messages relating to the prevention of cardiovascular diseases may not have been heard, understood or absorbed by substantial proportions of people in black and minority ethnic groups.

Notes

1. Department of Health, *Nutritional aspects of cardiovascular disease: report of the Cardiovascular Review Group, Committee on Medical Aspects of Food Policy* (HMSO, London, 1994).

2. Health Education Authority, *Nutrition in minority ethnic groups: Asians and African-Caribbeans in the United Kingdom* (Health Education Authority, London, 1991).

3. Health Education Authority, *Nutrition in minority ethnic groups.*

9 Body image and body shape

Summary of the main findings

- Most men and women in all ethnic groups felt that people could be responsible for their own weight control, and that (in most cases) weight could be reduced. There was less likelihood of believing that they could 'put weight on' as they might wish.

- African-Caribbean women were the only group surveyed who were very likely to feel that they weighed 'a lot more' than they wished, and Bangladeshis, notably men, were rather more likely to feel that they were in fact underweight. In general, men were more likely than women to believe they were underweight.

- People in the survey reported that they were doing a variety of possibly contradictory things to control their body weight, but overall, most people saw exercise and control over the quantity eaten as being the key activity.

- Very few people, despite objective measures showing considerable levels of obesity, reported that they had been actively advised to lose weight.

- Reasons for wanting to lose weight were very general and mostly health related: very few people in the survey referred to issues of personal appearance.

- Despite the previous finding, one in three men and more than half the women, most notably the African-Caribbean females, stated that they would like to alter their body shape in some manner. The body area giving rise to most concern was the stomach, but women were also interested in changing their bottoms or hips.

- The physique of the different ethnic groups, including height, varies considerably. Using the BMI ratio to correct for height, and the waist–hip ratio, provides valuable additional information.

- Very substantial numbers, about two in five, of older women are obese in terms of BMI ratios, with the exception of Bangladeshis. Among males, Pakistani and African-Caribbean men are the most likely to be obese on this measure.

9.1 Introduction

In this chapter, we focus upon the perceptions of the members of black and minority ethnic groups who were interviewed in respect of their 'body image', that is, their height, weight and shape. This is not necessarily the same as their beliefs about fitness and health, although there are in some cultures beliefs that 'bigger is healthier', which may conflict with the 'Western' (or at least, commercial advertisers') preoccupation with slimness. We have chosen to start with the beliefs and values of the interviewees before examining the measured data relating to their height and weight, since we believe that those working in the field of health promotion need first of all to understand the perceptions of their clients, rather than relying on their own values and interpretations of 'objective' data. It is clear from studies in the USA that there are 'ethnic' differences in perceptions of weight and size which are related to what people actually do.[1] The data presented here provide the first clear evidence of this process in Britain.

9.2 Perceptions of body weight

There is no simple relationship between body shape and health. Anorexia and obesity are equally unhealthy. While in terms of perception there is a degree of cultural stereotype and fashion affecting the 'ideal' body shape, it is clear that (other things being equal) a very thin person may be seen as sickly, unless she is a fashion model. On the other hand, a very 'fat' person may be regarded (possibly at the same time) as both probably wealthy or poor and 'working class', and at risk of heart disease. Modern medical evidence has shown that there is a close relationship between excess body weight or certain patterns of physique and enhanced risks of particular diseases, including heart failure, diabetes and even some cancers.[2] However, it is evident that there will not always be a direct correspondence between what medical science would assert and what people feel is attractive to them and their peers. The survey therefore asked both about people's actual weight and height and their self-perception, as well as about the medical advice they had been given in relation to their weight.

I weigh ...	African-Caribbean	Indian	Pakistani	Bangladeshi
Females				
Less than I would wish	6	7	8	10
My weight is about right	25	38	37	51
A little more than I would wish	37	37	34	28
A lot more than I would wish	33	18	21	11
Base	*621*	*561*	*468*	*535*
Males				
Less than I would wish	16	15	17	23
My weight is about right	53	50	44	54
A little more than I would wish	24	29	30	21
A lot more than I would wish	7	7	8	3
Base	*416*	*460*	*612*	*536*

Note: 'Don't know' and similar replies excluded from this figure: see also Table 9.1.

Q22 'Which of these (phrases) best describes you: "I weigh ... than I would wish to".'

Figure 9.1: Q22 Perceptions of own body weight (percentages selecting answers)

The obsession with 'body image' and weight frequently apparent in fashion and other magazines appears in the problem pages of ethnic minority publications just as much as in those of the majority population. It is therefore of interest to note that the majority of respondents (especially the men) seemed relatively content with their weight. However, perhaps as expected, women were somewhat more likely than men to agree with the statement that they weighed 'a lot more than I would wish to'. We had not expected to find that people would feel that they weighed less than their ideal size, but in fact there was a substantial group who chose this response, among the Bangladeshi group in particular. It was the case that men were generally twice as likely as women to indicate a desire to be heavier. One in five Bangladeshi men reported that they felt either a little or 'a lot' less than their desired amount. Two explanations might suit this finding. Firstly, evidence from this and other surveys[3] consistently demonstrates that the Bangladeshi community is relatively speaking the most impoverished out of all the main ethnic minority groups in Britain. A desire for more weight may therefore reflect a feeling of poverty or even actual malnourishment, and an association of size and well-being. There is certainly scope to explore through qualitative research why men across all ethnic groups are so much more likely to see themselves as underweight.

Certain other patterns emerge from these data. It is apparent that Bangladeshi women were most content with their weight, while those of African-Caribbean origin were most likely to see themselves as overweight. Research has demonstrated that black women in America do tend to be larger and heavier than white women, because of bone and muscle structures, which gives certain advantages in resisting osteoporosis in later life.[4] Equally, however, this will place them at a disadvantage when comparing themselves with mainstream advertising of conventional images of acceptable or desirable size – and also at a disadvantage when seeking to buy clothing. Otherwise, we cannot explain the considerable range of variation in self-image in terms of 'ethnic grouping'. Indian and Pakistani females' replies indicate very similar levels of reported satisfaction with their weight, quite different from the views of Bangladeshi women.

Those who weighed more than they thought desirable were asked if they felt people could lose weight, while those who weighed less than they wanted were asked if it was possible to put on weight 'when they want to', and those whose weight was 'about right' were asked, 'As far as you know, is there anything people can do to control or maintain their weight when they want to?' From the replies to these three questions (Q23, Q26, Q29; Tables 9.2, 9.5, 9.8) it is clear that weight is seen as something that most people are able to control. The overwhelming majority of those whose weight was satisfactory felt this to be true. Only a small number, 8% of men overall and 12% of women, disagreed. Curiously, Bangladeshi men were least likely to disagree while Bangladeshi women were most likely to say 'no', and both sexes from this community were also the most likely to reply 'don't know'. However, nearly 90% of all those who felt they were overweight, and nearly 80% of both Bangladeshi 'overweight' men and women, felt it was possible to reduce one's weight. While women were notably less likely to be sure if it was possible to put on weight if desired, more than half, and nearly three-quarters of the men who said they were underweight, felt that it would be possible to increase it. On the other hand, one in four women said that it would *not* be possible to put on weight 'to order'. This group included 42% of the 'underweight' African-Caribbean women, more than actually felt that it was possible to do so. It would not, however, be safe to conclude from this that they did not feel any responsibility or ability to watch their weight. In general, and aside from questions of desirability, it is clear that most people from all the minority ethnic groups felt that weight was personally controllable. In view of this, it is of particular interest to consider also their responses to questions asking 'why' they personally were seeking to take such action (if indeed they were).

9.3   Action to alter body weight and shape

As part of these questions on 'ideal body weight', respondents were asked whether they were doing anything to put on, control (maintain) or actively lose weight. Those who felt they were above their desired weight were asked about losing weight; those who felt they were underweight were asked about increasing weight, and those who were satisfied with their weight, about 'controlling' it (see Appendix, Tables 9.3, 9.6, 9.9). A number of possible actions were recorded, including a number of dietary options: in some cases the answers were clearly potentially contradictory. Thus, in order to control their weight, similar numbers of people were eating *more* and *less* starchy and fibre-rich foods; others were eating less generally (or more, in order to put on weight), while others again were varying the content of their diet. In reply to all three questions, a significant number of people were recorded as saying that they were 'doing nothing'. In terms of 'putting on weight', while a number of areas of the diet were mentioned, the majority of responses (38%) referred simply to 'eating more', and a further 15% to doing exercise. In order to 'control or maintain' weight, the most common single response was to report 'taking exercise' (27%) or to 'limit the total amount of food eaten' (20%): a significant number also reported reducing the amount of fatty, oily or fried foods in their diet. To lose weight, one in four replies (25%) referred to exercise, and nearly as many to 'eating less generally' (24%). Very few people referred to a 'calorie-controlled diet' or cutting down on alcohol, but a significant number of replies (5%) mentioned eating more vegetables and fruit. The complexity of the responses cannot be fully explored in this analysis.

Possibly the most important single response was related to exercise, but again this was seen as a means of both losing and gaining weight, perhaps in different ways (Figure 9.2). Irrespective of the patterns shown above, about 1 in 20 of all ethnic groups and genders had been advised to take exercise in respect of their weight, either to put it on or to reduce it. Rather more than those advised to do so in fact reported that they were exercising because of this issue. Men were somewhat more likely to say that they were doing exercise to put on or 'maintain' their weight compared to women. While in absolute terms more men were actually 'doing exercise' to lose weight than to gain it, a very much larger proportion of women were doing exercise for this reason. Certain 'ethnically different' patterns seemed to emerge from the data: notably that that Pakistanis of both genders were least likely to be using exercise as a means of weight control, and that nearly one in four Indian males said they were exercising to 'control' their weight. Overall, the pattern of replies from the Indian group seems to differ from the three other groups, in that more men in this ethnic group suggested that they were exercising to 'control' their weight. It is also clear that Bangladeshis were least likely to be seeking to lose weight through exercise.

	African-Caribbean %	Indian %	Pakistani %	Bangladeshi %
Female				
To put on weight	–	–	0	–
To control weight	6	10	7	6
To lose weight	25	19	16	10
Advised to do more to lose it	5	6	6	5
Male				
To put on weight	2	1	1	2
To control weight	15	23	15	15
To lose weight	12	14	14	5
Advised to do more to lose it	4	7	5	6

Note: Rows of data in this figure are derived from four separate questions:

Q24 Are you doing anything at the moment to put weight on? If yes what?

Q27 Do you do anything at the moment to control or maintain your weight or not? If yes what?

Q30 Are you doing anything at the moment to lose weight? If yes what?

Q33 Did (a doctor or nurse) give you any specific advice about how to lose weight or not? If yes what?

NB: Respondents could give any number of replies to each of these questions. Percentages were calculated on the basis of the number of respondents asked the question, following the earlier filter about perception of their own weight except Q33, which was asked of everyone.

Figure 9.2: Responses to questions on exercising or weight training in connection with weight change (Q24, Q27, Q30, Q33) (proportion mentioning exercise)

In addition to being asked what (they) were doing to raise, lower or control their weight, respondents were also asked the reason for this. All those in the survey were asked if they had ever been advised by a doctor or nurse to lose or gain weight (Q33 in Figure 9.2), and around 15% of the men and 25% of the women said that they had been given such advice. African-Caribbean women were the most likely to have been advised to lose weight, and Bangladeshi women the least likely: there were no apparent differences in this respect between men. A small number (about 3%) of Asian men reported being advised to gain some weight, as did slightly under 1 in 20 women. Again, there were no other ethnic differentials to be identified in the replies to this question. All respondents were also asked why (if appropriate) they were seeking to change their weight (Q25 increase, Q28 control, Q31 lose weight). Nearly all the replies referred to 'good health' (recorded as 'for the good of my health generally') or some similar phrase, such as 'to feel better about myself'. A small number mentioned specific health risks that they were seeking to avoid (the particular nature of which was not recorded) but the most common other reply was 'to feel better about myself generally' (or 'to be more confident'). Extremely few people suggested that they were doing it in order to be able to wear more attractive clothes, be a different shape or as a result of peer pressures. The majority of such answers were given by those aged under 30, and more frequently by female than male respondents. On the other hand, reducing the risk of specific health problems was more frequently the reply of older men (Tables 9.4, 9.7, 9.11).

9.4 Body image and appearance

Further evidence that people from minority ethnic groups are also likely to see their body shape as part of their overall self-presentation is located in the answers to a more general question (Q35), 'Would you like to lose weight from or alter the shape of any particular part of your body?' Nearly one-third of the men in the survey, and just over half of the women, said that there was some change that they would like. Among men, there were few differences between the ethnic groups, although Bangladeshi men were slightly less likely to want this (Table 9.14). Bangladeshi women too were very much less likely to wish to alter their physical appearance, but nearly two-thirds of African-Caribbean women, and only slightly fewer Indian and Pakistani women, answered in the affirmative. The question did not distinguish between those wishing to reduce or enlarge (or otherwise modify) the body part, although the assumption in its phrasing was clearly that it would be a reduction in size: in view of the earlier responses to questions 23–25, this may with hindsight have been a mistake.

A subsequent question (Q36) asked respondents, 'Which parts would you like to lose weight from or alter the shape of?' Respondents were allowed to mention more than one answer, and so it is not possible to identify precisely what the 'ideal body shape' might be from this question, especially since the phrasing did not distinguish between 'losing weight from' and 'altering the shape of' any part. In so far as any pattern can be discerned from the data, it is clear that the majority of men, with little difference between ethnic groups, were concerned to reduce (or change) the size of their belly, while a small number of Bangladeshi men mentioned their hips or bottom, and some African-Caribbean men were concerned about their legs (Figure 9.3). Women were slightly less concerned about their stomach area, but this was still the zone of greatest concern, closely followed by the hips or bottom – particularly in the case of Indian women. African-Caribbean women, like the men, were rather more likely to mention the legs, while Bangladeshi women were more concerned with the stomach and less with other parts of the body.

	African-Caribbean	Indian	Pakistani	Bangladeshi
Females				
Legs/thighs	37	25	15	19
Hips/bottom	34	45	39	33
Stomach etc.	67	65	72	75
Other	20	12	12	9
Base	414	344	293	173
Males				
Legs/thighs	10	5	4	7
Hips/bottom	5	5	7	10
Stomach etc.	79	85	87	86
Other	16	13	15	8
Base	123	148	202	132

Base: Those answering 'yes' to Q35, 'Would you like to lose weight from or alter the shape of any particular part of your body?' (See Table 9.14.)

Figure 9.3: Q36 Which parts (of the body) would you like to lose weight from or alter the shape of? (percentage mentioning each part).

While (Table 9.16) the majority of all those asked, particularly among the older groups, felt that 'it doesn't matter how much you weigh as long as you feel well' (Q37a), it is clear that there is still some possibility of persuading these populations that there is something to be gained by taking account of one's weight. Indeed, around nine out of every ten, irrespective of age, sex or ethnic group, felt that 'controlling your weight is an important part of looking after your health' (Q37b). There would appear to be a distinction drawn between 'reducing' and controlling weight. Indeed, as far as men are concerned, and possibly for some women, the phrasing of advice in terms of giving 'control' over weight would appear to have some advantages in terms of its acceptability. Given the proportions actually 'doing' exercise for weight-related reasons (Figure 9.2 above), it is perhaps surprising that so few seemed (or at least, reported) that they have been advised to do more exercise to lose weight. Furthermore, while the 'healthy living' message about the value of exercise has been heard, there would seem to be some scope to increase the degree to which this is followed up by medical advice on the same lines.

9.5 Measures of body shape: BMI, WHR and other physique measurements

In the following sections, we shall examine the 'objective' situation in respect of the body shape of the sampled population, in so far as it can be expressed through averages of measures of height, weight and girth. The figures on which these analyses were based included height (to the nearest centimetre), weight (in kilograms and tenths), and waist and hip circumference (the average of two measures). Details of the protocol followed for these measurements are given in Section 2.4, on p.16 . These were standardised as far as possible to resemble the definitions used by other similar surveys (HSE, ADNFS), while explicitly taking into account the sensitivities of the minority ethnic groups. Thus, 'if the respondent is wearing a turban or has a hairstyle which interferes with the measurement', this was noted. In analysis, certain cases where improbable data were recorded (such as heights over 2 m, weight under 20 kg) have been excluded from calculations. Tables 9.17–9.22 give the mean values for each of these measures. It is clear that there are important differences in the physical build of the four ethnic groups represented in this study. Pakistani women would appear – on average – to be bigger than either Indian or Bangladeshi women, and Bangladeshi men and women in the survey were demonstrably smaller (again, on average) than all other groups. These group labels will conceal other variations, and it is also clear that the younger generation of minority ethnic groups is, like that of the white majority population, growing bigger than its parents.

Two major indicators of obesity can be calculated from the data collected in the HEA Health and Lifestyle Survey: the well-known 'body mass index' (BMI, which is the weight in kilograms divided by the square of the height in metres, or kgs/m^2), and waist–hip ratio (WHR) calculated as a ratio of the measured circumference of the waist and hip (see Section 2.4). These measures (BMI, WHR) are used instead of a simple measure of girth or weight because they allow for the fact that there are very significant variations in height and bone structure, which may affect body mass. Indeed, as the data show, there are differences between ethnic groups in respect of the average height and hip measurement (see Figure 9.4). Taller people might expect to be able to 'manage' greater girth, through having larger frames, and indeed, would also be expected to be heavier. However, the use of a single measure is insufficient: 'those people who are not obese on the basis of their BMI may still have a high WHR and associated health risks'.[5] The nationwide Allied Dunbar study (ADNFS) found that overall, 11% (one in nine) men had a WHR of 1 or more, that is their waist was as great as their hip or greater, and were deemed to be at significantly increased risk of cardiovascular disease. It is important to note, however, that there are significant sex differences: men and women are different in shape. As recorded in the ADNFS, the national average WHR for men was 0.92, while that for women was 0.81. At the same time, the significance of this also varies. While only a small proportion of men were seriously over the target level, their risk was considerably increased, and there is a close relationship *for men* between risks and increase in BMI from an 'optimal' level of around 22.[6] The cardiovascular risk for women does not appear to rise at anything like the same rate, although aesthetic considerations may be more influential in taking action. In both sexes, it is probable that obesity may predispose to diabetes, a disease which has many other consequences, and which demonstrates very much higher prevalences amongst all minority ethnic groups compared to the majority white population.[7]

	BMI	WHR	Waist cms	Hip cms	Height cms	Weight kgs
Women						
ADNFS National	25.1	0.81	80.6	99.8	1.62	65.4
HEA Survey						
African-Caribbean	27.5	0.81	84.2	104.3	1.63	73.6
Indian	25.6	0.80	80.5	100.7	1.56	62.6
Pakistani	26.1	0.83	84.3	101.3	1.58	63.8
Bangladeshi	23.9	0.85	80.6	94.6	1.53	55.4
Men						
ADNFS National	25.2	0.92	90.3	98.2	1.75	77.2
HEA Survey						
African-Caribbean	25.5	0.89	86.6	96.9	1.74	76.9
Indian	24.6	0.91	88.2	96.7	1.70	71.3
Pakistani	24.9	0.92	87.6	95.0	1.71	72.6
Bangladeshi	23.4	0.92	84.7	92.3	1.65	64.0

Note: Figures represent group means for the ratios BMI and WHR, and mean values for measurements in centimetres (waist, hip and height) or kilogrammes (weight). A more detailed analysis is given in the appendix, Tables 9.17–9.22.

Figure 9.4: ADNFS 1992 National physical size findings compared to HEA 1994 data

It can be seen that (in broad terms and on average) despite the fact that African-Caribbean women tended to be considerably larger than the national figures for adults, their WHR data suggest that in proportionate terms their body shape was not significantly different from that of the national average. However, their BMI was considerably higher. Equally, however, Asian women tended to have rather higher WHRs, particularly in the case of the otherwise apparently slender and light Bangladeshis. Pakistani women, while generally having larger waists, were less broad in the hip and slightly taller, affecting their BMI score. Asian men, particularly the

Bangladeshis, were much smaller than the national average, but while having slightly advantageous BMI scores, had WHR figures very close to the mean.

Equally, however, these measurements of body shape are related to age. It can easily be observed that people tend to thicken and put on weight as they get older, until the age of about 70, when a slight decrease may be noted. Fuller detail of these statistics is presented in Tables 9.17–9.22), where it can be seen that the male African-Caribbean BMI average rises from 23.4 at age 16–24 to 27.5 in those aged 55–64. It is therefore customary to analyse the data within age bands and to set 'cut-offs' for desirable and undesirable levels of the key ratios. When this is done, some clear messages about the risks associated with the body shapes of people in the minority communities are shown.

The following break-points were taken for this analysis, using the categories defined for the HSE and in common use in general practice and hospital medicine:[8]

	Men	Women
Underweight	Up to 20.0	Up to 20.0
Acceptable	20.01–25.0	20.01–25.0
Mildly overweight	25.01–30.0	25.01–30.0
Obese	Over 30.0	Over 30.0

Figure 9.5: BMIs for men and women

	African-Caribbean %	Indian %	Pakistani %	Bangladeshi %
Female				
Overall	30	19	22	8
16–29	20	7	14	5
30–49	29	20	24	11
50+	44	39	39	7
Male				
Overall	11	10	12	5
16–29	4	9	8	4
30–49	11	10	11	6
50+	20	9	22	6

Note: Figures rounded to nearest percentage point.

Figure 9.6: Proportion of (age group) 'obese' (HEA age group categories)

According to the HSE, 16% of men and 18% of women were obese, that is, had a BMI in excess of 30 (Figure 9.6). In addition to the expected age differences, which nationally showed a variation between 8% of women aged 16–24 (6% men) to 26% of women aged 55–64 (18% men in the same age range), there are clearly very important differences between the patterns in the four main ethnic groups analysed here. The two different tables in Figures 9.6 and 9.7 are presented to permit a wider comparison of the data, since most of the analysis of the HEA surveys refers to three broad age bands, while the HSE and ADFNS reported an analysis in six age groups. Less confidence should be placed in the data for the 65–74 age band since the HEA sampling strategy reduced the number of possible respondents in this age range (see 'Selection of households and individual respondents', p.18). While the rates of obesity for African-Caribbean women were high, as noted above, these may be of less significance than the pattern among men, where a steady increase (after virtually no evidence of overweight in the youngest age group) can be seen up to 55–64. Indian men were an exception to this pattern, where more of those aged 25–34 appeared to be overweight and in the broader age group analysis appeared to have a fairly constant rate. The greatest risk, however, appears to have been demonstrated among Pakistani males in their later 40s and early 50s.

	African-Caribbean %	Indian %	Pakistani %	Bangladeshi %	HSE 94 %
Female					
16–24	14	6	8	4	8
25–34	26	13	25	11	13
35–44	26	14	29	8	17
45–54	48	38	26	14	18
55–64	47	41	37	5	26
65–74	34	33	(33)	(–)	25
Male					
16–24	–	6	8	3	6
25–34	9	15	8	8	10
35–44	8	8	12	6	16
45–54	16	14	29	4	17
55–64	24	4	22	10	18
65-74	17	9	7	–	18

N.B.: Figures rounded to whole numbers; () = less than 20 people in age category.

Figure 9.7: Proportion in each age group 'obese'

There are grounds for concern in that the average BMI score for African-Caribbean women aged over 50 was in excess of 30, the accepted cut-off value for clinical obesity. While it is important to be aware of ethnic variations in physique, which require standard tables and healthy living advice to be adjusted, it is also necessary to consider the implications of such differences for health outcomes.

9.6 Conclusions

There are clear physical differences between ethnic groups. African-Caribbean men and women are both taller and heavier than Asians, though they may have lower WHRs (on average). Within Asian categories, while Bangladeshi men and women are considerably smaller than people of either Indian or Pakistani origin (who do not appear to differ greatly in shape or size), Bangladeshi women have the highest WHRs. When age is taken into account, it is clear that a considerable increase in 'risk' appears after age 50. This will require intervention, in the light of clinical evidence of strong links between obesity and ill health among black and minority ethnic groups.

The notion of 'control' of weight and body shape seems to be widely used among minority ethnic groups, and the link with health is generally accepted. There is some dissatisfaction with personal appearance or form, but less concern or positive action to lose weight for health reasons than might seem desirable in the light of the objective measures reported. (Tables 9.17–9.22 in the Appendix give details of BMI and other measured data.)

Notes

1. G.L. Burke, D.E. Bild, J.E. Hilner, A.R. Folsom, L.E. Wagenknecht and S.Sidney, 'Differences in weight gain in relation to race, gender, age and education in young adults: the CARDIA study', *Ethnicity and Health* 1(4): 327–35

2. Obesity has been recognised as a major problem in the Caribbean, where recent research has found that it can increase the risk of having high blood pressure by a factor of three to six times; for those who are 25% or more overweight, fatal heart attacks are five times more common and overweight women have significantly higher rates of several cancers: D.P. Sinha, *Food, nutrition and health in the Caribbean* (Caribbean Food and Nutrition Institute, Kingston, Jamaica, 1995).

3. See, for example, the findings of the PSI survey in T. Modood *et al.*, *Ethnic minorities in Britain: diversity and disadvantage* (Policy Studies Institute, London, 1997).

4. J. Gasperino, 'Ethnic differences in body composition and their relation to health and disease in women', *Ethnicity and Health* 1(4): 337–47; D.A. Schoeller and R.F. Kushner, 'Expert review: increased rates of obesity among African Americans confirmed', *Ethnicity and Health* 1(4): 313–15.

5. See ADNFS 1992, p. 72.

6. A.G. Shaper, S.G. Wannamethree and M. Walker, 'Body weight: implications for the prevention of coronary heart disease, stroke and diabetes mellitus in a cohort study of middle aged men', *British Medical Journal* 314: 1311–17.

7. A. Stevens and J. Raftery, *Health care needs assessment* (Radcliffe Medical Press, Oxford, 1994), vol. 1, p. 48, shows relative risk rates for diabetes of between 3 (Asian:white males aged 40–59) and 14 (African-Caribbean: white males aged 45–74). Associated pathology includes poor peripheral circulation, eye disease and increased need for kidney replacement.

8. The ADNFS presents data in its analysis (Tables 4.1.1 and 4.1.2, p. 69) based upon an earlier set of cut-offs published by the Royal College of General Practice in 1983. While for men the obesity level was determined by a BMI score of 30, for women they used a cut-off of 28.6. The following table is presented to facilitate comparison with that data:

Proportion in each age group 'obese' after ADFNS

	African-Caribbean %	Indian %	Pakistani %	Bangladeshi %	National HSE %
Female					
16–24	16	14	11	5	8
25–34	34	16	30	24	13
35–44	31	25	42	19	17
45–54	70	52	39	21	18
55–64	61	45	41	33	26
65–74	55	36	(33)	(–)	25

Note: Cells in brackets based on very small sample size: <20 cases.

Chapter 3

Table 3.1a: Sample numbers by age and ethnic group (all respondents)

Category	African-Caribbean Women	African-Caribbean Men	Indian Women	Indian Men	Pakistani Women	Pakistani Men	Bangladeshi Women	Bangladeshi Men
Base	*641*	*428*	*598*	*463*	*517*	*627*	*603*	*567*
Age distribution								
16–29	178	114	208	129	281	235	307	213
30–49	270	140	283	227	186	268	233	183
50–74	193	174	107	107	50	124	63	171
Marital status								
Single	244	144	93	92	107	128	119	152
Married	160	161	429	352	345	476	418	409
Other partnership	98	62	13	12	9	10	4	5
Separated, widowed, divorced	138	60	63	7	56	13	61	1
Employment status								
In work	278	185	242	273	79	276	60	183
Unemployed	46	101	24	76	26	172	32	165
Economically inactive	305	138	331	110	409	171	509	214
Social class								
I	4	7	9	23	2	12	0	3
II	118	46	33	66	21	46	17	25
III non-manual	168	44	120	54	62	52	41	48
III manual	59	159	42	114	9	172	12	193
IV	150	112	188	123	93	181	69	186
V	61	26	15	23	4	54	2	27
Not classified	81	34	191	60	326	110	462	85
Housing tenure								
Owner-occupied	261	176	501	398	392	529	216	183
Local authority rented	244	184	28	29	47	30	296	281
Housing association rented	86	28	20	7	12	19	38	44
Private rented	37	23	37	22	55	37	51	50
Other	5	5	11	6	8	11	2	7

Table 3.1b: Weighting for region, age, sex and ethnic group (all respondents, mean weight)

	African-Caribbean Women	African-Caribbean Men	Indian Women	Indian Men	Pakistani Women	Pakistani Men	Bangladeshi Women	Bangladeshi Men
Greater London								
16–29	3.54	3.55	3.93	6.60	6.58	11.56	3.37	4.23
30–49	2.01	2.27	3.40	3.94	8.25	9.79	3.65	2.69
50–74	2.27	2.40	4.72	6.34	11.68	11.32	6.47	3.94
Outside Greater London								
16–29	2.32	3.27	2.66	3.70	2.89	3.01	2.90	4.19
30–49	1.38	2.71	2.52	3.00	3.91	2.53	3.09	4.60
50–74	1.39	2.31	2.50	2.77	5.39	3.13	3.55	3.62

Table 3.2: Weighted sample numbers by age and ethnic group (all respondents)

Age group	African-Caribbean Women	African-Caribbean Men	Indian Women	Indian Men	Pakistani Women	Pakistani Men	Bangladeshi Women	Bangladeshi Men
16–29	383	325	531	499	731	699	798	771
30–49	372	273	669	666	666	669	655	536
50–74	288	331	292	332	244	384	228	552
All ages	1043	928	1491	1497	1641	1752	1681	1860

Table 3.2a: Distribution of the sample population by age and sex (percentages of all respondents)

Age group	African-Caribbean Women	African-Caribbean Men	Indian Women	Indian Men	Pakistani Women	Pakistani Men	Bangladeshi Women	Bangladeshi Men
16–29	37	35	36	33	45	40	47	41
30–49	36	29	45	44	41	38	39	29
50–74	28	36	20	22	15	22	14	30
Base (= 100%)	641	428	598	463	517	627	603	567

Table 3.3: Mean number of persons per household (means of all respondents)

Age group	African-Caribbean Women	African-Caribbean Men	Indian Women	Indian Men	Pakistani Women	Pakistani Men	Bangladeshi Women	Bangladeshi Men
16–29	3.5	3.2	4.8	4.5	5.9	5.7	6.1	6.5
30–49	3.5	3.6	5.0	4.8	6.2	5.6	6.9	6.2
50–74	2.4	2.6	4.2	4.3	4.5	5.1	5.3	6.3
All ages	3.2	3.1	4.8	4.6	5.8	5.5	6.3	6.3
Base	641	428	598	463	517	627	603	567

Table 3.4: Mean number of persons aged 16 and over per household (means of all respondents)

Age group	African-Caribbean Women	African-Caribbean Men	Indian Women	Indian Men	Pakistani Women	Pakistani Men	Bangladeshi Women	Bangladeshi Men
16–29	2.6	2.8	3.7	3.9	3.9	4.2	3.9	4.2
30–49	2.1	2.3	3.2	2.9	3.3	3.0	3.3	2.7
50–74	2.2	2.3	3.5	3.7	3.7	3.7	4.1	3.9
All ages	2.3	2.5	3.4	3.4	3.6	3.7	3.7	3.7
Base	641	428	598	463	517	627	603	567

Table 3.5: Mean number of persons aged between 16 and 74 (inclusive) per household (means of all respondents)

Age group	African-Caribbean Women	African-Caribbean Men	Indian Women	Indian Men	Pakistani Women	Pakistani Men	Bangladeshi Women	Bangladeshi Men
16–29	2.6	2.8	3.6	3.9	3.8	4.2	3.9	4.1
30–49	2.0	2.3	3.1	2.8	3.2	3.0	3.2	2.7
50–74	2.2	2.3	3.5	3.7	3.7	3.6	4.0	3.8
All ages	2.3	2.5	3.4	3.4	3.6	3.6	3.6	3.6
Base	641	428	598	463	517	627	603	567

Table 3.6: Marital status of respondents (percentages of all respondents)

Marital/partnership status	African-Caribbean Women	Men	Indian Women	Men	Pakistani Women	Men	Bangladeshi Women	Men
16–29								
Married	14	8	45	24	44	40	53	24
Living with partner	9	13	2	4	1	2	1	1
Regular partner but not cohabiting	16	9	3	2	2	0	0	0
Single	62	69	48	69	49	57	45	75
Separated	0	0	1		3		1	
Divorced	0	0	1	0	2	0	0	
Widowed								
Base (= 100%)	*178*	*114*	*208*	*129*	*281*	*235*	*307*	*213*
30–49								
Married	35	56	91	94	93	97	89	99
Living with partner	6	11	1		0			1
Regular partner but not cohabiting	9	6	0	0	0	0		
Single	35	22	2	5	0	2	1	0
Separated	6	4	3	0	3	1	1	
Divorced	8	1	2	1	1		0	
Widowed	1		1	0	2		8	
Base (= 100%)	*269*	*140*	*283*	*227*	*186*	*268*	*233*	*183*
50–74								
Married	52	68	76	96	79	92	72	99
Living with partner	1	5						
Regular partner but not cohabiting	1	2				2		
Single	9	8	2	2		1		
Separated	7	2	1		5	2		
Divorced	13	11	1		2	0		
Widowed	17	5	21	2	14	2	27	1
Base (= 100%)	*193*	*173*	*107*	*107*	*50*	*124*	*62*	*171*
All ages								
Married	32	43	72	71	69	73	70	68
Living with partner	6	10	1	1	0	1	0	1
Regular partner but not cohabiting	9	6	1	1	1	1	0	0
Single	38	33	18	26	22	24	22	31
Separated	4	2	2	0	3	1	1	
Divorced	6	4	1	0	1	0	0	
Widowed	5	2	5	1	3	1	7	0
Base (= 100%)	*640*	*427*	*598*	*463*	*517*	*627*	*602*	*567*

Table 3.7: Respondents living in households containing children (0–15 years) (percentages of all respondents)

All or own dependent children	African-Caribbean		Indian		Pakistani		Bangladeshi	
	Women	Men	Women	Men	Women	Men	Women	Men
16–29								
Dependent children in household	58	24	65	40	84	65	87	79
Living with own children	41	11	37	15	43	29	44	23
Base (= 100%)	*178*	*114*	*208*	*129*	*281*	*235*	*307*	*213*
30–49								
Dependent children in household	75	52	77	85	90	85	93	98
Living with own children	72	51	71	83	86	81	93	97
Base (= 100%)	*270*	*140*	*283*	*227*	*186*	*268*	*233*	*183*
50–74								
Dependent children in household	14	17	37	32	39	59	65	84
Living with own children	6	11	13	19	20	46	43	79
Base (= 100%)	*193*	*174*	*107*	*107*	*50*	*124*	*63*	*171*
All ages								
Dependent children in household	52	30	65	58	80	72	86	86
Living with own children	42	23	48	46	57	53	63	61
Base (= 100%)	*641*	*428*	*598*	*463*	*517*	*627*	*603*	*567*

Table 3.8: Characteristics of respondents' dependent children (aged 0–15 years) (means of all respondents with their own dependent children)

Mean	African-Caribbean		Indian		Pakistani		Bangladeshi	
	Women	Men	Women	Men	Women	Men	Women	Men
16–29								
Mean number of children	1.6	1.6	1.7	1.8	2.1	1.9	2.2	2.5
Mean age of youngest (years)	2.5	1.9	2.0	2.5	1.6	1.9	2.0	2.9
Mean age of oldest (years)	4.8	4.5	4.2	4.3	4.8	4.4	5.6	6.7
Base (respondents living with dependent children)	*91*	*14*	*94*	*26*	*153*	*84*	*160*	*54*
30–49								
Mean number of children	2.0	2.4	2.2	2.3	3.3	3.0	3.9	3.6
Mean age of youngest (years)	5.7	4.6	7.3	5.9	5.8	5.0	5.2	2.8
Mean age of oldest (years)	10.0	9.7	11.3	10.1	12.0	10.5	13.0	9.8
Base (respondents living with dependent children)	*201*	*66*	*216*	*194*	*165*	*227*	*217*	*176*
50–74								
Mean number of children	1.4	1.9	1.7	1.6	1.3	2.3	2.1	3.0
Mean age of youngest (years)	9.0	9.7	5.7	10.4	9.3	9.5	9.0	7.2
Mean age of oldest (years)	11.1	11.6	9.7	11.9	11.9	13.5	13.3	12.9
Base (respondents living with dependent children)	*10*	*15*	*12*	*21*	*11*	*51*	*27*	*128*
All ages								
Mean number of children	1.8	2.2	2.1	2.2	2.8	2.6	3.2	3.2
Mean age of youngest (years)	4.7	5.1	5.8	5.9	4.6	5.2	4.5	4.5
Mean age of oldest (years)	8.3	9.2	9.4	9.6	9.7	9.8	10.8	10.5
Base (respondents living with dependent children)	*302*	*95*	*322*	*241*	*329*	*362*	*404*	*358*

Table 3.9: Relationship of household head to respondent (percentages of all respondents)

Relationship	African-Caribbean Women	Men	Indian Women	Men	Pakistani Women	Men	Bangladeshi Women	Men
16–29								
Self	33	36	8	16	7	24	5	17
Partner	14	2	33	3	28	2	30	0
Parent or parent-in-law	46	52	55	75	59	66	62	72
Child or child-in-law	1	2				1		2
Other relative	2	5	3	5	6	6	3	9
No relation	4	4	0	1		2		
Base (= 100%)	*178*	*114*	*208*	*129*	*281*	*235*	*307*	*213*
30–49								
Self	62	86	12	83	10	87	17	96
Partner	32	8	84	4	84	3	83	
Parent or parent-in-law	4	6	3	11	2	6	0	3
Child or child-in-law			0		0			
Other relative	1	3	0	1				
No relation	0		0	1				
Base (= 100%)	*270*	*140*	*283*	*227*	*186*	*268*	*233*	*183*
50–74								
Self	53	99	18	97	17	98	38	97
Partner	46	1	67	2	71		53	
Parent or parent-in-law	1				2		2	
Child or child-in-law			12	1	8		8	
Other relative			2		2	2		1
No relation			1					
Base (= 100%)	*193*	*174*	*107*	*107*	*50*	*124*	*63*	*171*
All ages								
Self	49	73	12	64	10	64	14	64
Partner	29	3	63	3	57	2	54	0
Parent or parent-in-law	19	20	21	30	28	28	30	31
Child or child-in-law	0	1	3	0	1	0	1	2
Other relative	1	2	2	2	4	5	1	4
No relation	2	1	0	1		1		
Base (= 100%)	*641*	*428*	*598*	*463*	*517*	*627*	*603*	*567*

Table 3.10: Economic status (percentages of all respondents)

Category	African-Caribbean		Indian		Pakistani		Bangladeshi	
	Women	Men	Women	Men	Women	Men	Women	Men
16–29								
Employed								
Full-time	25	24	23	33	15	31	12	21
Part-time	14	6	13	6	7	5	4	9
Self-employed								
Employing others	0	2	2	4	0	1	0	6
Without employees	2	1	1	2	4	1		
On government scheme	0	1	1	2	2	1	2	
Unemployed	8	30	5	17	8	23	8	16
Temporarily sick	1	1				2	1	1
In full-time education	26	28	26	34	21	27	25	39
Permanently sick	2	3			2	2		0
Retired							0	
Looking after a home/family	21	1	26	0	40	1	45	1
Other	1	3	4	2	3	2	3	3
Base (= 100%)	*176*	*112*	*208*	*127*	*280*	*234*	*306*	*211*
30–49								
Employed								
Full-time	42	50	33	60	3	38	1	37
Part-time	16	8	14	2	5	3	2	4
Self-employed								
Employing others	1	4	2	9		11		7
Without employees	0	8	3	6	3	7		2
On government scheme				0				
Unemployed	9	26	4	13	2	22	1	38
Temporarily sick		0	1	3		4	1	0
In full-time education	3		1	0	1	2	1	
Permanently sick	3	2	2	3	1	8	1	8
Retired	0	0	0	0	0	0	0	0
Looking after a home/family	25	2	39	2	81	2	94	2
Other	1	0	2	1	5	2		2
Base (= 100%)	*266*	*140*	*283*	*226*	*185*	*266*	*232*	*182*
50–74								
Employed								
Full-time	21	31	8	31	3	16		7
Part-time	10	2	12		3	1		
Self-employed								
Employing others	1	1		5	1	1		1
Without employees	1			5		3		
On government scheme	0	0		0	0	0	0	0
Unemployed	1	10		8		18		17
Temporarily sick		3		3		2		9
In full-time education	0				2			
Permanently sick	13	12	8	14	7	26	17	38
Retired	35	39	12	30	4	28		24
Looking after a home/family	16	1	49	2	78	0	81	3
Other	2	1	12	1	2	5	2	1
Base (= 100%)	*187*	*172*	*106*	*106*	*49*	*119*	*63*	*169*
All Ages								
Employed								
Full-time	30	34	25	45	8	31	6	21
Part-time	14	5	13	3	6	3	3	5
Self-employed								
Employing others	0	2	1	6	0	5	0	5
Without employees	1	3	1	4	1	5		1
On government scheme	0	0		1	1	1	0	1
Unemployed	7	22	4	13	5	22	4	23
Temporarily sick	0	1	0	2		3	1	3
In full-time education	11	10	10	11	10	12	12	16
Permanently sick	5	6	3	5	2	10	2	14
Retired	10	14	2	7	1	6	0	7
Looking after a home/family	21	1	36	1	62	1	69	2
Other	1	1	5	1	4	3	2	2
Base (= 100%)	*455*	*314*	*389*	*334*	*235*	*386*	*296*	*353*

Table 3.11: Economic status of household head (percentages of all respondents)

Category	African-Caribbean		Indian		Pakistani		Bangladeshi	
	Women	Men	Women	Men	Women	Men	Women	Men
16–29								
Employed								
Full-time	28	22	16	30	8	17	3	10
Part-time	11	7	13	6	3	1	1	3
Self-employed								
Employing others	3	4	9	9	3	2	5	2
Without employees	4	6	7	8	7	8	4	2
On government scheme	0	0		1	0		0	1
Unemployed	10	23	16	13	21	23	18	20
Temporarily sick	2	3	1	2	2	6	4	5
In full-time education	6	7	8	3	1	3	1	1
Permanently sick	5	3	7	10	23	9	23	10
Retired	6	9	15	11	12	16	14	20
Looking after a								
home/family	24	12	6	5	13	9	22	22
Other	1	2		1	1	1	3	3
Base (= 100%)	*149*	*96*	*149*	*102*	*213*	*214*	*222*	*200*
30–49								
Employed								
Full-time	38	46	34	55	4	35	2	34
Part-time	14	8	11	2	5	3	1	4
Self-employed								
Employing others	2	3	8	7	10	7	3	9
Without employees	2	8	8	6	10	8	1	2
On government scheme				0				
Unemployed	16	24	15	13	30	22	17	37
Temporarily sick		0	5	4	1	4	9	0
In full-time education	3		0		1	1	1	
Permanently sick	5	2	8	5	19	8	26	8
Retired	3	6	3	4	6	3	15	
Looking after a								
home/family	16	2	7	1	11	4	19	4
Other	0	0	0	2	1	2	1	2
Base (= 100%)	*258*	*137*	*229*	*218*	*126*	*261*	*195*	*179*
50–74								
Employed								
Full-time	18	30	7	31	3	16		7
Part-time	8	2	8		1	1		
Self-employed								
Employing others	1	1	1	5	5	1		1
Without employees	0		5	7	6	2		
On government scheme	0	0	0	0	0	0	0	0
Unemployed	7	10	3	9	9	18	5	16
Temporarily sick	2	2	4	3	4	2	5	9
In full-time education	0							
Permanently sick	10	12	19	14	25	26	36	37
Retired	42	39	37	28	30	26	25	25
Looking after a								
home/family	7	1	7		9	0	29	4
Other	3	1	9	1	2	5	0	1
Base (= 100%)	*184*	*171*	*88*	*103*	*45*	*122*	*61*	*168*
All ages								
Employed								
Full-time	29	32	23	42	6	24	2	16
Part-time	11	5	11	3	3	2	1	2
Self-employed								
Employing others	2	3	7	7	6	4	3	4
Wthout employees	2	4	7	7	8	6	2	1
On government scheme	0	0		0	0		0	0
Unemployed	11	19	13	12	22	21	16	24
Temporarily sick	1	2	4	3	2	4	6	5
In full-time education	3	2	3	1	1	2	1	1
Permanently sick	6	6	10	9	22	12	26	18
Retired	16	20	14	12	13	13	16	15
Looking after a								
home/family	16	5	6	2	12	5	22	11
Other	1	1	2	1	1	2	1	2
Base (= 100%)	*591*	*404*	*466*	*423*	*384*	*597*	*478*	*547*

Table 3.12: Occupation breakdown of persons in work (percentages of all working respondents)

SOC* major group	African-Caribbean		Indian		Pakistani		Bangladeshi	
	Women	Men	Women	Men	Women	Men	Women	Men
16–29								
Managers and administrators	2	7	8	10		4	3	10
Professional occupations	3	2	5	6	2	6	3	2
Associate professional and technical	13	5	4	12	4	3	1	1
Clerical and secretarial	44	32	35	17	29	14	44	9
Craft and skilled manual	3	26	3	11	14	7	20	15
Personal and protective services	21	1	16	5	17	13	14	44
Sales	12	8	16	15	23	15	9	9
Plant and machine operatives		6	8	21	9	28	4	5
Other occupations	2	12	4	4	2	8	2	5
Base (= 100%)	*58*	*37*	*73*	*56*	*52*	*103*	*49*	*83*
30–49								
Managers and administrators	7	5	4	12	21	17		12
Professional occupations	6	8	4	13	3	6	11	2
Associate professional and technical	22	15	2	3	5	4	33	7
Clerical and secretarial	29	5	17	10	20	4		4
Craft and skilled manual	2	29	19	25	9	17		24
Personal and protective services	18	7	6	3	27	4	39	38
Sales	4	2	10	3	5	4	9	4
Plant and machine operatives	6	20	32	26		37	9	6
Other occupations	8	9	7	4	9	7		2
Base (= 100%)	*153*	*88*	*137*	*169*	*20*	*143*	*9*	*85*
50–74								
Managers and administrators	1	2	5	20		5		7
Professional occupations	4	3	5	5				
Associate professional and technical	25	6		5		4		
Clerical and secretarial		2	19	6	40			34
Craft and skilled manual	4	21	18	15		3		34
Personal and protective services	29	8	5	3	34	7		24
Sales	1					5		
Plant and machine operatives	9	43	27	35	17	62		24
Other occupations	27	15	20	10	9	13		10
Base (= 100%)	*55*	*50*	*18*	*37*	*4*	*27*	*0*	*13*
All ages								
Managers and administrators	4	5	5	13	5	11	3	10
Professional occupations	4	5	4	10	2	5	4	2
Associate professional and technical	20	10	3	6	4	4	6	4
Clerical and secretarial	28	11	24	11	28	8	38	7
Craft and skilled manual	2	26	13	20	12	12	17	20
Personal and protective services	22	6	9	3	21	8	18	40
Sales	6	3	11	6	17	9	9	6
Plant and machine operatives	5	23	23	26	7	36	5	7
Other occupations	10	11	7	5	4	8	2	4
Base (= 100%)	*266*	*175*	*228*	*262*	*76*	*273*	*58*	*181*

*SOC: Standard Occupational Classification

Table 3.13: Occupation breakdown of persons not in work (percentages of all)

SOC* major group	African-Caribbean		Indian		Pakistani		Bangladeshi	
	Women	Men	Women	Men	Women	Men	Women	Men
16–29								
Managers and administrators	4	2	2	3		0	0	5
Professional occupations	1	2	0	0	1	1	0	0
Associate professional and technical	4	5	1	3	6	12	5	3
Clerical and secretarial	29	12	25	19	26	12	18	7
Craft and skilled manual	4	25	17	19	29	13	33	12
Personal and protective services	10	7	14	7	6	8	18	52
Sales	30	16	30	17	12	17	12	11
Plant and machine operatives		18	10	22	16	26	11	2
Other occupations	11	13	2	9	4	11	2	8
Base (= 100%)	*80*	*56*	*61*	*33*	*78*	*59*	*66*	*62*
30–49								
Managers and administrators	2	15	1	5	6	6		2
Professional occupations	2	8	0	3	5	1	0	2
Associate professional and technical	5	0	3	7	0	5	8	0
Clerical and secretarial	29	5	15	12	16	0		2
Craft and skilled manual	2	30	33	24	39	18		37
Personal and protective services	22	7	6	4	12	10	40	39
Sales	10	4	4	8	2	1	0	1
Plant and machine operatives	12	18	36	28		48	0	11
Other occupations	15	15	2	8	10	11		8
Base (= 100%)	*91*	*44*	*83*	*47*	*32*	*108*	*11*	*92*
50–74								
Managers and administrators	2	1	0	13		7		3
Professional occupations	1	2	4	1				
Associate professional and technical	8	0		0		1		
Clerical and secretarial		6	1	4	0			
Craft and skilled manual	8	24	27	26		14		22
Personal and protective services	35	3	8	3	0	0		15
Sales	0					2		
Plant and machine operatives	18	48	52	32	6	49		47
Other occupations	26	16	8	19	0	22		11
Base (= 100%)	*124*	*118*	*39*	*67*	*7*	*96*	*3*	*152*
All ages								
Managers and administrators	2	4	1	8	4	5		3
Professional occupations	1	3	1	1	3	1		1
Associate professional and technical	6	2	2	3	3	5	5	1
Clerical and secretarial	19	8	15	11	21	5	14	2
Craft and skilled manual	5	26	26	24	35	15	33	24
Personal and protective services	23	5	9	5	8	5	19	29
Sales	13	6	12	8	8	5	9	3
Plant and machine operatives	13	32	31	28	14	43	16	28
Other occupations	18	15	3	13	6	16	4	9
Base (=100%)	*295*	*218*	*183*	*147*	*117*	*263*	*80*	*306*

*SOC: Standard Occupational Classification

Table 3.14: Economic activity of persons not in work (percentages of all respondents unemployed or economically inactive, but not retired)

SOC* major group	African-Caribbean Women	Men	Indian Women	Men	Pakistani Women	Men	Bangladeshi Women	Men
16–29								
Waiting to start a job	1	4			1	1	0	
Unemployed								
Previously worked	10	41	5	22	5	31	4	24
Never worked	5	2	3	10	5	12	7	6
Inactive								
Previously worked	61	29	39	19	25	13	19	19
Never worked	24	24	53	50	64	43	70	51
Base (= 100%)	*112*	*72*	*131*	*70*	*226*	*130*	*254*	*128*
30-49								
Waiting to start a job	1							
Unemployed								
Previously worked	20	85	9	69	2	59	1	74
Never worked	1	1	1	2		5	1	3
Inactive								
Previously worked	71	9	48	24	17	28	4	23
Never worked	6	4	42	4	80	7	94	1
Base (= 100%)	*108*	*47*	*138*	*49*	*164*	*121*	*223*	*96*
50–74								
Waiting to start a job	0	0	0	0	0	0	0	0
Unemployed								
Previously worked	2	47		40		39		37
Never worked								1
Inactive								
Previously worked	89	51	33	56	5	61	2	59
Never worked	8	3	67	4	95	0	98	3
Base (= 100%)	*56*	*49*	*72*	*33*	*43*	*60*	*63*	*115*
All ages								
Waiting to start a job	1	2			0	0	0	
Unemployed								
Previously worked	12	52	5	39	3	41	2	40
Never worked	3	1	2	6	2	7	3	3
Inactive								
Previously worked	70	30	41	27	19	29	10	33
Never worked	15	15	52	28	76	22	84	23
Base (= 100%)	*276*	*168*	*341*	*152*	*433*	*311*	*540*	*339*

*SOC: Standard Occupational Classification

Table 3.15: Duration of unemployment (percentages of all respondents waiting to start a job, looking for work or unable to seek work due to temporary sickness)

Duration of Unemployment	African-Caribbean		Indian		Pakistani		Bangladeshi	
	Women	Men	Women	Men	Women	Men	Women	Men
16–29								
Less than 6 months	34	19	56	60	51	31	28	56
6–12 months	6	12	21	15	13	12	24	16
1–2 years	19	36		8	26	23	15	21
2+ years	41	33	23	17	10	33	34	7
Base (= 100%)	*19*	*37*	*10*	*26*	*21*	*65*	*28*	*47*
30–49								
Less than 6 months	17	23	53	28	8	10	100	28
6–12 months	9	6	17	19	19	7		21
1–2 years	7	17	5	11	8	18		13
2+ years	66	54	25	42	65	64		38
Base (= 100%)	*26*	*40*	*14*	*36*	*5*	*83*	*4*	*74*
50–74								
Less than 6 months		27				9		13
6–12 months		5		11				3
1–2 years	100	10		13				6
2+ years		58		77		91		78
Base (= 100%)	*1*	*24*	*0*	*14*	*0*	*24*	*0*	*44*
All ages								
Less than 6 months	24	22	54	33	37	17	38	30
6–12 months	8	8	18	16	15	7	20	14
1–2 years	15	24	3	10	20	16	13	13
2+ years	53	46	24	40	29	59	29	42
Base (= 100%)	*46*	*101*	*24*	*76*	*26*	*172*	*32*	*165*

Table 3.16: Socio-economic group of respondents
(percentages of all respondents)

Socio-economic group	African-Caribbean		Indian		Pakistani		Bangladeshi	
	Women	Men	Women	Men	Women	Men	Women	Men
16–29								
Employers								
Large establishments	1		1	1		1		
Small establishments	1	3	7	8	1	4	9	7
Managers								
Large establishments	2	1	2	1				
Small establishments	4	2	3	5	1	0	1	1
Professional workers								
Self-employed			1		0			
Employees	4	1	1	1	1	5	1	
Ancillary workers and artists	7	12	3	3	4	1	2	1
Foremen and supervisors (non-manual)			2		1	1		
Junior non-manual	19	16	16	11	10	4	6	4
Personal service workers	9	5	1		5	4	28	27
Foremen and supervisors (manual)	4	6	5	7	4	1	1	3
Skilled manual workers	16	18	19	14	23	24	17	20
Semi-skilled manual workers	19	18	26	29	19	25	18	22
Unskilled manual workers	7	12	3	12	11	11	10	8
Own account workers	4	6	7	7	10	12	3	2
Farmers								
Employers								
Own account								
Agricultural workers								
Armed forces								
Inadequately described	4	1	2	1	10	5	3	4
Base (= 100%)	*135*	*97*	*175*	*115*	*217*	*195*	*236*	*155*
30–49								
Employers								
Large establishments	1							
Small establishments	6	5	1	3	3	1	1	
Managers								
Large establishments	1	2	9	5	4	9	7	10
Small establishments	2	4	2	1	3	1		2
Professional workers								
Self-employed			0	1	1	2		
Employees	2	2	4	8	1	1	2	
Ancillary workers and artists	13	18	4	5	21	4	2	4
Foremen and supervisors (non-manual)	1	1	2	1	1	1		
Junior non-manual	26	7	7	7	8	4	2	4
Personal service workers	7	2	0	1	1	3	20	34
Foremen and supervisors (manual)	3	5	5	7	0	4	0	
Skilled manual workers	10	24	21	21	19	23	19	17
Semi-skilled manual workers	21	14	28	26	27	29	27	21
Unskilled manual workers	5	7	6	6	16	8	13	4
Own account workers	1	8	8	7	10	9	4	3
Farmers								
Employers								
Own account								
Agricultural workers								
Armed forces							0	
Inadequately described	1	2	2	1	4	0	2	0
Base (= 100%)	*238*	*134*	*250*	*213*	*154*	*239*	*170*	*174*

Continued on next page

Table 3.16: *continued*

Socio-economic group	African-Caribbean		Indian		Pakistani		Bangladeshi	
	Women	Men	Women	Men	Women	Men	Women	Men
50–74								
Employers								
Large establishments								1
Small establishments	2	0	3	8	9	2	5	2
Managers								
Large establishments	1	1	4			4		
Small establishments	2	0	3	8	9	2	5	2
Professional workers								
Self-employed				2				
Employees	0	2	1	1				2
Ancillary workers and artists	11	2	4	2	2	2		1
Foremen and supervisors (non-manual)		2				0		
Junior non-manual	1	2	8	3	4	2		1
Personal service workers	7	0	2	1		0	8	10
Foremen and supervisors (manual)	6	5	3	3	2	4		3
Skilled manual workers	22	37	25	16	17	26	24	21
Semi-skilled manual workers	26	39	31	40	37	37	38	50
Unskilled manual workers	18	9	7	12	13	20	26	8
Own account workers	2	0	5	8	7	3		0
Farmers								
Employers								
Own account								
Agricultural workers	0							
Armed forces								
Inadequately described	3		6	1	2			2
Base (= 100%)	*178*	*168*	*78*	*102*	*36*	*118*	*38*	*166*
All ages								
Employers								
Large establishments	1		0	0		0		0
Small establishments	1	2	7	7	4	5	8	7
Managers								
Large establishments	3	2	2	2		1	2	0
Small establishments	2	2	2	3	3	0	0	7
Professional workers								
Self-employed			1	1	0	1		
Employees	2	2	2	4	1	2	1	1
Ancillary workers and artists	11	10	4	3	3	2	2	2
Foremen and supervisors (non-manual)	0	1	2	0	1	1		
Junior non-manual	16	8	10	7	8	3	4	3
Personal service workers	8	2	1	1	3	3	22	23
Foremen and supervisors (manual)	4	5	6	6	2	3	1	2
Skilled manual workers	16	27	21	17	20	24	19	31
Semi-skilled manual workers	22	25	28	30	25	29	24	31
Unskilled manual workers	10	9	5	9	14	12	13	7
Own account workers	2	4	7	7	9	9	3	2
Farmers								
Employers								
Own account								
Agricultural workers	0					0		
Armed forces								
Inadequately described	2	1	3	1	6	2	2	2
Base (= 100%)	*551*	*399*	*503*	*431*	*407*	*552*	*444*	*495*

Table 3.17: Social class of respondents (percentages of all respondents)

Registrar-General's social class group		African-Caribbean		Indian		Pakistani		Ba...	
		Women	Men	Women	Men	Women	Men	Women	...
16–29									
I	Professional etc.	0		2	2	0	2		0
II	Intermediate	10	8	8	11	4	7	3	4
IIINM	Skilled non-manual	44	24	32	21	20	14	15	15
IIIM	Skilled manual	7	23	3	15	2	16	3	22
IV	Partly skilled	12	19	17	16	19	25	16	22
V	Unskilled	4	3	1	3	0	2	0	2
	Not classified	23	23	37	33	54	35	64	35
	Base (= 100%)	*178*	*114*	*208*	*129*	*281*	*235*	*307*	*213*
30–49									
I	Professional etc.	1	3	2	8	0	3		
II	Intermediate	24	22	4	15	4	13	2	8
IIINM	Skilled non-manual	32	9	18	12	5	7	1	8
IIIM	Skilled manual	6	36	10	32	1	33	1	45
IV	Partly skilled	23	16	39	22	12	29	4	31
V	Unskilled	4	6	2	5	1	7	1	5
	Not classified	10	8	25	6	75	8	92	4
	Base (= 100%)	*270*	*140*	*283*	*227*	*186*	*268*	*233*	*183*
50–74									
I	Professional etc.	0	3		2				1
II	Intermediate	25	3	3	18	4	6		2
IIINM	Skilled non-manual	3	3	4	4	3	2		2
IIIM	Skilled manual	12	42	5	21	2	32		33
IV	Partly skilled	33	37	33	37	8	36	10	50
V	Unskilled	19	8	6	11	1	19		8
	Not classified	8	4	49	7	83	4	90	4
	Base (= 100%)	*193*	*174*	*107*	*107*	*50*	*124*	*63*	*171*
All ages									
I	Professional etc.	0	2	1	5	0	2		0
II	Intermediate	19	11	5	14	4	9	2	4
IIINM	Skilled non-manual	28	12	20	13	12	9	7	9
IIIM	Skilled manual	8	34	7	24	2	26	2	32
IV	Partly skilled	22	24	30	23	15	29	10	33
V	Unskilled	8	6	3	6	1	8	0	5
	Not classified	14	12	34	15	67	18	78	17
	Base (= 100%)	*641*	*428*	*598*	*463*	*517*	*627*	*603*	*567*

Table 3.18: Social class of respondents' households (percentages of all respondents)

Social class of household head		African-Caribbean		Indian		Pakistani		Bangladeshi	
		Women	Men	Women	Men	Women	Men	Women	Men
16–29									
I	Professional etc.	3	1	2	1	1	4	0	0
II	Intermediate	11	14	11	16	6	8	4	2
IIINM	Skilled non-manual	14	13	14	10	9	4	10	8
IIIM	Skilled manual	20	26	28	25	29	27	28	30
IV	Partly skilled	19	17	26	28	17	23	22	24
V	Unskilled	5	10	3	12	9	9	8	6
Not classified		28	18	15	9	29	25	29	30
Base (= 100%)		178	114	208	129	281	235	307	213
30–49									
I	Professional etc.	2	2	4	8	1	3	1	
II	Intermediate	18	26	13	13	11	9	4	8
IIINM	Skilled non-manual	23	9	10	8	10	6	5	9
IIIM	Skilled manual	14	34	29	33	21	36	30	43
IV	Partly skilled	24	14	26	25	25	28	27	31
V	Unskilled	5	7	5	6	14	8	10	4
Not classified		14	8	13	8	18	11	23	6
Base (= 100%)		270	140	283	227	186	268	233	183
50–74									
I	Professional etc.	1	2	1	2				1
II	Intermediate	13	3	9	16	7	6		2
IIINM	Skilled non-manual	1	3	8	5	9	2	2	3
IIIM	Skilled manual	33	41	24	21	17	32	21	31
IV	Partly skilled	25	37	25	38	28	35	27	50
V	Unskilled	18	8	5	11	9	19	17	8
Not classified		10	5	28	7	30	4	32	5
Base (= 100%)		193	174	107	107	50	124	63	171
All ages									
I	Professional etc.	2	2	3	4	1	3	1	0
II	Intermediate	14	14	11	14	8	8	4	4
IIINM	Skilled non-manual	14	9	11	8	9	4	7	7
IIIM	Skilled manual	22	34	28	28	24	32	28	34
IV	Partly skilled	22	23	26	29	22	27	25	33
V	Unskilled	8	8	4	9	11	11	10	6
Not classified		18	10	16	8	25	15	27	16
Base (= 100%)		641	428	598	463	517	627	603	567

Table 3.19: Housing tenure of respondents (percentages of all respondents)

Tenure type	African-Caribbean		Indian		Pakistani		Bangladeshi	
	Women	Men	Women	Men	Women	Men	Women	Men
16–29								
Owned outright	10	17	36	37	41	36	15	12
Owned/being bought on mortgage	30	22	45	52	39	47	21	25
Bought from council/ under right to buy	2	1			0	0	2	1
Rented from								
council	34	44	4	4	5	5	50	46
housing association	12	7	4	1	2	2	7	5
private landlord	12	7	9	4	11	8	5	9
Other		3	2	2	1	2	0	2
Base (= 100%)	*176*	*114*	*206*	*129*	*281*	*235*	*307*	*213*
30–49								
Owned outright	7	12	36	25	36	28	12	7
Ownedl/being bought on mortgage	35	32	56	61	47	60	20	32
Bought from council/ under right to buy	0		0	1	0		5	1
Rented from								
council	42	42	3	8	10	4	49	43
housing association	12	6	2	1	2	2	6	9
private landlord	3	7	2	3	4	3	7	6
Other	1	1	1	1	0	2	0	1
Base (=100%)	*270*	*140*	*283*	*227*	*186*	*268*	*233*	*183*
50–74								
Owned outright	31	36	69	48	51	40	6	9
Owned/being bought on mortgage	27	22	22	39	34	48	18	17
Bought from council/ under right to buy	1	1						2
Rented from								
council	32	33	2	6	4	5	60	53
housing association	5	5	0	1	1	2	2	9
private landlord	3	2	6	3	10	4	14	10
Other	1	1	1	4	1	1		
Base (=100%)	*193*	*174*	*107*	*107*	*50*	*124*	*63*	*171*
All ages								
Owned outright	15	22	42	34	40	34	13	10
Owned/being bought on mortgage	31	25	45	53	42	52	20	25
Bought from council/ under right to Buy	1	1	0	0	0	0	3	1
Rented from								
council	36	40	3	6	7	5	51	47
housing association	10	6	2	1	1	2	6	7
private landlord	6	5	5	3	8	5	7	9
Other	1	2	1	2	1	2	0	1
Base (=100%)	*641*	*428*	*598*	*463*	*517*	*627*	*603*	*567*

Table 3.20: Car availability (percentages of all respondents)

Tenure type	African-Caribbean		Indian		Pakistani		Bangladeshi	
	Women	Men	Women	Men	Women	Men	Women	Men
16–29								
Own car	32	26	37	39	32	36	18	24
Use of car								
(e.g. company car)	5	8	10	12	8	9	1	1
No car	63	66	54	49	61	55	80	75
Base (= 100%)	*178*	*114*	*208*	*129*	*281*	*234*	*307*	*213*
30–49								
Own car	44	61	65	82	50	67	15	47
Use of car								
(e.g. company car)	2	6	3	1	4	4	2	3
No car	54	33	32	17	47	30	82	50
Base (= 100%)	*269*	*140*	*282*	*227*	*185*	*267*	*233*	*182*
50–74								
Own car	21	35	35	52	26	30	3	4
Use of car								
(e.g. company car)	5	1	5	2	7	5		2
No car	74	64	60	46	67	65	97	95
Base (= 100%)	*193*	*174*	*105*	*105*	*49*	*122*	*63*	*170*
All ages								
Own car	33	39	49	61	38	47	15	25
Use of car								
(e.g. company car)	4	5	6	5	6	6	1	2
No car	63	56	45	34	56	47	84	73
Base (= 100%)	*640*	*428*	*595*	*461*	*515*	*623*	*603*	*565*

Table 3.21: Country of birth and age at entry (percentages and means of all respondents)

Place of birth/ age at entry	African-Caribbean		Indian		Pakistani		Bangladeshi	
	Women	Men	Women	Men	Women	Men	Women	Men
16–29								
Percentage born outside the UK	8	5	40	26	47	52	82	74
Mean age of entry (years)	1.2	1.1	12.3	10.2	11.3	11.3	11.3	9.6
Base (= 100%)	*178*	*114*	*207*	*129*	*281*	*235*	*307*	*211*
30–49								
Percentage born outside the UK	62	57	96	94	97	97	98	98
Mean age of entry (years)	8.3	8.2	18.6	18.8	19.4	17.3	25.8	18.7
Base (= 100%)	*268*	*138*	*282*	*227*	*185*	*268*	*233*	*182*
50–74								
Percentage born outside the UK	100	92	100	99	98	98	100	100
Mean age of entry (years)	25.2	24.0	35.0	32.4	32.1	28.9	40.2	26.8
Base (= 100%)	*193*	*173*	*107*	*107*	*50*	*123*	*63*	*170*
All ages								
Percentage born outside the UK	52	51	77	72	75	79	91	89
Mean age of entry (years)	10.3	11.3	21.5	21.9	19.4	18.8	21.6	18.2
Base (= 100%)	*639*	*425*	*596*	*463*	*516*	*626*	*603*	*563*

Table 3.22: Ability in the English language (percentages of South Asian respondents)

Language ability	Indian		Pakistani		Bangladeshi	
	Women	Men	Women	Men	Women	Men
16–29						
Able to speak English	96	99	93	96	85	96
Able to read English	98	100	93	95	86	95
Able to read another language	59	37	68	71	69	56
(Base = 100%)	*208*	*129*	*281*	*235*	*307*	*213*
30–49						
Able to speak English	89	98	72	95	39	94
Able to read English	78	98	55	82	37	87
Able to read another language	62	77	45	69	31	46
(Base = 100%)	*282*	*227*	*185*	*268*	*233*	*183*
50–74						
Able to speak English	57	90	51	68	17	80
Able to read English	43	79	31	55	13	62
Able to read another language	36	69	26	51	3	35
(Base = 100%)	*107*	*107*	*50*	*124*	*63*	*169*
All ages						
Able to speak English	85	97	78	89	58	91
Able to read English	79	94	68	81	57	83
Able to read another language	56	62	52	66	45	47
(Base = 100%)	*597*	*463*	*516*	*627*	*603*	*565*

Table 3.23: Self-assessed degree of ability in spoken English (percentages of South Asian respondents who can speak English)

Degree of ability	Indian		Pakistani		Bangladeshi	
	Women	Men	Women	Men	Women	Men
16–29						
Can speak English very well	87	89	72	64	56	61
Can speak English fairly well	10	8	19	30	30	32
Can speak just a little English	3	3	9	6	13	7
Don't know					1	
Base (= 100%)	*197*	*127*	*255*	*225*	*256*	*202*
30–49						
Can speak English very well	49	52	31	31	8	16
Can speak English fairly well	27	35	34	37	16	41
Can speak just a little English	25	14	34	31	76	42
Don't know			1			0
Base (= 100%)	*254*	*222*	*131*	*249*	*88*	*171*
50–74						
Can speak English very well	18	45	17	17		2
Can speak English fairly well	41	31	16	38		31
Can speak just a little English	41	24	67	46	100	64
Don't know						2
Base (= 100%)	*63*	*95*	*23*	*86*	*5*	*133*
All ages						
Can speak English very well	60	63	51	43	41	32
Can speak English fairly well	22	25	25	34	25	35
Can speak just a little English	18	12	24	23	33	32
Don't know			0		1	1
Base (= 100%)	*514*	*444*	*409*	*560*	*349*	*506*

Table 3.25: Language best understood (percentages of all South Asian respondents)

Language	Indian Women	Indian Men	Pakistani Women	Pakistani Men	Bangladeshi Women	Bangladeshi Men
16–29						
English	70	86	57	58	40	34
Bengali					41	38
Gujerati	19	8				
Hindi	3					0
Kutchi		1	0			
Punjabi	6	5	28	16		1
Sylheti			1		19	26
Urdu	2	1	13	26		
Other	0	0	0	0	0	1
Base (= 100%)	*208*	*129*	*281*	*233*	*307*	*212*
30–49						
English	25	36	10	22	1	2
Bengali					62	49
Gujerati	36		31	1		
Hindi	3	3		0		
Kutchi	0	0	0			
Punjabi	32	25	60	26		
Sylheti			2	2	36	48
Urdu	1	3	25	47		1
Other	2	3	2	2	1	1
Base (= 100%)	*282*	*226*	*185*	*266*	*233*	*180*
50–74						
English	8	19	3	9		1
Bengali	1	1			54	42
Gujerati	43	41	2			
Hindi	3	3				
Kutchi	0	0	0	0	0	0
Punjabi	45	30	80	30		1
Sylheti				9	46	56
Urdu		2	15	49		1
Other	1	4		2		
Base (= 100%)	*106*	*105*	*50*	*124*	*63*	*170*
All ages						
English	38	49	30	33	19	15
Bengali	0	0			51	42
Gujerati	31	25	0	0		
Hindi	3	2		0		0
Kutchi	0	0	0			
Punjabi	25	19	49	23		1
Sylheti			1	3	29	41
Urdu	1	2	18	39		0
Other	1	2	1	1	0	0
Base (= 100%)	*596*	*460*	*516*	*623*	*603*	*562*

Table 3.26: Education outside the UK (percentages of respondents born outside the UK)

Highest educational level	African-Caribbean		Indian		Pakistani		Bangladeshi	
	Women	Men	Women	Men	Women	Men	Women	Men
16–29								
Attended school in country of birth	92	81	70	60	65	56	72	62
Level higher than school			9		8	7		3
Sixth form/A-level equivalent	0	0	0	0	0	0	0	0
Matriculation/higher	33	11	21	37	20	28	13	3
Secondary school		5						3
Class 7–10	0	0	19	25	17	18	29	20
Class 1–6	30	60	15	12	33	26	53	62
Infant school					2	2	0	1
Other	33		13	5	13	12	2	4
Don't know	5	23	23	22	7	6	3	4
Base (= 100%)	14	7	57	24	91	76	188	102
30–49								
Attended school in country of birth	84	90	88	87	62	87	77	96
Level higher than school	0		1	3	5	5	2	3
Sixth Form/A-level equivalent		1	1	1				
Matriculation/Higher	15	10	31	41	28	15	4	16
Secondary school	2		0	0		2		3
Class 7–10	6	4	21	24	23	33	20	24
Class 1–6	22	42	26	15	31	33	71	41
Infant school	5	2		1	1		2	3
Other	17	13	9	8	7	8	1	6
Don't know	32	27	10	7	6	5	1	4
Base (= 100%)	128	71	229	166	116	223	169	166
50–74								
Attended school in country of birth	97	98	62	89	36	72	54	79
Level higher than school	0	1		5		2		
Sixth Form/A-level equivalent	1							
Matriculation/Higher	15	9	26	33	19	30		15
Secondary school	0	1				3		1
Class 7–10	16	15	32	20	52	28	5	18
Class 1–6	36	57	34	22	30	34	95	51
Infant school		4						5
Other	7	5	3	10		4		3
Don't know	24	8	5	10				7
Base (= 100%)	178	157	67	90	16	96	29	126
All ages								
Attended school in country of birth	91	94	78	84	58	75	72	78
Level higher than school	0	1	2	3	5	5	1	2
Sixth Form/A-level equivalent	1	0	0	0				
Matriculation/Higher	16	9	29	38	24	22	7	12
Secondary school	1	1	0	0		2		2
Class 7–10	11	11	23	23	24	28	22	21
Class 1–6	30	53	26	17	31	32	66	50
Infant school	2	3		1	1	0	1	3
Other	13	7	8	9	9	8	2	5
Don't know	26	14	11	9	5	4	1	5
Base (= 100%)	320	235	353	300	223	395	386	394

Table 3.27: Highest qualification held (percentages of all respondents)

Qualification	African-Caribbean		Indian		Pakistani		Bangladeshi	
	Women	Men	Women	Men	Women	Men	Women	Men
16–29								
Degree (or degree level)	6	3	8	10	4	8	1	2
Teaching qualification	15	11	14	16	4	12	8	10
A-levels/SCE higher	15	14	10	19	11	13	8	13
O-level passes or equivalent	35	42	36	32	22	30	27	31
CSE Grades 2–5 or equivalent	15	7	7	6	15	8	9	4
Ungraded	0	0	1	0	1			3
Other qualifications	2	1	5	5	4	6	5	6
None	11	21	18	11	38	23	43	31
Base (= 100%)	*178*	*113*	*204*	*127*	*277*	*232*	*302*	*210*
30–49								
Degree (or degree level)	6	8	11	17	6	11	0	3
Teaching qualification	15	21	3	10	1	5	1	1
A-levels/SCE higher	8	8	5	4	2	4	0	
O-level passes or equivalent	30	18	17	12	14	6	1	4
CSE Grades 2–5 or equivalent	14	13	5	5	5	6		1
Ungraded	1	0		1		1		2
Other qualifications	4	3	4	6	3	8	3	13
None	23	31	55	45	70	60	94	77
Base (= 100%)	*267*	*139*	*281*	*221*	*181*	*266*	*232*	*180*
50–74								
Degree (or degree level)	1	2	2	12		4		1
Teaching qualification	8	1	4	2	1	1		1
A-levels/SCE higher	1	2		1				
O-level passes or equivalent	5	6	8	13	11	5		2
CSE Grades 2–5 or equivalent	7	7	2	0		2		
CSE ungraded			1					1
Other qualifications	8	3	7	5		6		4
None	69	79	76	66	88	81	100	93
Base (= 100%)	*190*	*172*	*106*	*106*	*48*	*121*	*63*	*171*
All ages								
Degree (or degree level)	5	4	8	13	4	8	1	2
Teaching qualification	13	10	7	10	3	7	4	4
A-levels/SCE higher	8	8	6	9	6	7	4	5
O-level passes or equivalent	25	22	22	19	17	16	13	15
CSE Grades 2–5 or equivalent	12	9	5	4	8	6	4	2
CSE ungraded	0	0	1	0	0	0		2
Other qualifications	4	2	5	6	3	7	3	7
None	31	45	46	39	58	49	71	63
Base (= 100%)	*635*	*424*	*591*	*454*	*506*	*619*	*597*	*561*

Table 3.28: Religious affiliation (percentages of all respondents)

Religion or church	African-Caribbean		Indian		Pakistani		Bangladeshi	
	Women	Men	Women	Men	Women	Men	Women	Men
16–29								
Baptist	5	5						
Buddhism					1		1	
Islam		0	25	21	95	95	98	98
Sikhism			34	32	0	1	0	
Hinduism			36	41				
Church of England/ Wales/Scotland/ Ireland	31	16	0		1			0
Roman Catholic	13	13	0	3				
Methodist	7	4						
Seventh Day Adventist	2	3						
Jehovah's Witness	3	2						
Pentecostal/Church of God/Church of Christ	13	11	0					
Cherubim and Seraphim								
Rastafarian	1							
Other	8	8	3	2	3	3	1	1
None	16	35	2	1	1	1	0	1
Don't know	0	2			1	0	0	
Base (= 100%)	177	112	207	129	280	234	305	207
30–49								
Baptist	7	3						
Buddhism	0			1	0			
Islam	0	1	20	23	93	97	98	99
Sikhism			32	29	2		0	1
Hinduism	1	1	45	38		2	1	
Church of England/ Wales/Scotland/ Ireland	31	17	2	1	1		1	
Roman Catholic	18	17	0	2	1			
Methodist	6	4			1			
Seventh Day Adventist	3	2						
Jehovah's Witness	3	6		0				
Pentecostal/Church of God/Church of Christ	11	4						
Cherubim and Seraphim		0						
Rastafarian	1	3						
Other	6	9	1	3	2	1		
None	11	31		1	1			
Don't know		2		0			0	
Base (= 100%)	269	139	281	226	184	266	230	178

Continued on next page

Table 3.28: *continued*

Religion or church	African-Caribbean Women	African-Caribbean Men	Indian Women	Indian Men	Pakistani Women	Pakistani Men	Bangladeshi Women	Bangladeshi Men
50–74								
Baptist	13	11						
Buddhism	0	0	0	0	0	0	0	0
Islam			13	15	95	97	98	98
Sikhism			40	31		1	2	
Hinduism	1	1	41	48	1			0
Church of England/ Wales/Scotland/ Ireland	27	28	0	2	1	0		
Roman Catholic	16	17	4	2	3	1		
Methodist	9	11	0					
Seventh Day Adventist	5	3						
Jehovah's Witness	1	1						
Pentecostal/Church of God/Church of Christ	15	9						
Cherubim and Seraphim	0	0	0	0	0	0	0	0
Rastafarian	0							
Other	11	6	2	2		1		1
None	1	14		0				
Don't know		1						
Base (= 100%)	*191*	*172*	*106*	*107*	*49*	*122*	*60*	*168*
All ages								
Baptist	8	7						
Buddhism	0			1	0		0	
Islam	0	1	20	21	94	96	98	98
Sikhism			34	30	1	0	0	0
Hinduism	0	1	41	41	0	1	0	0
Church of England/ Wales/Scotland/ Ireland	30	20	1	1	1	0	0	0
Roman Catholic	16	16	1	2	1	0		
Methodist	7	6	0		0			
Seventh Day Adventist	3	3						
Jehovah's Witness	3	3		0				
Pentecostal/Church of God/Church of Christ	13	8	0					
Cherubim and Seraphim		0						
Rastafarian	1	1						
Other	8	7	2	3	2	2	0	1
None	10	26	1	1	1	1	0	1
Don't know	0	1		0	0	0	0	
Base (= 100%)	*637*	*423*	*594*	*462*	*513*	*622*	*595*	*553*

Table 3.29: Receipt of benefits by respondent or spouse/partner (percentages of all respondents)

Type of benefit	African-Caribbean		Indian		Pakistani		Bangladeshi	
	Women	Men	Women	Men	Women	Men	Women	Men
16–29								
Income support or social security	40	35	16	15	29	29	38	25
Family credit	3	2	4	4	7	8	18	7
Housing benefit	30	21	5	3	10	11	25	14
Any of the above	46	39	20	19	36	37	54	31
Base (= 100%)	*178*	*114*	*208*	*129*	*281*	*235*	*307*	*213*
30–49								
Income support or social security	37	31	22	19	43	42	71	52
Family credit	8	8	10	12	21	15	19	23
Housing benefit	39	21	10	11	15	20	58	35
Any of the above	48	37	32	28	59	55	88	71
Base (= 100%)	*270*	*140*	*283*	*227*	*186*	*268*	*233*	*183*
50–74								
Income support or social security	36	30	45	43	60	57	94	93
Family credit	1		2	3	1	10	6	5
Housing benefit	29	14	14	16	16	25	68	59
Any of the above	45	34	46	44	61	66	97	95
Base (= 100%)	*193*	*174*	*107*	*107*	*50*	*124*	*63*	*171*
All ages								
Income support or social security	38	32	25	23	39	40	59	53
Family credit	4	3	7	7	12	11	17	11
Housing benefit	33	19	9	10	13	17	44	33
Any of the above	46	37	30	28	49	50	73	62
Base (= 100%)	*641*	*428*	*598*	*463*	*517*	*627*	*603*	*567*

Chapter 4: General health status

Table 4.1: Prevalence of health problems (Q15) (percentages of all respondents in sample)

Condition diagnosed by doctor or nurse	African-Caribbean		Indian		Pakistani		Bangladeshi	
	Women	Men	Women	Men	Women	Men	Women	Men
16–29								
Diabetes	1		1		1	1	5	0
High blood pressure	11	1	9	1	7		4	1
Angina							1	0
Heart attack (and related)			0		0		1	
Any other kind of heart trouble	1	2	1		2	0	1	
Stroke	0			1	0		1	
Base (= 100%)	*178*	*114*	*208*	*129*	*281*	*235*	*307*	*213*
30–49								
Diabetes	2	1	5	3	10	10	15	11
High blood pressure	29	6	17	12	12	7	16	6
Angina	2	1	2	3	1	0	5	7
Heart attack (and related)			1	1		2	1	2
Any other kind of heart trouble	3	1	1	2	1	1	7	7
Stroke	0			1	1	0		1
Base (= 100%)	*270*	*140*	*283*	*227*	*186*	*268*	*233*	*183*
50–74								
Diabetes	30	15	14	24	19	25	21	30
High blood pressure	53	40	22	29	24	31	21	30
Angina	10	7	4	6	7	8	16	21
Heart attack (and related)	3	8	2	8	3	14		11
Any other kind of heart trouble	5	8		0	2	11	1	15
Stroke	3	5	5	8	3	4	1	7
Base (= 100%)	*193*	*174*	*107*	*107*	*50*	*124*	*63*	*171*
All ages								
Diabetes	9	5	5	7	7	10	11	12
High blood pressure	29	17	15	12	12	9	11	11
Angina	3	3	2	3	1	2	5	8
Heart attack (and related)	1	3	1	2	1	4	1	4
Any other kind of heart trouble	3	4	1	1	2	3	3	7
Stroke	1	2	1	2	1	1	0	2
Base (= 100%)	*641*	*428*	*598*	*463*	*517*	*627*	*603*	*567*

Table 4.2a: Diabetes and pregnancy (Q16–18) (percentages of women who had ever been told by a doctor or nurse that they had diabetes)

Pregnant or not	African-Caribbean	Indian	Pakistani	Bangladeshi
16–29				
Pregnant when diagnosed	65	75	86	100
(*If so, ever had diabetes when* not *pregnant*)			14	21
Not pregnant	35	25	14	
Base (= 100%)	3	3	7	14
30–49				
Pregnant when diagnosed	51	37	57	74
(*If so, ever had diabetes when* not *pregnant*)		5	19	18
Not pregnant	49	63	43	26
Base (= 100%)	4	14	20	31
50–74				
Pregnant when diagnosed	5			
(*If so, ever had diabetes when* not *pregnant*)	1			
Not pregnant	95	100	100	100
Base (= 100%)	60	15	13	8
All ages				
Pregnant when diagnosed	10	21	39	65
(*If so, ever had diabetes when* not *pregnant*)	1	2	12	15
Not pregnant	90	79	61	35
Base (= 100%)	67	32	40	53

Table 4.2b: High blood pressure and pregnancy (Q18–19) (percentages of women who had ever been told by a doctor or nurse that they had high blood pressure)

Pregnant or not	African-Caribbean	Indian	Pakistani	Bangladeshi
16–29				
Pregnant when diagnosed	78	81	81	93
(*If so, ever had high blood*				
pressure when not *pregnant*)	14	16	39	3
Not pregnant	22	19	19	7
Base (= 100%)	20	19	22	13
30–49				
Pregnant when diagnosed	64	38	48	70
(*If so, ever had high blood*				
pressure when not *pregnant*)	23	11	23	33
Not pregnant	36	62	52	30
Base (= 100%)	75	43	24	32
50–74				
Pregnant when diagnosed	22	1	3	22
(*If so, ever had high blood*				
pressure when not *pregnant*)	22	1	3	10
Not pregnant	78	99	97	78
Base (=100%)	97	25	14	11
All ages				
Pregnant when diagnosed	45	37	43	64
(*If so, ever had high blood*				
pressure when not *pregnant*)	21	9	21	24
Not pregnant	55	63	57	36
Base (=100%)	192	87	60	56

Table 4.3: Ever had blood pressure measured by a doctor or nurse (Q67)
(percentages of all respondents)

Response	African-Caribbean		Indian		Pakistani		Bangladeshi	
	Women	Men	Women	Men	Women	Men	Women	Men
16–29								
Yes	90	78	77	62	74	61	68	47
No	8	22	23	36	25	37	31	45
Don't know	2	0	0	2	1	2	1	8
Base (= 100%)	*178*	*114*	*208*	*129*	*281*	*235*	*307*	*213*
30–49								
Yes	99	95	88	83	89	83	91	80
No	1	5	12	17	11	16	8	18
Don't know		1			0	0	0	2
Base (= 100%)	*270*	*140*	*283*	*227*	*186*	*268*	*233*	*183*
50–74								
Yes	96	96	92	91	85	93	90	93
No	4	4	8	9	12	7	8	4
Don't know					3		2	3
Base (= 100%)	*193*	*174*	*107*	*107*	*50*	*124*	*63*	*171*
All ages								
Yes	95	89	85	78	82	77	80	70
No	4	10	15	22	17	22	19	25
Don't know	1	0	0	1	1	1	1	5
Base (= 100%)	*640*	*428*	*597*	*463*	*517*	*625*	*603*	*566*

Table 4.4: Result of last measurement of blood pressure (Q68)
(percentages of all those whose blood pressure had been measured)

Result recalled	African-Caribbean		Indian		Pakistani		Bangladeshi	
	Women	Men	Women	Men	Women	Men	Women	Men
16–29								
Blood pressure all right fine/normal	84	90	78	88	83	91	92	89
Higher than normal	7	3	9	2	5	5	4	1
Lower than normal	7	2	5		7		3	1
Not told anything	1	3	4	3	3	2		6
Don't know/can't remember	2	2	5	7	2	3	0	3
Base (= 100%)	163	89	160	83	218	138	222	105
30–49								
Blood pressure all right fine/normal	79	89	86	82	86	87	82	90
Higher than normal	13	5	8	11	8	7	9	6
Lower than normal	6		4	4	5	3	6	2
Not told anything	2	4	2	2	1	2	0	
Don't know/can't remember		1	0	2	0	2	2	1
Base (= 100%)	266	131	251	185	164	219	214	151
50–74								
Blood pressure all right fine/normal	71	80	81	78	68	75	78	75
Higher than normal	27	17	10	19	17	14	16	20
Lower than normal	2		7		10	1	6	2
Not told anything	0	2	0	2	2	8		
Don't know/can't remember		1	1	1	3	2		3
Base (= 100%)	183	166	100	97	43	113	55	154
All ages								
Blood pressure all right fine/normal	79	86	82	83	82	85	86	84
Higher than normal	15	9	8	10	8	8	8	10
Lower than normal	5	1	5	2	7	2	5	2
Not told anything	1	3	2	2	2	3	0	2
Don't know/can't remember	1	1	2	3	1	2	1	2
Base (= 100%)	612	386	511	365	425	470	491	410

Table 4.5: Pregnant at the time the last blood pressure test was taken (Q69)
(percentages of women whose blood pressure was higher than normal at the time of the last test)

Response	African-Caribbean	Indian	Pakistani	Bangladeshi
16–29				
Pregnant last time	21	72	50	92
Not pregnant last time	79	28	50	8
Base (= 100%)	*8*	*14*	*15*	*8*
30–49				
Pregnant last time	26	12	36	58
Not pregnant last time	74	88	64	42
Base (= 100%)	*37*	*19*	*15*	*19*
50–74				
Pregnant last time	1			
Not pregnant last time	99	100	100	100
Base (= 100%)	*48*	*10*	*9*	*5*
All ages				
Pregnant last time	12	30	29	57
Not pregnant last time	88	70	71	43
Base (= 100%)	*93*	*43*	*39*	*33*

Table 4.6: Understanding of the term 'high blood pressure' (Q118)
(percentages of all respondents)

Response	African-Caribbean		Indian		Pakistani		Bangladeshi	
	Women	Men	Women	Men	Women	Men	Women	Men
16–29								
Yes	77	86	66	68	66	66	63	71
No	22	10	28	27	29	28	25	21
Don't know	1	4	6	6	5	5	12	8
Base (= 100%)	*178*	*114*	*208*	*125*	*281*	*235*	*307*	*213*
30–49								
Yes	80	83	70	81	66	74	51	75
No	17	13	22	15	27	19	25	18
Don't know	3	4	6	4	7	7	24	8
Base (= 100%)	*270*	*140*	*283*	*227*	*186*	*268*	*233*	*183*
50–74								
Yes	79	73	55	77	66	62	40	73
No	19	18	35	20	26	31	31	17
Don't know	2	9	9	3	8	7	29	11
Base (= 100%)	*193*	*174*	*107*	*107*	*50*	*124*	*63*	*171*
All ages								
Yes	79	81	66	76	66	68	55	72
No	19	14	27	20	28	25	26	19
Don't know	2	6	7	4	6	6	19	9
Base (= 100%)	*641*	*428*	*598*	*463*	*517*	*627*	*603*	*567*

Table 4.7: Awareness of the causes of high blood pressure (Q118) (percentages of all respondents who understood the meaning of the term 'high blood pressure')

Cause	African-Caribbean		Indian		Pakistani		Bangladeshi	
	Women	Men	Women	Men	Women	Men	Women	Men
16–29								
Eating too much salt	33	19	27	29	46	46	23	19
Drinking too much alcohol	6	3	14	9	9	14	9	4
Being overweight/obese	21	14	19	20	21	24	26	16
Stress/worry/pressure	64	56	57	57	40	38	40	29
Runs in families/genetic/hereditary	4		1	1	2	11	7	2
Hardened arteries/clogged-up arteries	4	3	5	3	2	6	3	2
Other	42	24	32	30	37	29	22	25
Nothing in particular					1			1
Don't know	6	19	17	9	15	11	30	27
Base (= 100%)	*131*	*98*	*139*	*88*	*182*	*154*	*189*	*152*
30–49								
Eating too much salt	32	30	29	29	31	46	16	14
Drinking too much alcohol	11	10	9	14	6	14	3	5
Being overweight/obese	27	21	24	28	26	18	12	22
Stress/worry/pressure	60	51	51	46	52	46	25	35
Runs in families/genetic/hereditary	13	4	5	4	4	4	4	2
Hardened arteries/clogged-up arteries	6	6	5	5	4	4		2
Other	44	43	26	27	26	19	3	17
Nothing in particular	0	0	2	2	1	0		
Don't know	3	7	16	17	23	18	59	41
Base (= 100%)	*215*	*117*	*198*	*181*	*119*	*186*	*116*	*137*
50–74								
Eating too much salt	22	22	21	27	32	31	16	8
Drinking too much alcohol	10	14	5	10	3	8		4
Being overweight/obese	19	22	27	21	20	25	20	25
Stress/worry/pressure	56	48	58	56	70	40	20	32
Runs in families/genetic/hereditary	11	5	3	3		5	2	4
Hardened arteries/clogged-up arteries	10	5	8	5	5	2		
Other	36	24	22	28	30	24		12
Nothing in particular		0	6	1	5			4
Don't know	13	17	17	12	7	20	58	43
Base (= 100%)	*152*	*127*	*61*	*78*	*33*	*76*	*24*	*124*
All ages								
Eating too much salt	30	23	27	29	38	43	20	14
Drinking too much alcohol	9	9	10	11	7	13	6	4
Being overweight/obese	23	19	23	24	23	22	20	20
Stress/worry/pressure	60	52	54	51	49	42	33	32
Runs in families/genetic/hereditary	9	3	3	3	3	7	5	2
Hardened arteries/clogged-up arteries	6	4	6	4	4	4	2	1
Other	41	30	27	28	31	24	13	19
Nothing in particular	0	0	2	1	2	0	0	1
Don't know	7	15	17	13	17	15	43	36
Base (= 100%)	*498*	*342*	*398*	*347*	*334*	*416*	*329*	*413*

Table 4.8: Awareness of risks associated with high blood pressure (Q118) (percentages of all respondents who understood the meaning of the term 'high blood pressure')

Increased risk of	African-Caribbean		Indian		Pakistani		Bangladeshi	
	Women	Men	Women	Men	Women	Men	Women	Men
16–29								
Overweight/obesity	6	2	12	12	12	18	12	6
Diabetes	9	7	12	10	10	11	14	6
Coronary heart disease	23	2	19	17	21	22	9	8
Heart attack	43	45	49	68	50	61	39	48
Stroke	34	20	23	19	21	26	19	13
Headaches or migraines	8	5	16	13	13	14	24	21
Other	29	34	31	15	22	21	18	17
No health risks	0		1		1			
Don't know	16	19	14	5	13	9	29	23
Base (= 100%)	*131*	*98*	*139*	*88*	*182*	*154*	*189*	*152*
30–49								
Overweight/obesity	9	11	11	11	10	16	12	8
Diabetes	10	6	8	10	12	8	7	5
Coronary heart disease	23	15	16	18	23	14	4	9
Heart attack	49	61	47	52	43	60	26	40
Stroke	60	22	24	31	14	31	16	15
Headaches or migraines	9	6	32	19	27	20	42	30
Other	39	29	24	31	18	24	8	20
No health risks			0		1			
Don't know	8	11	12	6	18	9	38	21
Base (= 100%)	*215*	*117*	*198*	*181*	*119*	*186*	*116*	*137*
50–74								
Overweight/obesity	8	12	16	12	35	10	2	9
Diabetes	6	5	6	12	11	6	7	2
Coronary heart disease	10	11	14	4	23	10	5	7
Heart attack	41	51	49	55	36	52	48	39
Stroke	60	37	36	39	25	28	8	11
Headaches or migraines	10	14	43	27	43	22	24	41
Other	24	22	17	21	17	23		22
No health risks	1		1			1		1
Don't know	9	12	4	10	11	17	37	17
Base (= 100%)	*152*	*127*	*61*	*78*	*33*	*76*	*24*	*124*
All ages								
Overweight/obesity	8	8	12	11	15	15	11	7
Diabetes	8	6	9	10	11	9	11	4
Coronary heart disease	19	9	17	14	22	16	7	8
Heart attack	44	52	48	57	45	59	35	43
Stroke	51	27	25	29	19	28	17	13
Headaches or migraines	9	8	28	19	23	18	30	30
Other	31	29	25	24	20	23	13	19
No health risks	0	0	1	0	1	0	0	0
Don't know	11	14	11	7	15	10	33	21
Base (= 100%)	*498*	*342*	*398*	*347*	*334*	*416*	*329*	*413*

Table 4.9: Advice offered to others to avoid high blood pressure (Q118) (percentages of all respondents who understood the meaning of the term 'high blood pressure')

Response	African-Caribbean Women	African-Caribbean Men	Indian Women	Indian Men	Pakistani Women	Pakistani Men	Bangladeshi Women	Bangladeshi Men
16–29								
(a) Lose weight/avoid becoming overweight	57	61	58	57	58	61	64	49
(b) Avoid fatty/oily foods and drinks	62	50	65	54	63	58	58	44
(c) Avoid sugary/sweet foods and drinks	39	27	37	21	24	34	34	29
(d) Avoid drinking alcohol/cut down	52	40	46	55	50	49	49	35
(e) Don't smoke/give up smoking	40	30	41	38	49	42	50	43
(f) Avoid salty foods	64	41	54	42	62	43	44	33
(g) Eat more of such foods as bread, rice, etc.	24	28	17	19	13	30	23	19
(h) Eat plenty of fresh fruit and vegetables	54	42	43	53	56	53	50	42
(i) Take (regular) exercise	57	38	59	53	55	56	43	38
Other	9	1	1	4	3	3	1	3
None of these							0	
There is nothing you can do to reduce risk			1				0	1
Don't know	2	8	6	3	4	4	10	11
Base (= 100%)	*131*	*98*	*139*	*88*	*182*	*154*	*189*	*152*
30–49								
(a) Lose weight/avoid becoming overweight	69	51	59	57	51	64	35	40
(b) Avoid fatty/oily foods and drinks	62	58	58	56	45	56	47	44
(c) Avoid sugary/sweet foods and drinks	39	37	38	33	28	35	28	20
(d) Avoid drinking alcohol/cut down	68	45	44	51	35	54	11	17
(e) Don't smoke/give up smoking	58	39	38	42	36	48	23	26
(f) Avoid salty foods	78	55	58	48	49	64	43	25
(g) Eat more of such foods as bread, rice, etc.	14	16	14	15	17	14	12	6
(h) Eat plenty of fresh fruit and vegetables	69	50	52	43	44	48	26	25
(i) Take (regular) exercise	64	44	46	41	36	39	12	23
Other	1	5	3	5	6	3	6	20
None of these		0		0	2			
There is nothing you can do to reduce risk	1		1			0		
Don't know	3	2	7	5	21	6	29	23
Base (= 100%)	*215*	*117*	*198*	*181*	*119*	*186*	*116*	*137*

Continued on next page

Table 4.9: *continued*

Response	African-Caribbean		Indian		Pakistani		Bangladeshi	
	Women	Men	Women	Men	Women	Men	Women	Men
50–74								
(a) Lose weight/avoid becoming overweight	62	45	54	63	68	53	31	34
(b) Avoid fatty/oily foods and drinks	59	52	55	52	47	45	46	37
(c) Avoid sugary/sweet foods and drinks	47	36	32	46	48	20	16	18
(d) Avoid drinking alcohol/cut down	54	50	32	54	41	40		17
(e) Don't smoke/give up smoking	50	34	28	51	46	38		26
(f) Avoid salty foods	69	48	56	50	53	56	24	14
(g) Eat more of such foods as bread, rice, etc.	18	14	16	20	23	20	5	4
(h) Eat plenty of fresh fruit and vegetables	63	51	38	54	42	43	10	22
(i) Take (regular) exercise	47	33	26	47	34	30	2	11
Other	7	2	20	4	13	11		21
None of these		0						
There is nothing you can do to reduce risk	1		1			1		5
Don't know	5	8	8	6	11	19	44	28
Base (= 100%)	*152*	*127*	*61*	*78*	*33*	*76*	*24*	*124*
All ages								
(a) Lose weight/avoid becoming overweight	63	53	58	59	57	60	50	42
(b) Avoid fatty/oily foods and drinks	61	53	60	54	53	54	53	42
(c) Avoid sugary/sweet foods and drinks	41	33	36	32	29	32	30	23
(d) Avoid drinking alcohol/cut down	58	45	43	53	42	49	30	24
(e) Don't smoke/give up smoking	49	34	38	43	43	44	35	33
(f) Avoid salty foods	70	48	56	47	56	54	42	25
(g) Eat more of such foods as bread, rice, etc.	19	20	16	17	16	21	17	11
(h) Eat plenty of fresh fruit and vegetables	62	47	46	49	49	49	37	31
(i) Take (regular) exercise	57	38	47	46	44	44	28	26
Other	3	3	6	4	6	4	4	16
None of these	0	0	0	0	1	0	0	0
There is nothing you can do to reduce risk	1	0	1	0	0	0	0	2
Don't know	3	6	7	5	12	8	20	19
Base (= 100%)	*498*	*342*	*398*	*347*	*334*	*416*	*329*	*413*

Chapter 5 Knowledge of health and health-promoting behaviour

Table 5.1: Respondents' perceptions of their own health (Q1) (percentages)

Assessment of own health	African-Caribbean Women	Men	Indian Women	Men	Pakistani Women	Men	Bangladeshi Women	Men
16–29								
Very good	31	52	35	45	35	41	42	42
Fairly good	58	41	55	46	53	49	48	50
Fairly poor	9	5	8	8	10	8	8	7
Very poor	2	2	2	1	3	2	1	2
Don't know							0	
Base (= 100%)	177	114	207	129	278	235	307	210
30–49								
Very good	42	55	28	41	23	34	21	23
Fairly good	48	38	57	50	55	48	42	58
Fairly poor	6	6	12	8	15	14	26	14
Very poor	3	0	2	1	7	3	11	5
Don't know	1		1		0	1	0	1
Base (= 100%)	270	139	281	225	186	268	231	183
50–74								
Very good	19	27	11	21	13	9	6	6
Fairly good	52	47	63	54	50	44	33	31
Fairly poor	17	16	16	20	25	25	48	36
Very poor	12	10	9	5	11	21	14	25
Don't know	0	1	1			0		1
Base (= 100%)	193	173	107	107	49	124	63	170
All ages								
Very good	32	44	27	38	27	32	29	26
Fairly good	53	42	58	50	53	48	44	47
Fairly poor	10	9	11	10	14	14	20	18
Very poor	5	4	3	2	6	6	7	10
Don't know	0	0	0	0	0	0	0	0
Base (= 100%)	640	426	595	461	513	627	601	563

Table 5.2: Respondents' awareness of things people can do to improve or maintain their health (Q2) (percentages)

Aware	African-Caribbean		Indian		Pakistani		Bangladeshi	
	Women	Men	Women	Men	Women	Men	Women	Men
16–29								
Yes	95	94	90	92	85	91	72	88
No	2	2	3	3	6	7	10	7
Don't know	3	4	7	5	10	2	19	6
Base (= 100%)	*178*	*114*	*208*	*128*	*280*	*234*	*303*	*209*
30–49								
Yes	93	96	77	87	73	82	55	81
No	3	3	9	10	14	13	16	8
Don't know	4	1	14	3	12	5	29	11
Base (= 100%)	*270*	*140*	*282*	*227*	*186*	*267*	*231*	*176*
50–74								
Yes	79	81	68	82	70	79	41	67
No	6	7	16	12	19	10	12	15
Don't know	14	12	16	6	11	11	47	19
Base (= 100%)	*191*	*174*	*107*	*106*	*50*	*124*	*62*	*165*
All ages								
Yes	90	90	80	88	78	85	61	79
No	4	4	8	8	11	10	13	9
Don't know	6	6	12	4	11	5	26	11
Base (= 100%)	*639*	*428*	*597*	*461*	*516*	*625*	*596*	*550*

Table 5.3: Respondents' perception of ways in which people could improve their health (percentages of all those who knew of ways which people could improve their health)

Method mentioned	African-Caribbean		Indian		Pakistani		Bangladeshi	
	Women	Men	Women	Men	Women	Men	Women	Men
16–29								
Eat a healthy diet	85	77	86	82	90	79	78	71
Take (regular) exercise	87	85	85	80	78	82	76	77
Not to								
Smoke	25	17	21	14	14	33	18	18
Drink (too much)								
alcohol	13	9	16	11	9	19	14	8
Work too hard	0		2	1	2	3	1	
Worry (too much)	4	1	7	3	10	6	7	3
Get a good night's sleep/								
plenty of rest	6	4	9	1	6	8	8	9
Avoid getting overweight	0	2	7	8	6	7	9	4
Don't take drugs	6	1	7	2	5	11	11	4
Avoid fatty foods	4	7	11	4	8	10	12	11
Regular check-ups	4	4	1	3	2	0	1	2
Other dietary								
recommendation								
(eat/drink)	4	2	4	4	3	2	4	2
Psycho-social factors								
(willpower, social)	9	3	5	5	6	4	4	9
Take vitamins/mineral								
supplements	3				0	1		
Other	12	6	15	11	14	6	7	7
Don't know		0	2	2	0	2	5	0
No answer	0							
Base (= 100%)	*167*	*108*	*179*	*114*	*228*	*207*	*208*	*180*
30–49								
Eat a healthy diet	91	76	84	77	79	81	75	77
Take (regular) exercise	80	82	68	79	55	77	39	55
Not to								
Smoke	19	26	12	17	6	15	21	15
Drink (too much)								
alcohol	13	16	12	13	6	15	16	4
Work too hard	1	1	3	2	5	4	3	0
Worry(too much)	5	2	9	7	19	5	8	8
Get a good night's sleep/								
plenty of rest	8	8	6	5	8	7	17	20
Avoid getting overweight	2	2	7	3	11	13	15	3
Don't take drugs	3	4	6	3	5	7	18	3
Avoid fatty foods	6	4	14	6	16	13	23	12
Regular check-ups	3	0	1	2	3	2	2	
Other dietary								
recommendation								
(eat/drink)	5	1	2	2	3	3	1	3
Psycho-social factors								
(willpower, social)	11	12	8	8	3	6	3	8
Take vitamins/mineral								
supplements	0		0					
Other	14	12	15	13	8	9	4	10
Don't know		0	2	3	4	1	6	6
No answer					1			
Base (= 100%)	*252*	*134*	*218*	*196*	*136*	*220*	*121*	*140*

Continued on next page

Table 5.3: *continued*

Method mentioned	African-Caribbean		Indian		Pakistani		Bangladeshi	
	Women	Men	Women	Men	Women	Men	Women	Men
50–74								
Eat a healthy diet	82	76	76	76	78	71	70	73
Take (regular) exercise	66	58	46	67	57	49	29	39
Not to								
Smoke	16	11	9	11	3	16	28	15
Drink(too much)								
alcohol	16	17	9	9		11	21	3
Work too hard	1	1	7	3	4	4		1
Worry (too much)	3	3	12	8	35	13	11	8
Get a good night's sleep/ plenty of rest	10	10	15	2	9	3	35	24
Avoid getting overweight	6	2	10		12	11	16	8
Don't take drugs		2	3		2	3	13	2
Avoid fatty foods	7	5	15	15	7	12	13	9
Regular check-ups	2	6		4		3		4
Other dietary recommendation (eat/drink)	9	4	4	3		2		7
Psycho-social factors (willpower, social)	10	10	16	15	9	17		7
Take vitamins/mineral supplements								
Other	21	16	9	25	18	18		5
Don't know	2	4	6	1	4	4	11	6
No answer					1	1		1
Base (= 100%)	*147*	*133*	*72*	*82*	*36*	*99*	*22*	*111*
All ages								
Eat a healthy diet	87	76	84	79	84	78	76	73
Take (regular) exercise	79	75	71	77	66	74	59	61
Not to								
Smoke	21	18	15	14	10	23	20	16
Drink(too much)								
alcohol	14	14	13	12	7	16	15	5
Work too hard	1	1	3	2	4	4	2	1
Worry (too much)	4	2	9	6	17	7	8	6
Get a good night's sleep/ plenty of rest	8	7	9	3	7	7	14	16
Avoid getting overweight	2	2	7	4	9	10	12	5
Don't take drugs	4	2	6	2	5	8	14	3
Avoid fatty foods	5	5	13	7	11	11	16	11
Regular check-ups	3	3	1	3	2	1	1	3
Other dietary recommendation (eat/drink)	6	2	3	3	3	2	3	4
Psycho-social factors (willpower, social)	10	8	8	8	6	8	3	8
Take vitamins/mineral supplements	1	0	0	0	0	0	0	0
Other	15	11	14	15	12	10	5	7
Don't know	0	1	3	2	2	2	6	3
No answer	0	0	0	0	1	0	0	0
Base(= 100%)	*148*	*133*	*72*	*82*	*37*	*99*	*22*	*111*

Table 5.4: Do you take action on a regular basis to maintain or improve your health? (percentages of all those who knew of ways in which people could improve their health)

Response	African-Caribbean		Indian		Pakistani		Bangladeshi	
	Women	Men	Women	Men	Women	Men	Women	Men
16–29								
Yes	65	80	62	83	60	74	61	70
No	34	20	37	17	40	26	37	30
Don't know	1		0				2	
Base (= 100%)	167	108	179	114	228	207	208	178
30–49								
Yes	74	78	57	72	55	75	44	48
No	26	21	42	27	43	25	54	52
Don't know		1	0	1	2		2	1
Base(= 100%)	251	134	218	196	133	219	121	139
50–74								
Yes	80	77	78	72	62	77	41	48
No	19	23	19	28	36	23	56	51
Don't know	1		4		2		3	1
Base (= 100%)	146	132	72	82	36	99	22	111
All ages								
Yes	72	78	63	76	58	75	53	58
No	28	21	36	24	41	25	45	41
Don't know	1	0	1	0	1	0	2	0
Base (= 100%)	564	374	469	392	396	525	351	428

Table 5.5: Actions taken on a regular basis to maintain or improve your health (percentages of all those who replied that they took regular action to maintain or improve their health)

Action	African-Caribbean Women	Men	Indian Women	Men	Pakistani Women	Men	Bangladeshi Women	Men
16–29								
Eat a healthy diet	52	35	55	37	59	41	61	35
Take (regular) exercise	87	83	74	81	67	86	64	84
Not to								
Smoke	10	4	8	8	7	13	18	10
Drink (too much)								
alcohol	8	3	5	7	6	13	17	8
Work too hard		1	0		0	3	1	
Worry (too much)	7		3	2	4	6	3	3
Get a good night's sleep/								
plenty of rest	1	1	7	0	5	8	7	7
Avoid getting overweight	2	2	7	5	8	6	8	5
Avoid fatty foods	5	5	17	8	10	10	21	5
Don't take drugs	6	4	5	2	3	3	15	2
Other dietary								
recommendations	1	6	1	3	3	2	5	0
Psycho-social factors	3	2		3	3	4	2	1
Other	11	11	11	23	14	13	7	7
Don't know					1	1	1	
Base (= 100%)	*109*	*85*	*112*	*94*	*135*	*152*	*125*	*120*
30–49								
Eat a healthy diet	57	46	65	50	70	54	46	58
Take (regular) exercise	73	79	68	74	45	67	43	60
Not to								
Smoke	13	9	2	9	3	9	32	10
Drink (too much)								
alcohol	6	9	5	8	4	8	29	2
Work too hard		0	1	2	4	2	9	2
Worry (too much)	3	1	7	2	7	2	4	10
Get a good night's sleep/								
plenty of rest	8	3	8	4	8	5	9	16
Avoid getting overweight	2	3	9	3	15	3	20	5
Avoid fatty foods	9	7	16	9	19	17	47	8
Don't take drugs	4	2	2	1	4	2	25	
Other dietary								
recommendations	7	4	2	4	1	5	5	7
Psycho-social factors	5	5	7	5	2	4		2
Take vitamins/mineral								
supplements			0		1			
Regular health checks	0	2	0					
Other	14	10	16	15	6	9	4	9
Don't know	0	1			1			
Base (= 100%)	*183*	*102*	*125*	*144*	*77*	*160*	*52*	*65*

Continued on next page

Table 5.5: *continued*

Action	African-Caribbean Women	Men	Indian Women	Men	Pakistani Women	Men	Bangladeshi Women	Men
50–74								
Eat a healthy diet	71	41	76	50	57	64	61	57
Take (regular) exercise	53	62	48	63	25	41	16	52
Not to								
Smoke	12	12	9	13		9	61	15
Drink (too much) alcohol	10	11	12	14		9	13	
Work too hard	1	2	2		5	2		
Worry (too much)	3	2	5	3	26	5		6
Get a good night's sleep/ plenty of rest	4	6	11	8	7	6	87	7
Avoid getting overweight	7	4	9	5	8	3	31	5
Avoid fatty foods	10	8	17	10	22	21	18	7
Don't take drugs	1	1	2	6	4	3	26	
Other dietary recommendations	8	4	5	2	4	6		3
Psycho-social factors	7	9	11	9	10	7		7
Take vitamins/mineral supplements		1	1					
Regular health checks	1							1
Other	22	24	18	37	18	31		14
Don't know		1		1	7			2
Base (= 100%)	*116*	*100*	*55*	*61*	*24*	*74*	*7*	*53*
All ages								
Eat a healthy diet	63	46	73	49	95	61	117	76
Take (regular) exercise	78	87	76	80	80	84	113	122
Not to								
Smoke	13	9	7	10	7	13	51	18
Drink (too much) alcohol	8	9	7	9	7	13	42	8
Work too hard	0	1	1	1	4	3	6	1
Worry (too much)	5	1	6	3	12	5	7	9
Get a good night's sleep plenty of rest	5	3	9	3	10	8	26	15
Avoid getting overweight	4	3	10	5	15	5	27	9
Avoid fatty foods	8	7	19	9	23	18	59	10
Don't take drugs	4	3	3	2	5	3	38	2
Other dietary recommendations	6	6	2	3	4	4	9	4
Psycho-social factors	5	6	6	5	6	6	3	4
Take vitamins/mineral supplements	4	5	5	10	11	7	9	6
Reguiar health checks	0	1	0	0	0	0	2	0
Other	12	12	12	15	8	12	2	10
Don't know	38	44	46	41	77	51	132	94
Base (= 100%)	*436*	*281*	*264*	*309*	*135*	*346*	*83*	*157*

Table 5.6: Which serious health problems are linked to diet and types of food eaten? (percentages of all respondents)

Illness or health problem	African-Caribbean		Indian		Pakistani		Bangladeshi	
	Women	Men	Women	Men	Women	Men	Women	Men
16–29								
Heart trouble/disease/ attack	67	44	53	48	52	41	34	31
Diabetes	17	12	20	16	30	24	23	12
Stroke	5	1	4	5	4	3	2	1
Overweight/obesity	22	20	17	18	14	21	12	16
High blood pressure	15	9	12	6	14	13	10	6
Constipation	1	1	4	4	1	2	1	2
Bowel cancer	1		2		1	4	0	2
Lung cancer	2		5		2	3	2	6
Breast cancer			1		0	1	0	1
Cancer in general/ unspecified type	9	8	7	8	6	1	3	4
Liver disease/cirrhosis of the liver	2	1	4	3	1	1	2	5
Kidney disease	1		5	3	2	1	1	2
Arthritis/rheumatism/ problems with joints	2	2	1	1	1	1	2	1
Cholesterol level	2			1	1	1	0	0
Anaemia	1	1	1		0	1		0
Stomach problems (including ulcers)	2	2	3	3	2	1	7	10
Underweight	4	2	2		1	2	1	2
Respiratory/breathing disorders (asthma)	3	3		1	1	4	1	
Skin diseases/problems	4	3	1	1	1	1	2	
Other	17	18	17	8	12	18	8	10
None (no serious illnesses are linked to diet)		1	2	2	4	2	5	2
Don't know	10	22	21	21	24	26	38	38
Base (= 100%)	*178*	*114*	*208*	*129*	*281*	*235*	*307*	*213*
30–49								
Heart trouble/disease/ attack	64	55	46	47	36	48	13	30
Diabetes	21	14	26	27	26	23	13	25
Stroke	4		3	2	3	3	1	4
Overweight/obesity	20	19	24	20	17	17	5	22
High blood pressure	25	13	17	15	13	16	6	7
Constipation	1	3	3	5	4	5	2	5
Bowel cancer	1	2		1	1	2		2
Lung cancer	0	4	1	1	1	2		2
Breast cancer	0		0		0	1		
Cancer in general/ unspecified type	11	1	2	3	4	1	1	3
Liver disease/cirrhosis of the liver	2	2	1	1		4	1	2
Kidney disease	2	4	3	1	1	2	1	0
Arthritis/rheumatism/ problems with joints	3	0	3	2	3	2	1	3
Cholesterol level	3		1					
Anaemia	1	0	1					
Stomach problems (including ulcers)	5	4	4	4	3	6	13	16
Underweight	2	1				1		0
Respiratory/breathing disorders (asthma)	3	1	3	2	3	5	1	0
Skin diseases/problems	2	2	1	1			0	
Other	18	15	17	10	11	17	11	14
None (no serious illnesses are linked to diet	1	1	3	6	4	2	10	1
Don't know	10	20	23	19	31	24	46	26
Base (= 100%)	*270*	*140*	*283*	*227*	*186*	*266*	*233*	*183*

Continued on next page

Table 5.6: *continued*

Illness or health problem	African-Caribbean		Indian		Pakistani		Bangladeshi	
	Women	Men	Women	Men	Women	Men	Women	Men
50–74								
Heart trouble/disease/ attack	44	28	26	34	27	36	15	18
Diabetes	24	19	17	28	20	18	16	21
Stroke	4	1	3	2	2	6		1
Overweight/obesity	14	17	15	15	17	23	14	20
High blood pressure	24	12	10	15	9	14	4	10
Constipation	1	1	11	2	2	6	2	3
Bowel cancer	1		3			5		
Lung cancer	1		1	0		3		1
Breast cancer			2			1		
Cancer in general/ unspecified type	6	5	6	1	1	3		
Liver disease/cirrhosis of the liver	3	1	2			1		0
Kidney disease	3		0	1		3		1
Arthritis/rheumatism/ problems with joints	5	3	11	0	2	0		2
Cholesterol level				0		0		
Anaemia			1					
Stomach problems (including ulcers)	4	3	3	6		6	4	14
Underweight	0		2					1
Respiratory/breathing disorders (asthma)	1	1	1	3		9	4	0
Skin diseases/problems	0	0	1	0				
Other	12	6	7	13	7	17	6	7
None (no serious illnesses are linked to diet	4	2	3	4	5	2	3	4
Don't know	24	37	35	28	43	27	68	32
Base (= 100%)	*193*	*174*	*107*	*107*	*50*	*124*	*63*	*171*
All ages								
Heart trouble/disease/ attack	60	41	45	44	42	42	23	27
Diabetes	20	15	22	23	27	22	18	19
Stroke	4	1	3	3	4	4	1	2
Overweight/obesity	19	19	20	18	16	20	10	19
High blood pressure	21	11	14	12	13	14	8	7
Constipation	1	1	5	4	3	4	2	3
Bowel cancer	1	1	1	0	1	3	0	1
Lung cancer	1	1	3	1	1	2	1	3
Breast cancer	0	0	1	0	0	1	0	0
Cancer in general/ unspecified type	9	5	5	4	4	1	2	2
Liver disease/cirrhosis of the liver	2	1	2	1	1	2	1	2
Kidney disease	2	1	3	2	1	2	1	1
Arthritis/rheumatism/ problems with joints	3	2	4	1	2	1	1	2
Cholesterol level	2	0	1	0	0	0	0	0
Anaemia	1	1	1	0	0	0	0	0
Stomach problems (including ulcers)	4	3	4	4	2	4	9	13
Underweight	2	1	1	0	0	1	0	1
Respiratory/breathing disorders (asthma)	2	2	1	2	1	6	1	0
Skin diseases/problems	2	2	1	1	0	1	1	0
Other	16	13	15	10	11	17	9	10
None (no serious illnesses are linked to diet	1	1	3	4	4	2	7	2
Don't know	14	27	25	22	30	25	45	33
Base (= 100%)	*641*	*428*	*598*	*463*	*517*	*627*	*603*	*567*

Table 5.7: Which serious health problems are linked to smoking? (percentages of all respondents)

Illness or health problem	African-Caribbean		Indian		Pakistani		Bangladeshi	
	Women	Men	Women	Men	Women	Men	Women	Men
16–29								
Heart trouble/disease/attack	30	19	32	16	35	26	34	27
Diabetes					1	3		1
Stroke	1	1	2	1	2	4	1	1
Overweight/obesity	2		2	1	1	1	0	1
High blood pressure	2	1	3	2	2	5	4	4
Constipation					1	1		
Bowel cancer	1	2	4	1	2	3	2	2
Lung cancer	62	53	52	66	48	59	43	57
Breast cancer	2	3	2	2	2	1	3	2
Cancer in general/unspecified type	45	42	30	40	30	37	29	28
Liver disease/cirrhosis of the liver	1	3	7	0	4	2	2	3
Kidney disease		2	4	2	5	1	1	1
Arthritis/rheumatism/problems with joints	0	1	1		0	0		1
Respiratory/breathing disorders	15	13	10	7	12	15	12	13
TB/tuberculosis	0		2		1	1	3	3
Throat cancer/mouth cancer	1	1			1			1
Other	19	14	25	11	18	16	14	15
None (no serious illnesses are linked to smoking)	0	1	2		1		2	
Don't know	1	7	6	4	12	4	17	5
Base (= 100%)	178	114	208	129	281	235	307	213
30–49								
Heart trouble/disease/attack	32	29	22	28	30	25	32	27
Diabetes	0		0	1	1	2	1	3
Stroke	1	1	1	2	2	3	1	
Overweight/obesity	0	0	2	1	2	2	1	
High blood pressure	2	2	1	3	6	5	1	4
Constipation	0					1		
Bowel cancer	1	1	1	0	2	6	1	0
Lung cancer	57	54	44	59	31	56	31	39
Breast cancer	1	1	3	4	3	2	1	2
Cancer in general/unspecified type	38	37	29	31	20	23	26	34
Liver disease/cirrhosis of the liver	1	3	7	2	3	3	5	3
Kidney disease	0	3	4	2	2		1	
Arthritis/rheumatism/problems with joints	1		1	1	0	2	1	0
Respiratory/breathing disorders	25	15	8	17	15	18	4	10
TB/tuberculosis	3	2	2	2	1	2	1	9
Throat cancer/mouth cancer	1		0	1	1	1	1	
Other	28	16	14	16	19	18	5	8
None (no serious illnesses are linked to smoking	0	1	1	1	1	1	2	
Don't know	3	3	15	6	28	10	31	10
Base (= 100%)	270	140	283	227	186	268	233	183

Continued on next page

Illness or health problem	African-Caribbean		Indian		Pakistani		Bangladeshi	
	Women	Men	Women	Men	Women	Men	Women	Men
50–74								
Heart trouble/disease/attack	24	24	18	13	15	21	20	16
Diabetes	1	1	2	3	2	3		0
Stroke	1		1	5		6		1
Overweight/obesity	0			3		2	1	0
High blood pressure	4		1	3	3	7		3
Constipation				3		0		
Bowel cancer	1	1	1	1	2	3		3
Lung cancer	41	44	36	51	23	49	25	34
Breast cancer	1	2	9	0	2	2		
Cancer in general/unspecified type	36	27	24	23	23	29	24	27
Liver disease/cirrhosis of the liver	1	3	5	2	5	5		1
Kidney disease	1	2	4	1	4	6	1	
Arthritis/rheumatism/problems with joints			3	0	5			1
Respiratory/breathing disorders	16	11	12	11	10	17	1	24
TB/tuberculosis	1		2	1		1	13	8
Throat cancer/mouth cancer								
Other	19	11	5	16	11	17		7
None (no serious illnesses are linked to smoking	2	2	3	1	3	1	3	2
Don't know	13	16	21	12	31	9	48	16
Base (= 100%)	*193*	*174*	*107*	*107*	*50*	*124*	*63*	*171*
All ages								
Heart trouble/disease/attack	29	24	25	21	30	25	31	24
Diabetes	0	0	0	1	1	3	0	1
Stroke	1	1	1	2	2	4	1	1
Overweight/obesity	1	0	1	1	1	2	0	1
High blood pressure	3	1	1	3	4	5	2	4
Constipation	0	0	0	1	0	1	0	0
Bowel cancer	1	1	2	1	2	4	1	2
Lung cancer	54	50	46	59	37	56	36	45
Breast cancer	1	2	4	3	2	2	2	1
Cancer in general/unspecified type	40	35	28	32	25	30	27	30
Liver disease/cirrhosis of the liver	1	3	7	2	4	3	3	2
Kidney disease	0	2	4	2	3	2	1	0
Arthritis/rheumatism/problems with joints	0	0	1	1	1	1	1	1
Respiratory/breathing disorders	19	13	9	12	13	17	7	15
TB/tuberculosis	1	0	2	1	1	1	4	6
Throat cancer/mouth cancer	1	0	0	0	0	0	0	1
Other	22	14	16	15	17	17	8	11
None (no serious illnesses are linked to smoking	1	2	1	1	1	0	2	1
Don't know	5	9	13	7	21	7	27	10
Base (= 100%)	*641*	*428*	*598*	*463*	*517*	*627*	*603*	*567*

Table 5.8: Which serious health problems are linked to not taking enough exercise? (percentages of all respondents)

Illness or health problem	African-Caribbean		Indian		Pakistani		Bangladeshi	
	Women	Men	Women	Men	Women	Men	Women	Men
16–29								
Heart trouble/disease/attack	48	34	39	37	40	35	27	23
Diabetes		2	5	3	2	6	2	4
Stroke	1	3	8	2	3	4	3	3
Overweight/obesity	41	38	42	45	50	56	43	44
High blood pressure	8	4	7	4	7	9	7	5
Constipation					0	1	0	
Bowel cancer			1			0		
Lung cancer	0			1	1	1		1
Breast cancer					1	1		
Cancer in general/unspecified type	1	1	2	0	1	2	1	1
Liver disease/cirrhosis of the liver		1		1	1			1
Kidney disease				1	2	1	0	
Arthritis/rheumatism/problems with joints	5	7	8	7	8	5	9	5
Tiredness, laziness, feeling dull, sluggish	2	3	3	2	2	8	4	10
Respiratory/breathing disorders (asthma)	3	2	3	1	1	3	1	1
Mental health problems, e.g. depression	1	1	1	1	0			0
Poor circulation	0	1				2		
Back problems/backache	1		0		0	1	1	2
Joint problems/stiffness	0		1		1		0	
Other	11	15	13	17	10	17	9	8
None (no serious illnesses are linked to exercise)		2	4	2	4	0	4	2
Don't know	19	16	16	15	16	13	29	22
QNA			0	2	1	1	0	
Base (= 100%)	178	114	208	129	281	235	307	213
30–49								
Heart trouble/disease/attack	47	44	31	36	23	35	11	14
Diabetes	1	1	3	2	4	7	1	3
Stroke	1	3	6	3	4	4	1	1
Overweigh/obesity	41	36	46	47	34	48	42	44
High blood pressure	8	5	6	9	6	10	3	5
Constipation	0		1	1	1	1		
Bowel cancer	0				0	1		
Lung cancer			1	1		0		
Breast cancer						1		
Cancer in general/unspecified type	0		1			1	0	
Liver disease/cirrhosis of the liver		1	0					
Kidney disease		1	1			0		1
Arthritis/rheumatism/problems with joints	12	10	13	11	10	8	14	20
Tiredness, laziness, feeling dull, sluggish	2	6	3	8	1	4	3	12
Respiratory/breathing disorders (asthma)	5	4	1	4	2	1	0	1
Mental health problems, e.g. depression	3	1	1	1		0		1
Poor circulation	1	2		0	1	1		1
Back problems/backache	0		0	0	2			
Joint problems/stiffness	1	1	0		0	0	1	
Other	14	22	10	17	6	12	3	10
None (no serious illnesses are linked to exercise)	2	1	2	3	4	3	4	1
Don't know	14	15	18	14	36	17	45	22
QNA	0	2	0	1	0	0	1	1
Base (= 100%)	270	140	283	227	186	266	233	183

Continued on next page

Table 5.8: *continued*

Illness or health problem	African-Caribbean		Indian		Pakistani		Bangladeshi	
	Women	Men	Women	Men	Women	Men	Women	Men
50–74								
Heart trouble/disease/attack	34	24	9	24	8	26	5	9
Diabetes	0	0		3	1	5	3	3
Stroke	2	3	2		4	9		2
Overweight/obesity	26	26	38	26	37	46	26	30
High blood pressure	5	3	5	6		5	0	2
Constipation	1	1	1	3		1		
Bowel cancer				0		1		
Lung cancer				0		1		
Breast cancer			3			1		
Cancer in general/ unspecified type			2				2	1
Liver disease/cirrhosis of the liver				3				
Kidney disease			2			0		0
Arthritis/rheumatism/ problems with joints	18	19	31	14	7	19	16	21
Tiredness, laziness, feeling dull, sluggish	3	5	3	6		9		9
Respiratory/breathing disorders (asthma)	1	2	1	2		3		1
Mental health problems, e.g. depression	0		1		1	0		1
Poor circulation	0		1			1		0
Back problems/backache			3					1
Joint problems/stiffness	4	2		0		1		
Other	10	11	11	18	6	11		9
None (no serious illnesses are linked to exercise	6	1	3	10	5	2	6	5
Don't know	21	29	27	19	38	22	61	36
Base (= 100%)	*193*	*174*	*107*	*107*	*50*	*124*	*63*	*171*
All ages								
Heart trouble/disease/attack	43	33	30	33	28	33	17	16
Diabetes	0	1	3	3	3	6	2	4
Stroke	1	3	6	2	4	5	2	2
Overweight/obesity	37	34	43	42	41	51	40	40
High blood pressure	7	4	6	7	5	8	5	4
Constipation	0	0	1	1	1	1	0	0
Bowel cancer	0	0	0	0	0	1	0	0
Lung cancer	0	0	0	1	1	1	0	0
Breast cancer	0	0	0	0	0	1	0	0
Cancer in general/ unspecified type	0	0	1	0	1	1	1	1
Liver disease/cirrhosis of the liver	0	0	0	1	0	0	0	0
Kidney disease	0	0	1	0	1	1	0	0
Arthritis/rheumatism/ problems with joints	11	12	15	10	9	9	12	14
Tiredness, laziness, feeling dull, sluggish	2	4	3	6	1	7	3	10
Respiratory/breathing disorders (asthma)	3	2	2	3	1	2	1	1
Mental health problems, e.g. depression	2	0	1	1	0	0	0	0
Poor circulation	1	1	0	0	0	2	0	0
Back problems/backache	0	0	1	0	1	0	0	1
Joint problems/stiffness	2	1	0	0	0	0	0	0
Other	12	16	11	17	8	14	5	9
None (no serious illnesses are linked to exercise	2	1	3	4	4	2	4	2
Don't know	18	20	19	15	28	17	39	26
Base (= 100%)	*641*	*428*	*598*	*463*	*517*	*627*	*603*	*567*

Table 5.9: Which serious health problems are linked to drinking too much alcohol? (percentages of all respondents)

Illness or health problem	African-Caribbean		Indian		Pakistani		Bangladeshi	
	Women	Men	Women	Men	Women	Men	Women	Men
16–29								
Heart trouble/disease/ attack	16	4	24	19	26	21	10	11
Diabetes	4	2	3	2	1	3	1	
Stroke	0		1	1	0	6	1	0
Overweight/obesity	4	3	6	4	4	17	3	4
High blood pressure	5	7	5	5	3	7	3	3
Constipation					1	1		
Bowel cancer		1	2		1	3		1
Lung cancer	1	1	5	3	6	4	3	2
Breast cancer			1		1	1		1
Cancer in general/ unspecified type	7	3	9	4	4	6	6	3
Liver disease/cirrhosis of the liver	53	46	37	45	20	40	14	26
Kidney disease	20	29	25	27	11	24	11	9
Arthritis/rheumatism/ problems with joints		1	1	1		0	0	
Addiction to alcohol/ alcoholism	5	4	1	3	0	1	1	2
Mental health problems/ brain damage	6	6	3	3	3	7	3	3
Stomach ulcer/ulcer	2	3	1	2		1	0	0
Other	19	18	13	13	10	7	8	9
None (no serious illnesses are linked to alcohol)			2		1	0	1	1
Don't know	12	19	21	14	39	23	60	43
Base (= 100%)	*178*	*114*	*208*	*129*	*281*	*235*	*307*	*213*
30–49								
Heart trouble/disease/ attack	18	12	25	20	23	18	4	8
Diabetes	3	1	3	7	2	7	0	1
Stroke	1		3	3	2	2		1
Overweight/obesity	1	10	4	5	2	7	1	
High blood pressure	5	4	6	12	3	6		1
Constipation	0			1		1		
Bowel cancer	0	1	1	1	1	2		
Lung cancer	3	3	12	4	10	7	0	1
Breast cancer			1	0	1	1		
Cancer in general/ unspecified type	3		6	1	4	3		1
Liver disease/cirrhosis of the liver	67	56	31	47	14	36	3	19
Kidney disease	21	31	13	21	6	28	1	5
Arthritis/rheumatism/ problems with joints	0					1		
Addiction to alcohol/ alcoholism	4	2	1	4	1	1	1	3
Mental health problems/ brain damage	4	4	1	8	0	2	2	4
Stomach ulcer/ulcer			0	1	1	1		4
Other	16	21	7	18	7	6	4	10
None (no serious illnesses are linked to alcohol)	0	1	1	1	0	1	3	
Don't know	8	7	30	16	49	35	87	58
Base (= 100%)	*270*	*140*	*283*	*227*	*186*	*268*	*233*	*183*

Continued on next page

Table 5.9: *continued*

Illness or health problem	African-Caribbean		Indian		Pakistani		Bangladeshi	
	Women	Men	Women	Men	Women	Men	Women	Men
50–74								
Heart trouble/disease/attack	23	23	28	13	18	21		3
Diabetes	4	2	3	0	1	4		
Stroke	1		1	1	1	3		1
Overweight/obesity	4	2	2			8		0
High blood pressure	7	7	4	11	4	6		2
Constipation				0				
Bowel cancer	0	1				3		
Lung cancer	0	1	11	7	10	9		1
Breast cancer			1		1	1		
Cancer in general/unspecified type	2	5	5	2	6	14		2
Liver disease/cirrhosis of the liver	45	38	21	37	8	27		14
Kidney disease	9	17	19	21	7	21		3
Arthritis/rheumatism/problems with joints		1	0	2		1		
Addiction to alcohol/alcoholism	3	1	3	3			0	3
Mental health problems/brain damage	4	5		9		6	1	2
Stomach ulcer/ulcer	0	2	3	2				
Other	20	12	6	23	5	11		3
None (no serious illnesses are linked to alcohol)	3	2	6	0	4	2	3	3
Don't know	16	20	34	19	52	35	96	67
Base (= 100%)	*193*	*174*	*107*	*107*	*50*	*124*	*63*	*171*
All ages								
Heart trouble/disease/attack	19	13	25	18	24	20	6	8
Diabetes	4	2	3	4	1	5	1	0
Stroke	1	0	2	2	1	4	0	1
Overweight/obesity	3	5	4	3	3	11	2	2
High blood pressure	6	6	5	9	3	6	2	2
Constipation	0	0	0	1	0	1	0	0
Bowel cancer	0	1	1	0	1	2	0	0
Lung cancer	2	1	9	4	8	6	1	2
Breast cancer	0	0	1	0	1	1	0	0
Cancer in general/unspecified type	4	3	7	2	5	7	3	2
Liver disease/cirrhosis of the liver	56	46	31	44	16	36	8	21
Kidney disease	17	25	18	23	8	25	6	6
Addiction to alcohol/alcoholism	0	1	0	1	0	1	0	0
Addiction to alcohol/alcoholism	4	2	1	3	1	1	1	2
Mental health problems/brain damage	5	5	1	7	1	5	2	3
Stomach ulcer/ulcer	1	2	1	2	0	1	0	1
Other	18	17	9	17	8	8	6	8
None (no serious illnesses are linked to alcohol)	1	1	2	0	1	1	2	1
Don't know	12	16	27	16	45	30	75	54
QNA								
Base (= 100%)	*641*	*428*	*598*	*463*	*517*	*627*	*603*	*567*

Table 5.10: What kinds of health problems are overweight people more likely to suffer from? (percentages of all respondents)

Illness or health problem	African-Caribbean		Indian		Pakistani		Bangladeshi	
	Women	Men	Women	Men	Women	Men	Women	Men
16–29								
Heart disease	54	43	41	54	50	43	36	28
Heart attack	39	50	40	37	35	52	38	31
Stroke	2	5	9	6	6	7	5	1
High blood pressure	14	8	20	14	26	20	27	18
Diabetes	9	2	10	4	15	12	21	13
Tiredness	4	5	0	3	3	4	2	4
Respiratory/breathing disorders (asthma)	14	5	5	7	7	4	5	8
Back problems/joint problems/arthritis	4	3	2	2	4	4	1	1
Poor circulation	1	1	0		0			
Depression		1	1		1	1		
High cholesterol	0		0	2	1	1		
Mobility problems/ difficulty walking	2	1	5	1	3	3	2	4
Other	25	14	25	18	22	14	11	19
None			1		1	0	1	1
Don't know	8	12	14	7	9	12	20	19
Base (= 100%)	*178*	*114*	*208*	*129*	*281*	*235*	*307*	*213*
30–49								
Heart disease	60	43	34	41	41	48	28	25
Heart attack	42	40	44	52	32	53	35	37
Stroke	7	6	6	6	2	5	2	2
High blood pressure	27	23	26	26	31	26	29	26
Diabetes	9	7	13	13	17	15	25	21
Tiredness	4	2	3	2	2	3	2	4
Respiratory/breathing disorders (asthma)	17	12	9	10	8	6	4	8
Back problems/joint problems/arthritis	8	7	5	5	5	7	3	5
Poor circulation	2	3	1	0	0			
Depression	2	1	0	1				
High cholesterol	1	2	0	0	1			1
Mobility problems/ difficulty walking	0		3	3	2	3	2	9
Other	29	28	25	19	24	17	5	14
None		1	0	1	1		1	1
Don't know	1	6	9	7	16	10	31	12
Base (= 100%)	*270*	*140*	*283*	*227*	*186*	*268*	*233*	*183*

Continued on next page

Table 5.10: *continued*

Illness or health problem	African-Caribbean		Indian		Pakistani		Bangladeshi	
	Women	Men	Women	Men	Women	Men	Women	Men
50–74								
Heart disease	45	39	32	33	35	41	24	22
Heart attack	36	39	35	30	39	48	18	21
Stroke	14	7	3	3	4	4		1
High blood pressure	19	19	22	28	29	17	21	24
Diabetes	12	2	11	12	18	16	21	14
Tiredness	1	4	3	6		6	2	5
Respiratory/breathing disorders (asthma)	4	5	9	12	4	8		11
Back problems/joint problems/arthritis	5	3	6	3	4	7	10	5
Poor circulation	1							
Depression					2			
High cholesterol								
Mobility problems/difficulty walking		0	5	4		7	3	7
Other	20	15	18	21	18	14	4	19
None	0			1	4			2
Don't know	10	10	19	13	17	10	45	21
Base (= 100%)	*193*	*174*	*107*	*107*	*50*	*124*	*63*	*171*
All ages								
Heart disease	54	41	36	43	44	45	31	25
Heart attack	39	43	41	42	35	51	34	30
Stroke	7	6	7	5	4	6	3	1
High blood pressure	20	16	23	22	29	22	27	22
Diabetes	10	4	12	10	16	14	22	16
Tiredness	3	4	2	3	2	4	2	4
Respiratory/breathing disorders (asthma)	13	7	7	9	7	6	4	9
Back problems/joint problems/arthritis	6	4	4	3	5	6	3	3
Poor circulation	1	1	0	0	0	0	0	0
Depression	1	1	0	1	1	1	0	0
High cholesterol	1	1	0	1	1	0	0	0
Mobility problems/difficulty walking	1	0	4	3	2	4	2	6
Other	25	19	24	19	22	15	8	18
None	0	0	1	1	1	0	1	1
Don't know	6	10	13	8	13	11	28	18
Base (= 100%)	*641*	*428*	*598*	*463*	*517*	*627*	*603*	*567*

Table 5.11: Is there anything people can do to reduce their risk of getting serious illnesses? (percentages of all respondents)

Response	African-Caribbean Women	African-Caribbean Men	Indian Women	Indian Men	Pakistani Women	Pakistani Men	Bangladeshi Women	Bangladeshi Men
16–29								
Yes	90	83	82	93	81	89	69	73
No	5	6	9	3	11	5	4	9
Don't know	5	11	9	5	9	6	27	18
Base (= 100%)	*176*	*114*	*208*	*128*	*280*	*234*	*305*	*208*
30–49								
Yes	90	88	66	80	54	80	54	69
No	6	8	11	11	20	9	9	9
Don't know	4	4	23	9	25	11	37	22
Base (= 100%)	*267*	*139*	*283*	*227*	*185*	*266*	*230*	*176*
50–74								
Yes	79	69	68	67	56	74	37	45
No	7	11	10	17	14	15	12	19
Don't know	13	21	21	16	30	11	51	37
Base (= 100%)	*189*	*174*	*107*	*106*	*48*	*123*	*63*	*164*
All ages								
Yes	87	79	72	81	66	82	59	63
No	6	8	10	10	15	8	7	12
Don't know	7	12	18	9	18	9	34	25
QNA								
Base (= 100%)	*632*	*427*	*598*	*461*	*513*	*623*	*599*	*548*

Table 5.12: Actions taken to enhance health (percentages of all respondents taking action)

Action	African-Caribbean Women	African-Caribbean Men	Indian Women	Indian Men	Pakistani Women	Pakistani Men	Bangladeshi Women	Bangladeshi Men
16–29								
1	47	62	46	54	43	46	37	58
2–4	50	35	46	46	53	46	49	39
5 or more	3	3	7		4	8	15	2
Base (= 100%)	*108*	*85*	*112*	*94*	*133*	*151*	*124*	*119*
30–49								
1	43	51	41	47	48	46	34	42
2–4	53	48	56	49	49	51	39	58
5 or more	5	1	3	4	3	3	27	
Base (= 100%)	*182*	*99*	*124*	*143*	*74*	*159*	*51*	*64*
50–74								
1	33	47	28	31	47	44	8	49
2–4	62	51	68	61	43	53	79	51
5 or more	5	2	4	9	10	3	13	
Base (= 100%)	*116*	*98*	*54*	*61*	*23*	*74*	*7*	*51*
All ages								
1	42	54	40	46	45	46	34	53
2–4	54	44	55	50	50	49	48	46
5 or more	4	2	5	3	5	5	18	1
Base (= 100%)	*406*	*282*	*290*	*298*	*230*	*384*	*182*	*234*

Chapter 6 Cigarette smoking and the use of chewing tobacco products

Table 6.1: Have you ever smoked a cigarette, cigar or pipe? (Q38)
(percentages of all respondents)

Response	African-Caribbean		Indian		Pakistani		Bangladeshi	
	Women	Men	Women	Men	Women	Men	Women	Men
16–29								
Yes	56	54	18	26	15	42	8	44
No	44	46	82	74	85	58	92	56
Base (= 100%)	*178*	*114*	*208*	*129*	*281*	*235*	*306*	*213*
30–49								
Yes	50	69	4	43	5	43	7	67
No	50	31	96	57	95	57	93	33
Base (= 100%)	*269*	*140*	*283*	*226*	*183*	*266*	*233*	*183*
50–74								
Yes	23	68	2	49	11	59	24	89
No	77	32	98	51	89	41	76	11
Base (= 100%)	*192*	*173*	*106*	*107*	*50*	*124*	*63*	*171*
All ages								
Yes	45	63	8	39	11	46	10	64
No	55	37	92	61	89	54	90	36
Base (= 100%)	*639*	*427*	*597*	*462*	*514*	*625*	*602*	*567*

Table 6.2: Do you smoke cigarettes at all, nowadays? (Q39)
(percentages of all who have ever smoked)

Response	African-Caribbean		Indian		Pakistani		Bangladeshi	
	Women	Men	Women	Men	Women	Men	Women	Men
16–29								
Yes	54	56	31	40	22	56	33	67
No	46	44	69	60	78	44	67	33
Base (= 100%)	*110*	*64*	*33*	*38*	*43*	*95*	*22*	*100*
30–49								
Yes	48	60	37	52	22	73	100	81
No	52	40	63	48	78	27		19
Base (= 100%)	*146*	*95*	*16*	*95*	*12*	*120*	*15*	*128*
50–74								
Yes	21	45	26	39	6	50	59	78
No	79	55	74	61	94	50	41	22
Base (= 100%)	*54*	*121*	*3*	*50*	*4*	*68*	*11*	*150*
All ages								
Yes	47	53	32	45	19	60	60	76
No	53	47	68	55	81	40	40	24
Base (= 100%)	*310*	*280*	*52*	*183*	*59*	*283*	*48*	*378*

Table 6.3: Have you ever smoked cigarettes regularly? (Q40)
(percentages of all who have ever smoked, but not currently smokers)

Response	African-Caribbean		Indian		Pakistani		Bangladeshi	
	Women	Men	Women	Men	Women	Men	Women	Men
16–29								
Yes	26	23	24	11	12	33	12	23
No	74	77	76	89	88	67	88	77
Base (= 100%)	*42*	*25*	*24*	*18*	*31*	*31*	*14*	*31*
30–49								
Yes	32	47	33	33		40		89
No	68	53	67	67	100	60		11
Base (= 100%)	*63*	*34*	*6*	*43*	*10*	*26*	*0*	*22*
50–74								
Yes	37	63	35	82	35	72	100	84
No	63	37	65	18	65	28		16
Base (= 100%)	*40*	*65*	*2*	*27*	*3*	*33*	*2*	*36*
All ages								
Yes	30	47	26	43	14	49	43	62
No	70	53	74	57	86	51	57	38
Base (= 100%)	*145*	*124*	*32*	*88*	*44*	*90*	*16*	*89*

Table 6.4: Mean number of cigarettes smoked per day, when a regular smoker (Q41)
(means of all who have ever smoked, but are not currently smokers)

Age group	African-Caribbean		Indian		Pakistani		Bangladeshi	
	Women	Men	Women	Men	Women	Men	Women	Men
16–29	6	8	4	6	6	9	10	10
30–49	9	17	13	13		14		17
50–74	15	12	2	18	20	6	50	4
All	*10*	*13*	*6*	*16*	*12*	*13*	*42*	*15*

Table 6.5: Years since ceased smoking (Q42)
(mean number of years of all ex-cigarette smokers)

Age group	African-Caribbean		Indian		Pakistani		Bangladeshi	
	Women	Men	Women	Men	Women	Men	Women	Men
16–29	4	5	4	5	4	3	2	2
30–49	13	13	6	10	8	7	0	4
50–74	19	18	13	15	1	11	14	9
All	*10*	*13*	*5*	*10*	*4*	*7*	*6*	*5*

Table 6.6: Do you smoke cigarettes regularly nowadays? (Q43)
(percentages of all who have ever smoked, and are currently smokers)

Age group	African-Caribbean Women	Men	Indian Women	Men	Pakistani Women	Men	Bangladeshi Women	Men
16–29								
Yes	86	78	78	71	65	92	100	89
No	14	22	22	29	35	8		11
Weighted base (= 100%)	*67*	*39*	*9*	*20*	*11*	*64*	*7*	*68*
30–49								
Yes	88	91	100	87	100	81	100	97
No	12	9		13		19		3
Weighted base (= 100%)	*82*	*61*	*7*	*51*	*2*	*94*	*15*	*106*
50–74								
Yes	76	87	100	100	100	93	100	93
No	24	13				7		7
Weighted base (= 100%)	*14*	*56*	*1*	*23*	*1*	*35*	*9*	*114*
All ages								
Yes	86	86	84	87	74	88	100	93
No	14	14	16	13	26	12	0	7
Weighted base (= 100%)	*163*	*156*	*17*	*94*	*14*	*193*	*31*	*288*

Table 6.7: How many cigarettes do you usually smoke on each weekday? (Q44)
(mean number of all who have ever smoked, and are currently smokers)

Age group	African-Caribbean Women	Men	Indian Women	Men	Pakistani Women	Men	Bangladeshi Women	Men
16–29	9	17	9	6	10	9	6	15
30–49	10	10	13	10	13	11	12	18
50–74	7	10	36	21	6	15	14	17
All	*9*	*12*	*11*	*12*	*11*	*11*	*11*	*17*

Table 6.8: How many cigarettes a day do you usually smoke on weekends? (Q45)
(mean number of cigarettes of all who have ever smoked, and are currently smokers)

Age group	African-Caribbean Women	Men	Indian Women	Men	Pakistani Women	Men	Bangladeshi Women	Men
16–29	13	13	13	8	11	12	6	12
30–49	13	14	10	10	18	11	5	15
50–74	7	11	36	18	8	15	5	12
All	*13*	*13*	*13*	*12*	*13*	*12*	*6*	*13*

Table 6.9: Have you ever attempted to give up smoking? (Q46)
(percentages of all current smokers)

Age group	African-Caribbean		Indian		Pakistani		Bangladeshi	
	Women	Men	Women	Men	Women	Men	Women	Men
16–29								
Yes	69	49	85	45	65	46	64	55
No	31	51	15	55	35	54	36	45
Base (= 100%)	62	36	9	19	11	64	7	68
30–49								
Yes	67	63	100	63	50	59	78	75
No	33	37		37	50	41	22	25
Base (= 100%)	79	58	7	51	2	89	14	101
50–74								
Yes	58	64	100	68		61	90	77
No	42	36		32	100	39	10	23
Base (= 100%)	14	54	1	23	1	33	8	110
All ages								
Yes	68	59	89	61	59	55	79	71
No	32	41	11	39	41	45	21	29
Base (= 100%)	155	148	17	93	14	186	29	279

Table 6.10: Have you ever attempted to give up smoking: regular and occasional smokers? (Q46) (percentages of all current smokers)

	African-Caribbean		Indian		Pakistani		Bangladeshi	
	Women	Men	Women	Men	Women	Men	Women	Men
Regular smokers								
16–29								
Yes	69	56	90	45	58	49	64	52
No	31	44	10	55	42	51	36	48
Base (= 100%)	*57*	*29*	*7*	*14*	*7*	*59*	*7*	*61*
30–49								
Yes	73	66	100	67	50	58	78	75
No	27	34		33	50	42	22	25
Base (= 100%)	*71*	*52*	*7*	*45*	*2*	*79*	*14*	*97*
50–74								
Yes	55	64	100	68		61	90	76
No	45	36		32	100	39	10	24
Base (= 100%)	*12*	*49*	*1*	*23*	*1*	*30*	*8*	*102*
All ages								
Yes	70	63	94	64	52	55	79	70
No	30	37	6	36	48	45	21	30
Base(= 100%)	*140*	*130*	*15*	*82*	*10*	*168*	*29*	*260*
Occasional smokers								
16–29								
Yes	66	26	67	46	79	17		75
No	34	74	33	54	21	83		25
Base (= 100%)	*4*	*7*	*2*	*5*	*4*	*5*	*0*	*7*
30–49								
Yes	21	39		33		61		75
No	79	61		67		39		25
Base (= 100%)	*8*	*6*	*0*	*6*	*0*	*10*	*0*	*4*
50–74								
Yes	67	68				60		100
No	33	32				40		
Base (= 100%)	*2*	*5*	*0*	*0*	*0*	*3*	*0*	*8*
All ages								
Yes	49	39	67	38	79	52		86
No	51	61	33	62	21	48		14
Base (= 100%)	*14*	*18*	*2*	*11*	*4*	*18*	*0*	*19*

Table 6.11: Have you ever used one of these substances? (Q47)
(percentages of all Asians)

Substance	Indian		Pakistani		Bangladeshi	
	Women	Men	Women	Men	Women	Men
16–29						
Betel nut/sopari						
Chewed with tobacco	3	7		17	26	34
Chewed without tobacco	29	32	59	63	75	81
Chewing tobacco on its own		2		6	3	8
Paan with tobacco	9	16	6	9	22	24
Paan without tobacco	90	76	64	69	59	61
Base (= 100%)	*46*	*30*	*21*	*31*	*145*	*118*
30–49						
Betel nut/sopari						
Chewed with tobacco	12	21	7	22	59	50
Chewed without tobacco	69	64	56	34	51	74
Chewing tobacco on its own		13	4	4	2	12
Paan with tobacco	4	23	18	10	53	42
Paan without tobacco	78	79	70	77	34	65
Base (= 100%)	*73*	*76*	*21*	*50*	*198*	*150*
50–74						
Betel nut/sopari						
Chewed with tobacco	14	20	19	13	88	56
Chewed without tobacco	65	72	49	53	26	83
Chewing tobacco on its own	10	10	19	12	6	17
Paan with tobacco	4	22	19	15	75	53
Paan without tobacco	70	75	51	77	22	79
Base (= 100%)	*27*	*36*	*5*	*25*	*61*	*133*
All ages						
Betel nut/sopari						
Chewed with tobacco	10	18	6	18	54	47
Chewed without tobacco	55	59	56	47	54	80
Chewing tobacco on its own	2	9	4	7	3	13
Paan with tobacco	6	21	13	11	47	40
Paan without tobacco	80	77	65	75	39	69
Base (= 100%)	*146*	*142*	*47*	*106*	*404*	*401*

Table 6.12: Have you used one of these substances in the last four weeks? (Q48) (percentages of all Asians)

Substance	Indian Women	Indian Men	Pakistani Women	Pakistani Men	Bangladeshi Women	Bangladeshi Men
16–29						
Betel nut/sopari						
Chewed with tobacco	8	26		25	26	29
Chewed without tobacco	21	48	75	55	73	81
Chewing tobacco on its own					1	6
Paan with tobacco					18	16
Paan without tobacco	92	52	66	35	49	51
Base (= 100%)	*8*	*4*	*4*	*4*	*120*	*98*
30–49						
Betel nut/sopari						
Chewed with tobacco	4	26	21	63	57	44
Chewed without tobacco	66	53	48	6	47	75
Chewing tobacco on its own		21			2	8
Paan with tobacco		20	10	9	54	34
Paan without tobacco	64	59	31	54	35	63
Base (= 100%)	*21*	*27*	*4*	*7*	*184*	*131*
50–74						
Betel nut/sopari						
Chewed with tobacco	32	23	50		91	46
Chewed without tobacco	32	71		65	26	79
Chewing tobacco on its own			50	11	5	5
Paan with tobacco	11	12	50	25	76	38
Paan without tobacco	28	34	50	11	21	68
Base (= 100%)	*7*	*15*	*2*	*5*	*58*	*116*
All ages						
Betel nut/sopari						
Chewed with tobacco	13	25	16	32	55	40
Chewed without tobacco	48	59	52	38	51	78
Chewing tobacco on its own	0	11	10	4	2	6
Paan with tobacco	3	15	13	12	48	30
Paan without tobacco	59	49	53	34	36	61
Base (= 100%)	*36*	*46*	*10*	*16*	*362*	*345*

Table 6.13a: Current smoking status (percentages of all respondents)

Status	African-Caribbean Women	African-Caribbean Men	Indian Women	Indian Men	Pakistani Women	Pakistani Men	Bangladeshi Women	Bangladeshi Men
16–29								
Current regular smoker	26	24	4	8	2	22	3	26
Ex-smoker	26	24	12	16	11	18	5	15
Never smoked/ occasional smoker	48	52	83	77	86	60	92	59
Base (= 100%)	*177*	*114*	*208*	*129*	*280*	*235*	*305*	*212*
30–49								
Current regular smoker	21	37	1	20	1	25	7	53
Ex-smoker	26	28	2	20	4	12		13
Never smoked/ occasional smoker	53	35	97	60	95	63	93	35
Base (= 100%)	*268*	*140*	*280*	*225*	*183*	*266*	*233*	*183*
50–74								
Current regular smoker	4	27	0	19	1	27	14	65
Ex-smoker	18	37	1	30	10	29	10	19
Never smoked/ occasional smoker	78	36	98	51	89	43	76	15
Base (= 100%)	*192*	*173*	*106*	*107*	*50*	*124*	*63*	*171*
All ages								
Current regular smoker	18	29	2	15	2	24	6	46
Ex-smoker	24	30	5	21	8	18	4	15
Never smoked/ occasional smoker	58	42	92	64	90	57	90	39
Base (= 100%)	*637*	*427*	*594*	*461*	*513*	*625*	*601*	*566*

Table 6.13b: Current smoking status (percentages of all respondents)

Status	African-Caribbean		Indian		Pakistani		Bangladeshi	
	Women	Men	Women	Men	Women	Men	Women	Men
16–29								
Current regular smoker	26	24	4	8	2	22	3	26
Current occasional smoker	4	7	1	3	1	2		3
Ex-smoker or never smoked	70	70	94	89	97	76	98	70
Base (= 100%)	*177*	*114*	*208*	*129*	*281*	*235*	*307*	*212*
30–49								
Current regular smoker	21	37	1	20	1	25	7	53
Current occasional smoker	3	4		3		6		2
Ex-smoker or never smoked	76	59	99	79	100	70	93	46
Base (= 100%)	*269*	*140*	*283*	*227*	*186*	*268*	*233*	*183*
50–74								
Current regular smoker	4	27	0	19	1	27	14	65
Current occasional smoker	1	4				2		5
Ex-smoker or never smoked	96	70	100	81	99	71	86	30
Base (= 100%)	*193*	*174*	*107*	*107*	*50*	*124*	*63*	*171*
All ages								
Current regular smoker	18	29	2	15	2	24	6	46
Current occasional smoker	3	5	0	2	1	3	0	3
Ex-smoker or never smoked	80	67	98	83	99	73	95	51
Base (= 100%)	*639*	*428*	*598*	*463*	*517*	*627*	*603*	*566*

Table 6.13c: Current smoking status (percentages of all respondents)

Status	African-Caribbean Women	African-Caribbean Men	Indian Women	Indian Men	Pakistani Women	Pakistani Men	Bangladeshi Women	Bangladeshi Men
16–29								
Current smoker	30	30	6	11	3	24	3	30
Former regular smoker	7	6	3	2	2	6	1	3
Never been a regular smoker	63	64	91	88	95	70	97	67
Base (= 100%)	*178*	*114*	*208*	*129*	*281*	*235*	*306*	*213*
30–49								
Current smoker	24	41	1	22	1	31	7	54
Former regular smoker	8	13	1	7		5		11
Never been a regular smoker	68	46	98	71	99	64	93	35
Base (= 100%)	*269*	*140*	*283*	*226*	*183*	*266*	*233*	*183*
50–74								
Current smoker	5	31	0	19	1	29	14	70
Former regular smoker	7	23	0	24	4	21	10	16
Never been a regular smoker	89	46	99	56	96	50	76	14
Base (= 100%)	*192*	*173*	*106*	*107*	*50*	*124*	*63*	*171*
All ages								
Current smoker	21	34	3	18	2	28	6	49
Former regular smoker	7	14	2	9	2	9	2	10
Never been a regular smoker	72	52	96	73	97	63	92	42
Base (= 100%)	*639*	*427*	*597*	*462*	*514*	*625*	*602*	*567*

Table 6.14: Mean number of cigarettes smoked per week (mean of all who have ever smoked and are currently smokers)

Age group	African-Caribbean Women	African-Caribbean Men	Indian Women	Indian Men	Pakistani Women	Pakistani Men	Bangladeshi Women	Bangladeshi Men
16–29	71	109	72	45	75	69	41	98
30–49	77	76	86	69	100	76	71	119
50–74	50	71	252	139	46	107	85	108
All	*72*	*85*	*81*	*81*	*79*	*81*	*69*	*109*

Table 6.15a: Mean number of cigarettes smoked per day
(percentages of all who have ever smoked and are currently smokers)

Age group	African-Caribbean Women	African-Caribbean Men	Indian Women	Indian Men	Pakistani Women	Pakistani Men	Bangladeshi Women	Bangladeshi Men
16–29								
0–19	88	73	90	100	91	93	93	72
20 or more	12	27	10		9	7	7	28
Base (= 100%)	*68*	*39*	*9*	*20*	*11*	*64*	*7*	*69*
30–49								
0–19	82	88	92	82	50	76	78	63
20 or more	18	12	8	18	50	24	22	37
Base (= 100%)	*83*	*61*	*7*	*51*	*2*	*94*	*15*	*106*
50–74								
0–19	95	85		58	100	74	75	73
20 or more	5	15	100	42		26	25	27
Base (= 100%)	*14*	*56*	*1*	*23*	*1*	*35*	*9*	*114*
All ages								
0–19	86	82	88	80	82	81	80	69
20 or more	14	18	12	20	18	19	20	31
Base (= 100%)	*165*	*156*	*17*	*94*	*14*	*193*	*31*	*289*

Table 6.15b: Mean number of cigarettes smoked per day
(mean of all who have ever smoked and are currently smokers)

Age group	African-Caribbean Women	African-Caribbean Men	Indian Women	Indian Men	Pakistani Women	Pakistani Men	Bangladeshi Women	Bangladeshi Men
16–29	10	16	10	6	11	10	6	14
30–49	11	11	12	10	14	11	10	17
50–74	7	10	36	20	7	15	12	15
All ages	10	12	12	12	11	12	10	16

Chapter 7 Activity and physical fitness

Table 7.1: Perceived health effects of lack of exercise (percentages of all respondents)

Health effects	African-Caribbean		Indian		Pakistani		Bangladeshi	
	Women	Men	Women	Men	Women	Men	Women	Men
16–29								
Get fat/overweight	52	53	64	68	67	74	69	64
Diabetes	1		2	5	5	5	6	2
Heart disease/heart attack	31	31	35	35	40	44	36	28
Stroke	3	4	4	6	5	6	6	4
Stiff joints/arthritis	17	10	19	13	8	14	21	9
Backache	4		8	4	5	5	7	1
Get out of breath easily	20	10	21	13	22	12	21	10
Less able to cope with worries/stress	7	2	7	5	4	3	5	4
Minor ailments such as colds, coughs	1	3	3	2	5	3	1	3
Feel tired all the time, feel weak, low	6	13	1	3	8	3	4	9
Become lazy	4	4	2	4	4	8	1	7
High blood pressure	2	2	2	8	4	8	6	4
Unfit/not healthy	6	5	5	2	1	1	2	5
Respiratory problems	1	1		2	1	0	1	
Circulatory problems		1	2		0	1		0
Other	16	20	22	20	23	17	14	19
None	2	4	2	1	2	1	1	1
Don't know	10	10	10	6	8	4	14	7
Base (= 100%)	*178*	*114*	*208*	*129*	*281*	*235*	*307*	*213*
30–49								
Get fat/overweight	55	56	66	64	62	65	70	66
Diabetes	0	1	3	6	9	7	6	6
Heart disease/heart attack	33	38	30	39	28	38	22	26
Stroke	2	3	2	5	3	5	3	2
Stiff joints/arthritis	13	16	23	20	18	18	31	17
Backache	3	3	4	3	10	5	9	2
Get out of breath easily	13	20	18	16	9	12	21	3
Less able to cope with worries/stress	4	7	5	5	4	5	3	6
Minor ailments such as colds, coughs	4	0	6	4	6	6	1	3
Feel tired all the time feel weak, low	17	8	6	7	5	2	2	11
Become lazy	5	2	2	8	2	7	1	11
High blood pressure	2	2	2	7	4	5		1
Unfit/not healthy	7	7	2	6	4	5	0	7
Respiratory problems	0	1		2		1		
Circulatory problems	1	1		1	1		1	
Other	27	26	20	21	15	19	2	13
None	2	3	1	2	2	3	1	0
Don't know	9	7	10	7	16	7	19	14
Base (= 100%)	*270*	*140*	*283*	*227*	*186*	*268*	*233*	*183*

Continued on next page

Table 7.1: *continued*

Health effects	African-Caribbean		Indian		Pakistani		Bangladeshi	
	Women	Men	Women	Men	Women	Men	Women	Men
50–74								
Get fat/overweight	46	38	66	49	65	62	58	48
Diabetes	1		2	6	3	4	6	4
Heart disease/heart attack	21	22	18	25	13	32	20	10
Stroke	2	3	2	5	2	5	1	
Stiff joints/arthritis	23	22	31	23	29	30	29	22
Backache	4	4	7	4	8	3		4
Get out of breath easily	10	8	17	11	9	5	16	8
Less able to cope with worries/stress	3	4	6	6	2	4	1	1
Minor ailments such as colds, coughs	3	1	3	6	5	4		3
Feel tired all the time, feel weak, low	11	7	5	9	7	5		6
Become lazy	4	8	3	9		11		6
High blood pressure	0	3	1	2	2	4	0	1
Unfit/not healthy	5	1	3	4		3		3
Respiratory problems						1		1
Circulatory problems	1		0			1		2
Other	27	14	9	25	9	18	2	11
None	2	3	3	1	3			2
Don't know	15	16	14	14	17	8	33	26
Base (= 100%)	*193*	*174*	*107*	*107*	*50*	*124*	*63*	*171*
All ages								
Get fat/overweight	51	48	65	62	65	68	68	60
Diabetes	1	0	3	6	7	6	6	4
Heart disease/heart attack	29	30	30	34	31	39	28	22
Stroke	2	3	3	5	4	5	4	2
Stiff joints/arthritis	17	16	23	18	15	19	26	15
Backache	4	2	6	4	7	5	7	2
Get out of breath easily	15	12	19	14	15	11	20	7
Less able to cope with worries/stress	5	4	6	5	4	4	4	4
Minor ailments such as colds, coughs	2	2	5	4	5	5	1	3
Feel tired all the time, feel weak, low	12	9	4	6	7	3	3	9
Become lazy	5	5	2	7	3	8	1	8
High blood pressure	1	2	2	6	3	6	3	2
Unfit/not healthy	6	4	3	4	2	3	1	5
Respiratory problems	1	0	1	1	1	1	0	0
Circulatory problems	1	1		0	0	0	1	1
Other	23	19	19	22	18	18	7	15
None	2	3	2	1	2	2	1	1
Don't know	11	11	10	8	13	6	19	15
Base (= 100%)	*641*	*428*	*598*	*463*	*517*	*627*	*603*	*567*

Table 7.2: Respondent's perception of their own level of physical activity, relative to people of the same age (percentages of all respondents)

Activity level	African-Caribbean		Indian		Pakistani		Bangladeshi	
	Women	Men	Women	Men	Women	Men	Women	Men
16–29								
Very physically active	18	38	15	22	18	22	19	34
Fairly physically active	57	49	61	65	58	57	61	57
Not very physically active	20	12	23	11	16	20	13	6
Not at all physically active	5	1	2	1	7	2	5	2
Don't know		1	0		1		1	1
Base (= 100%)	*176*	*111*	*208*	*129*	*281*	*235*	*307*	*212*
30–49								
Very physically active	28	39	17	20	20	15	17	15
Fairly physically active	50	46	67	62	50	66	51	59
Not very physically active	19	13	13	14	21	15	29	18
Not at all physically active	3	2	2	4	8	4	3	7
Don't know		1	1	0	1		1	1
Base (= 100%)	*266*	*135*	*283*	*227*	*186*	*268*	*232*	*183*
50–74								
Very physically active	24	27	10	17	11	8	5	7
Fairly physically active	52	52	65	57	41	49	28	35
Not very physically active	14	15	15	17	33	25	53	37
Not at all physically active	9	5	8	9	10	18	14	20
Don't know	1		2	1	5	0		1
Base (= 100%)	*193*	*166*	*107*	*107*	*50*	*124*	*63*	*171*
All ages								
Very physically active	23	34	15	20	18	16	16	20
Fairly physically active	53	49	64	62	52	59	53	51
Not very physically active	18	13	17	14	21	19	25	19
Not at all physically active	5	3	3	4	8	6	5	9
Don't know	0	1	1	0	2	0	1	1
Base (= 100%)	*635*	*412*	*598*	*463*	*517*	*627*	*602*	*566*

Table 7.3: Respondent's perception of their own level of physical fitness, relative to people of the same age (percentages of all respondents)

Fitness level	African-Caribbean		Indian		Pakistani		Bangladeshi	
	Women	Men	Women	Men	Women	Men	Women	Men
16–29								
Very fit	8	29	13	15	16	17	22	27
Fairly fit	68	63	64	69	60	68	62	65
Not very fit	20	8	16	14	21	13	14	6
Not at all fit	4		6	1	3	2	2	2
Don't know			1		0		1	0
Base (= 100%)	*178*	*114*	*208*	*129*	*281*	*235*	*307*	*213*
30–49								
Very fit	22	33	16	20	19	16	15	19
Fairly fit	61	58	68	65	58	64	54	58
Not very fit	14	8	14	13	20	16	27	19
Not at all fit	3	1	1	2	3	3	4	3
Don't know			1	0	0		0	1
Base (= 100%)	*270*	*139*	*283*	*227*	*186*	*268*	*233*	*183*
50–74								
Very fit	19	30	13	17	9	14	6	8
Fairly fit	52	46	59	62	41	45	36	38
Not very fit	18	19	20	12	44	21	45	33
Not at all fit	10	4	5	9	7	18	13	21
Don't know	1	0	3	1		1		1
Base (= 100%)	*193*	*174*	*107*	*107*	*50*	*124*	*63*	*171*
All ages								
Very fit	16	31	15	18	16	16	17	19
Fairly fit	61	56	65	66	56	61	56	55
Not very fit	17	12	16	13	24	16	23	18
Not at all fit	5	2	3	3	4	6	4	8
Don't know	0	0	1	0	0	0	0	1
Base (= 100%)	*641*	*427*	*598*	*463*	*517*	*627*	*603*	*567*

Table 7.4: Respondent's perception as to whether they get enough exercise in order to keep fit (percentages of all respondents)

Response	African-Caribbean		Indian		Pakistani		Bangladeshi	
	Women	Men	Women	Men	Women	Men	Women	Men
16–29								
Yes	42	58	53	59	59	60	47	59
No	56	41	45	38	40	39	47	37
Don't know	2	2	2	2	1	1	6	4
Base (= 100%)	178	114	208	129	281	234	303	212
30–49								
Yes	51	56	67	62	57	59	28	32
No	49	43	30	36	33	40	62	60
Don't know	1	1	3	2	10	1	10	8
Base (= 100%)	270	138	283	227	186	267	233	182
50–74								
Yes	62	67	72	67	58	56	11	36
No	37	29	21	32	34	44	74	52
Don't know	2	4	8	1	8		15	12
Base (= 100%)	193	173	107	106	50	123	63	171
All ages								
Yes	50	60	63	62	58	59	35	44
No	48	37	34	36	36	41	56	48
Don't know	2	2	4	2	6	1	9	8
Base (= 100%)	641	425	598	462	517	624	599	565

Table 7.5: Opinions as to whether most people get enough exercise in everyday life in order to keep themselves fit (percentages of all respondents)

Response	African-Caribbean		Indian		Pakistani		Bangladeshi	
	Women	Men	Women	Men	Women	Men	Women	Men
16–29								
Yes	13	8	31	18	33	23	44	40
No	72	66	54	67	48	59	32	47
Don't know	15	26	15	15	19	17	24	13
Base (= 100%)	175	112	206	128	279	232	303	212
30–49								
Yes	18	13	40	17	37	22	56	40
No	71	73	36	54	32	53	6	33
Don't know	11	13	24	29	31	25	38	27
Base (= 100%)	270	140	283	227	186	268	233	182
50–74								
Yes	28	15	32	30	43	28	39	33
No	45	46	32	42	8	52	16	34
Don't know	27	39	36	28	50	20	45	33
Base (= 100%)	192	174	107	107	50	124	63	171
All ages								
Yes	19	12	35	20	36	24	48	38
No	64	61	41	56	35	55	20	39
Don't know	17	27	23	24	28	21	32	23
Base (= 100%)	637	426	596	462	515	624	599	565

Table 7.6: Taking vigorous exercise (makes the respondent out of breath/sweaty) at least three times a week for 20 minutes or more each (percentages of all respondents)

Response	African-Caribbean		Indian		Pakistani		Bangladeshi	
	Women	Men	Women	Men	Women	Men	Women	Men
16–29								
Yes	31	54	21	55	21	46	20	51
No	69	46	79	45	79	54	80	49
Base (= 100%)	*176*	*113*	*208*	*129*	*280*	*230*	*304*	*213*
30–49								
Yes	24	34	15	31	10	24	7	22
No	76	66	85	69	90	76	93	78
Base (= 100%)	*270*	*140*	*283*	*226*	*186*	*265*	*230*	*182*
50–74								
Yes	11	18	13	12	18	18		14
No	89	82	87	88	82	82	100	86
Base (= 100%)	*192*	*174*	*107*	*107*	*50*	*123*	*63*	*170*
All ages								
Yes	23	35	17	35	16	32	12	32
No	77	65	83	65	84	68	88	68
Base (= 100%)	*638*	*427*	*598*	*462*	*516*	*618*	*597*	*565*

Table 7.7: Taking vigorous exercise (makes the respondent out of breath/sweaty for 20 minutes or more each time) at least once a week (percentages of respondents who did not take vigorous exercise at least three times a week)

Response	African-Caribbean		Indian		Pakistani		Bangladeshi	
	Women	Men	Women	Men	Women	Men	Women	Men
16–29								
Yes	35	44	29	42	27	31	14	36
No	65	56	71	58	73	69	86	64
Base (= 100%)	*115*	*50*	*164*	*52*	*219*	*124*	*244*	*92*
30–49								
Yes	26	28	13	18	13	17	3	7
No	74	72	87	82	87	83	97	93
Base (= 100%)	*201*	*90*	*234*	*151*	*163*	*197*	*209*	*130*
50–74								
Yes	14	9	5	11	10	11	0	2
No	86	91	95	89	90	89	100	98
Base (= 100%)	*167*	*142*	*90*	*87*	*44*	*103*	*62*	*135*
All ages								
Yes	25	23	17	21	18	20	7	13
No	75	77	83	79	82	80	93	87
Base (= 100%)	*483*	*282*	*488*	*290*	*426*	*424*	*515*	*357*

Table 7.8a: Importance of different types of advice for persons of the respondent's age who wishes to be healthy (percentages of all respondents)

Advice and response	African-Caribbean Women	African-Caribbean Men	Indian Women	Indian Men	Pakistani Women	Pakistani Men	Bangladeshi Women	Bangladeshi Men
16–29								
(a) To get out and about								
Very important	62	62	64	50	66	53	64	53
Fairly important	31	36	30	40	30	41	29	39
Not very important	8	3	5	7	3	5	5	6
Not at all important					1	0	1	
Don't know			1	3	0	1	1	1
(b) To get a good night's sleep								
Very important	74	67	79	67	79	67	85	75
Fairly important	23	33	16	29	19	28	13	22
Not very important	3		4	3	1	3	2	2
Not at all important					0	0		
Don't know	1		2	1	0	1		1
(c) To avoid getting overweight								
Very important	70	72	70	66	67	64	66	63
Fairly important	27	25	25	29	29	29	25	32
Not very important	3	3	2	3	3	6	8	2
Not at all important				2	1		0	1
Don't know			3	1	0	1	1	2
(d) To avoid worrying too much								
Very important	63	54	61	39	62	47	64	50
Fairly important	32	37	31	49	28	38	28	37
Not very important	5	7	7	8	8	14	7	9
Not at all important	1	2		3	1	0	1	2
Don't know			1	1	2	1	1	2
(e) Not to smoke								
Very important	76	68	83	70	77	72	82	74
Fairly important	20	22	12	25	17	22	12	18
Not very important	3	9	1	4	2	5	4	5
Not at all important	1	1	1		1	1	1	1
Don't know	0		2	1	2	1	1	1
(f) To exercise regularly								
Very important	59	64	62	61	54	63	58	57
Fairly important	39	31	32	37	36	34	35	41
Not very important	2	4	5	2	9	2	6	0
Not at all important					0		0	
Don't know		1	2	1	1	1	1	2
(g) Not to drink much alcohol								
Very important	50	53	66	47	71	66	73	58
Fairly important	44	37	27	43	19	26	11	22
Not very important	5	7	3	8	5	3	2	4
Not at all important		1	1	1	0	2	4	5
Don't know		2	4	1	5	3	10	10
(h) To avoid fatty foods								
Very important	61	54	65	39	64	56	66	56
Fairly important	37	32	32	55	29	35	27	37
Not very important	2	9	2	4	5	5	5	4
Not at all important		2	1		0	2	2	1
Don't know		3	1	2	1	2	2	3
Base (=100%)	*178*	*114*	*208*	*129*	*281*	*235*	*307*	*213*

Continued on next page

Table 7.8a: *continued*

Advice and response	African-Caribbean Women	African-Caribbean Men	Indian Women	Indian Men	Pakistani Women	Pakistani Men	Bangladeshi Women	Bangladeshi Men
30–49								
(a) To get out and about								
Very important	62	50	65	61	62	72	62	56
Fairly important	33	43	30	34	35	26	32	30
Not very important	4	6	3	4	1	2	3	12
Not at all important			1	0			1	0
Don't know	0	1	1	0	2		2	2
(b) To get a good night's sleep								
Very important	82	73	77	72	73	72	87	71
Fairly important	17	20	21	26	24	27	11	26
Not very important	1	4	1	2	1	1		0
Not at all important	0	1				0		
Don't know	0	2	0	0	2	0	2	3
(c) To avoid getting overweight								
Very important	77	67	71	65	62	72	63	64
Fairly important	19	29	24	26	26	25	30	31
Not very important	3	3	3	7	6	2	4	3
Not at all important	1	0		2	1		1	
Don't know	0	1	1	0	5	0	2	1
(d) To avoid worrying too much								
Very important	72	71	66	58	69	66	76	61
Fairly important	19	25	28	30	23	28	20	34
Not very important	6	1	3	9	4	4	1	2
Not at all important	1	2	1	3	1	0	0	
Don't know	2	1	2	0	2	1	2	3
(e) Not to smoke								
Very important	84	66	84	71	75	79	67	67
Fairly important	12	24	6	19	13	17	21	25
Not very important	2	6	2	8	3	3	4	7
Not at all important	1	2	1	1	2	0	3	0
Don't know	1	3	6	1	7	1	5	1
(f) To exercise regularly								
Very important	60	53	59	57	48	62	43	48
Fairly important	35	41	34	37	37	32	44	45
Not very important	5	6	6	4	9	5	7	3
Not at all important				1	3		0	
Don't know	0	1	2	1	3	0	6	4
(g) Not to drink much alcohol								
Very important	62	49	73	51	68	74	47	59
Fairly important	31	39	16	38	16	15	7	16
Not very important	4	10	4	8	1	4	3	4
Not at all important	1	1	0	1	2	2	10	2
Don't know	2	2	7	2	14	4	34	19
(h) To avoid fatty foods								
Very important	75	66	73	53	64	74	66	72
Fairly important	23	28	24	37	27	25	27	25
Not very important	1	4	2	8	7	1	5	2
Not at all important				2	1	0	1	0
Don't know	1	2	1		2	0	1	1
Base (=100%)	*270*	*140*	*283*	*227*	*186*	*268*	*233*	*183*

Continued on next page

Advice and response	African-Caribbean Women	Men	Indian Women	Men	Pakistani Women	Men	Bangladeshi Women	Men
50–74								
(a) To get out and about								
Very important	77	70	53	50	66	74	62	52
Fairly important	20	24	43	39	30	23	32	40
Not very important	2	5	2	7			3	7
Not at all important	0	1		0		1		
Don't know	1	1	2	4	5	2	3	1
(b) To get a good night's sleep								
Very important	84	77	62	70	62	70	86	72
Fairly important	14	19	36	25	26	26	13	26
Not very important		3		2	8	3		1
Not at all important								
Don't know	2	2	2	3	4	1	0	1
(c) To avoid getting overweight								
Very important	76	76	62	64	67	74	62	51
Fairly important	19	20	29	29	20	21	34	38
Not very important	3	2	6	3	8	3	2	6
Not at all important	0	1		0	1	1		
Don't know	2	1	2	3	3	2	3	4
(d) To avoid worrying too much								
Very important	78	74	69	48	70	69	68	56
Fairly important	16	20	27	42	23	24	29	39
Not very important	3	2	1	6	5	4	1	2
Not at all important	0	0	1	1	2			1
Don't know	3	4	3	3		3	2	2
(e) Not to smoke								
Very important	85	72	80	66	69	73	77	59
Fairly important	11	19	13	19	19	23	15	32
Not very important	2	4		10	4	2	2	9
Not at all important		1		3	5	1	1	0
Don't know	2	5	7	2	3	2	5	
(f) To exercise regularly								
Very important	70	54	47	46	47	66	31	47
Fairly important	25	39	42	41	38	29	53	40
Not very important	3	5	7	8	7	4	3	8
Not at all important	0			1	2			2
Don't know	1	3	3	4	7	1	13	3
(g) Not to drink much alcohol								
Very important	77	57	77	53	58	77	46	45
Fairly important	15	34	11	34	18	9	7	10
Not very important	5	5	1	8	3	1	1	3
Not at all important		1	1	2	5	1	4	8
Don't know	3	3	11	4	16	11	42	35
(h) To avoid fatty foods								
Very important	87	65	68	61	57	79	63	58
Fairly important	9	29	25	31	31	18	31	27
Not very important	1	2	4	5	4	1	3	8
Not at all important	0	1		1	1	0	1	4
Don't know	2	4	3	3	8	1	2	4
Base (= 100%)	193	174	107	107	50	124	63	171

Continued on next page

Table 7.8a: *continued*

Advice and response	African-Caribbean		Indian		Pakistani		Bangladeshi	
	Women	Men	Women	Men	Women	Men	Women	Men
All ages								
(a) To get out and about								
Very important	66	61	63	55	64	65	63	54
Fairly important	29	33	33	37	32	31	31	37
Not very important	5	4	3	6	2	3	4	8
Not at all important	0	0	0	0	0	0	1	0
Don't know	0	1	1	2	1	1	1	2
(b) To get a good night's sleep								
Very important	80	72	75	70	74	70	86	73
Fairly important	18	24	22	27	22	27	12	24
Not very important	1	2	2	2	2	2	1	1
Not at all important	0	0	0	0	0	0	0	0
Don't know	1	1	1	1	2	1	1	2
(c) To avoid getting overweight								
Very important	74	72	69	65	65	69	64	60
Fairly important	22	24	25	28	26	26	28	34
Not very important	3	3	3	5	5	4	5	4
Not at all important	0	0	0	1	1	0	0	0
Don't know	1	1	2	1	3	1	2	3
(d) To avoid worrying too much								
Very important	70	66	65	49	66	59	69	55
Fairly important	23	27	29	39	26	31	25	37
Not very important	5	4	4	8	6	8	4	5
Not at all important	1	1	1	2	1	0	0	1
Don't know	1	2	2	1	1	1	1	2
(e) Not to smoke								
Very important	81	68	83	70	75	75	75	68
Fairly important	15	22	10	21	16	20	16	24
Not very important	2	7	1	7	3	3	4	7
Not at all important	0	1	1	1	2	0	2	1
Don't know	1	2	5	1	4	1	3	1
(f) To exercise regularly								
Very important	62	57	58	56	50	63	49	51
Fairly important	34	37	35	38	37	32	41	42
Not very important	3	5	6	4	8	4	6	3
Not at all important	0	0	0	1	2	0	0	1
Don't know	0	2	2	1	3	1	5	3
(g) Not to drink much alcohol								
Very important	62	53	71	50	68	72	59	55
Fairly important	31	36	19	39	17	18	9	17
Not very important	5	7	3	8	3	3	2	4
Not at all important	0	1	1	1	2	2	7	5
Don't know	2	2	7	2	10	5	24	20
(h) To avoid fatty foods								
Very important	73	62	69	50	63	68	66	61
Fairly important	24	30	27	42	29	27	27	30
Not very important	1	5	2	6	6	2	4	4
Not at all important	0	1	0	1	1	1	1	1
Don't know	1	3	1	1	2	1	2	3
Base (=100%)	*641*	*428*	*598*	*463*	*517*	*627*	*603*	*567*

Table 7.8b: Advice regarded as very important for persons of the respondent's age who wish to be healthy (percentages of all respondents)

Advice	African-Caribbean		Indian		Pakistani		Bangladeshi	
	Women	Men	Women	Men	Women	Men	Women	Men
16–29								
To get out and about	62	62	64	50	66	53	64	53
To get a good night's sleep	74	67	79	67	79	67	85	75
To avoid getting overweight	70	72	70	66	67	64	66	63
To avoid worrying too much	63	54	61	39	62	47	64	50
Not to smoke	76	68	83	70	77	72	82	74
To exercise regularly	59	64	62	61	54	63	58	57
Not to drink much alcohol	50	53	66	47	71	66	73	58
To avoid fatty foods	61	54	65	39	64	56	66	56
Base (= 100%)	*174*	*114*	*205*	*124*	*270*	*226*	*305*	*208*
30–49								
To get out and about	62	50	65	61	62	72	62	56
To get a good night's sleep	82	73	77	72	73	72	87	71
To avoid getting overweight	77	67	71	65	62	72	63	64
To avoid worrying too much	72	71	66	58	69	66	76	61
Not to smoke	84	66	84	71	75	79	67	67
To exercise regularly	60	53	59	57	48	62	43	48
Not to drink much alcohol	62	49	73	51	68	74	47	59
To avoid fatty foods	75	66	73	53	64	74	66	72
Base (= 100%)	*268*	*136*	*276*	*225*	*178*	*264*	*231*	*178*
50–74								
To get out and about	77	70	53	50	66	74	62	52
To get a good night's sleep	84	77	62	70	62	70	86	72
To avoid getting overweight	76	76	62	64	67	74	62	51
To avoid worrying too much	78	74	69	48	70	69	68	56
Not to smoke	85	72	80	66	69	73	77	59
To exercise regularly	70	54	47	46	47	66	31	47
Not to drink much alcohol	77	57	77	53	58	77	46	45
To avoid fatty foods	87	65	68	61	57	79	63	58
Base (= 100%)	*184*	*168*	*105*	*103*	*45*	*119*	*63*	*166*
All ages								
To get out and about	66	61	63	55	64	65	63	54
To get a good night's sleep	80	72	75	70	74	70	86	73
To avoid getting overweight	74	72	69	65	65	69	64	60
To avoid worrying too much	70	66	65	49	66	59	69	55
Not to smoke	81	68	83	70	75	75	75	68
To exercise regularly	62	57	58	56	50	63	49	51
Not to drink much alcohol	62	53	71	50	68	72	59	55
To avoid fatty foods	73	62	69	50	63	68	66	61
Base (=100%)	*626*	*418*	*586*	*452*	*493*	*609*	*599*	*552*

Table 7.9: Physical activity at work (percentages of respondents in paid employment or self-employed during the previous four weeks)

Response	African-Caribbean		Indian		Pakistani		Bangladeshi	
	Women	Men	Women	Men	Women	Men	Women	Men
16–29								
Very physically active	22	37	24	19	21	31	40	38
Fairly physically active	53	39	45	58	53	50	49	48
Not very physically active	10	11	24	16	15	15	8	11
Not at all physically active	15	12	7	7	11	5	3	3
Base (= 100%)	*63*	*41*	*73*	*55*	*54*	*99*	*53*	*83*
30–49								
Very physically active	42	54	31	36	13	30	58	34
Fairly physically active	29	19	50	38	69	43	33	48
Not very physically active	19	23	16	16	8	21	9	14
Not at all physically active	10	4	3	10	11	6		4
Base (= 100%)	*158*	*93*	*138*	*175*	*21*	*143*	*9*	*88*
50–74								
Very physically active	52	61	16	17	41	29		23
Fairly physically active	46	29	84	64		49		70
Not very physically active	2	7		16	59	12		6
Not at all physically active		2		3		9		
Base (= 100%)	*56*	*54*	*19*	*37*	*4*	*32*		*11*
All ages								
Very physically active	37	52	27	29	20	30	43	36
Fairly physically active	40	27	51	47	54	46	47	49
Not very physically active	13	16	17	16	15	18	8	12
Not at all physically active	10	6	4	8	10	6	3	4
Base (= 100%)	*277*	*188*	*230*	*267*	*78*	*274*	*62*	*181*

Table 7.10: Have you done any housework in the last four weeks? (percentages of all respondents)

Advice	African-Caribbean		Indian		Pakistani		Bangladeshi	
	Women	Men	Women	Men	Women	Men	Women	Men
16–29								
Yes	95	82	94	65	94	46	93	42
No	5	18	6	35	6	54	7	58
Base (= 100%)	*177*	*113*	*206*	*128*	*280*	*232*	*307*	*212*
30–49								
Yes	98	87	95	59	94	50	91	48
No	2	13	5	41	6	50	9	52
Base (= 100%)	*270*	*139*	*283*	*226*	*186*	*267*	*232*	*183*
50–74								
Yes	92	73	89	52	80	31	75	36
No	8	27	11	48	20	69	25	64
Base (= 100%)	*193*	*172*	*106*	*106*	*50*	*124*	*62*	*171*
All ages								
Yes	95	80	94	60	92	44	90	42
No	5	20	6	40	8	56	10	58
Base (= 100%)	*640*	*424*	*595*	*460*	*516*	*623*	*601*	*566*

Table 7.11a: Have you done any heavy housework in the last four weeks? (percentages of all respondents who had done housework within the last four weeks)

Response	African-Caribbean		Indian		Pakistani		Bangladeshi	
	Women	Men	Women	Men	Women	Men	Women	Men
16–29								
Yes	74	73	70	59	70	71	71	80
No	26	27	30	41	30	29	29	20
Base (= 100%)	*168*	*94*	*195*	*77*	*268*	*108*	*284*	*90*
30–49								
Yes	79	77	69	71	57	67	76	93
No	21	23	31	29	43	33	24	7
Base (= 100%)	*261*	*119*	*271*	*142*	*173*	*115*	*212*	*90*
50–74								
Yes	59	54	55	65	59	51	56	90
No	41	46	45	35	41	49	44	10
Base (= 100%)	*175*	*128*	*93*	*53*	*38*	*38*	*47*	*52*
All ages								
Yes	72	68	67	66	63	67	71	87
No	28	32	33	34	37	33	29	13
Base (= 100%)	*604*	*341*	*559*	*272*	*479*	*261*	*543*	*232*

Table 7.11b: Number of days on which heavy housework undertaken in the last four weeks (mean number of days for all respondents who had done heavy housework within the last four weeks)

Response	African-Caribbean		Indian		Pakistani		Bangladeshi	
	Women	Men	Women	Men	Women	Men	Women	Men
16–29	8	5	8	7	8	7	11	7
30–49	9	7	9	7	12	8	12	5
50–74	9	8	9	7	10	15	11	7
All ages	9	7	9	7	10	8	11	7

Table 7.11c: Time spent on heavy housework on most recent day (mean number of minutes for all respondents who had done heavy housework within the last four weeks)

Response	African-Caribbean		Indian		Pakistani		Bangladeshi	
	Women	Men	Women	Men	Women	Men	Women	Men
16–29	113	83	105	121	112	86	88	65
30–49	117	92	130	130	146	146	92	86
50–74	113	71	138	89	147	86	81	81
All ages 115	84	122	119	129	112	89	76	

Table 7.12: Have you done any gardening, DIY or building work in the last four weeks? (percentages of all respondents)

Response	African-Caribbean		Indian		Pakistani		Bangladeshi	
	Women	Men	Women	Men	Women	Men	Women	Men
16–29								
Yes	28	22	17	38	18	33	6	11
No	72	78	83	62	82	67	94	89
Base (= 100%)	*177*	*113*	*204*	*126*	*281*	*234*	*307*	*210*
30–49								
Yes	35	53	31	46	25	41	4	21
No	65	47	69	54	75	59	96	79
Base (= 100%)	*269*	*140*	*283*	*224*	*186*	*267*	*232*	*181*
50–74								
Yes	26	40	22	40	28	25	4	8
No	74	60	78	60	72	75	96	92
Base (= 100%)	*193*	*173*	*107*	*106*	*50*	*122*	*63*	*169*
All ages								
Yes	30	38	24	42	22	34	5	13
No	70	62	76	58	78	66	95	87
Base (=100%)	*639*	*426*	*594*	*456*	*517*	*623*	*602*	*560*

Table 7.13: Have you done any heavy gardening, DIY or building work in the last four weeks? (percentages of all respondents who had undertaken gardening/DIY/building in last four weeks)

Response	African-Caribbean		Indian		Pakistani		Bangladeshi	
	Women	Men	Women	Men	Women	Men	Women	Men
16–29								
Yes	71	86	74	79	59	76	54	90
No	29	14	26	21	41	24	46	10
Base (= 100%)	*50*	*24*	*35*	*48*	*53*	*71*	*22*	*21*
30–49								
Yes	64	71	55	74	51	71	51	88
No	36	29	45	26	49	29	49	12
Base (= 100%)	*97*	*66*	*83*	*104*	*38*	*104*	*9*	*31*
50–74								
Yes	59	62	31	68	46	68	100	54
No	41	38	69	32	54	32		46
Base (= 100%)	*49*	*64*	*21*	*41*	*11*	*26*	*3*	*11*
All ages								
Yes	66	70	56	74	53	72	58	82
No	34	30	44	26	47	28	42	18
Base (= 100%)	*196*	*154*	*139*	*193*	*102*	*201*	*34*	*63*

Table 7.14: On how many days did you undertake heavy gardening, DIY or building work in the last four weeks? (mean of all respondents who had undertaken heavy gardening/DIY/building work in last four weeks)

Age group	African-Caribbean		Indian		Pakistani		Bangladeshi	
	Women	Men	Women	Men	Women	Men	Women	Men
16–29	3	5	3	4	2	3	4	3
30–49	3	5	2	4	3	5	4	5
50–74	4	7	3	6	2	6	5	8
All ages	3	5	3	4	3	4	4	5

Table 7.15: On the most recent day on which you undertook heavy gardening, how long did you spend on it? (mean hours of all respondents who had undertaken heavy gardening/DIY/building work in last four weeks)

Age group	African-Caribbean		Indian		Pakistani		Bangladeshi	
	Women	Men	Women	Men	Women	Men	Women	Men
16–29	3	3	2	3	2	3	2	2
30–49	2	3	3	3	2	3	5	2
50–74	2	2	2	3	2	2	1	2
All ages	2	3	3	3	2	3	2	2

Table 7.16: Have you taken any walks of a quarter of a mile or more in the last four weeks? (percentages of all respondents)

Response	African-Caribbean		Indian		Pakistani		Bangladeshi	
	Women	Men	Women	Men	Women	Men	Women	Men
16–29								
Yes	87	84	85	85	80	79	85	87
No	13	16	15	15	20	21	14	13
Can't walk at all							1	
Base (= 100%)	*178*	*113*	*206*	*128*	*281*	*235*	*307*	*212*
30–49								
Yes	85	81	78	76	83	75	81	85
No	15	19	21	24	17	25	19	15
Can't walk at all			0				1	
Base (= 100%)	*269*	*140*	*283*	*227*	*186*	*268*	*232*	*183*
50–74								
Yes	84	73	71	75	83	73	80	89
No	15	27	28	24	14	27	18	11
Can't walk at all	1		1	2	2		3	
Base (= 100%)	*193*	*173*	*107*	*107*	*50*	*124*	*63*	*170*
All ages								
Yes	85	79	79	79	82	76	83	87
No	14	21	21	21	18	24	17	13
Can't walk at all	0	0	0	0	0	0	1	0
Base (= 100%)	*640*	*426*	*596*	*462*	*517*	*627*	*602*	*565*

Table 7.17: Did you take any walks of a mile or more in the last four weeks (continuous walking for 20 minutes or more)? (percentages of all respondents who had taken a walk of a quarter-mile or more in the last four weeks)

Response	African-Caribbean		Indian		Pakistani		Bangladeshi	
	Women	Men	Women	Men	Women	Men	Women	Men
16–29								
Yes	74	82	79	76	68	86	65	82
No	26	18	21	24	32	14	35	18
Base (= 100%)	*156*	*95*	*174*	*105*	*226*	*183*	*264*	*179*
30–49								
Yes	71	79	74	78	74	75	60	81
No	29	21	26	22	26	25	40	19
Base (= 100%)	*228*	*112*	*224*	*175*	*157*	*195*	*182*	*160*
50–74								
Yes	61	80	67	87	66	80	49	75
No	39	20	33	13	34	20	51	25
Base (= 100%)	*153*	*129*	*72*	*82*	*39*	*90*	*50*	*147*
All ages								
Yes	69	80	75	79	71	81	61	80
No	31	20	25	21	29	19	39	20
Base (= 100%)	*537*	*336*	*470*	*362*	*422*	*468*	*496*	*486*

Table 7.18: How many times did you take a walk of a mile or more in the last four weeks? (mean of all respondents who had taken a walk of a mile or more in the last four weeks)

Age group	African-Caribbean		Indian		Pakistani		Bangladeshi	
	Women	Men	Women	Men	Women	Men	Women	Men
18–29	13	9	14	13	10	11	12	13
30–49	13	11	11	13	14	15	10	17
50–74	9	11	12	21	11	15	13	19
All ages	12	11	13	15	12	13	12	18

Table 7.19: How many walks of two miles or more did you take during the last four weeks? (mean of all respondents who had taken a walk of a mile or more in the last four weeks)

Age group	African-Caribbean		Indian		Pakistani		Bangladeshi	
	Women	Men	Women	Men	Women	Men	Women	Men
16–29	2	4	3	4	3	5	3	7
30–49	3	4	4	6	3	6	1	8
50–74	2	5	1	6	3	3	2	10
All ages	3	4	3	6	3	5	2	8

Table 7.20: What best describes your walking pace? (percentages of all respondents who had taken a walk of a mile or more in the last four weeks)

Walking speed	African-Caribbean		Indian		Pakistani		Bangladeshi	
	Women	Men	Women	Men	Women	Men	Women	Men
16–29								
A slow pace	5	2	6	9	8	4	7	6
A steady average pace	48	42	58	47	58	55	54	57
A fairly brisk pace	41	38	29	26	25	29	30	25
A fast pace	6	17	7	18	9	12	9	12
Don't know	0	0	0	0	0	0	0	0
Base (= 100%)	120	79	133	80	151	154	170	149
30–49								
A slow pace	8	8	13	17	14	12	23	10
A steady average pace	41	47	61	58	67	72	55	72
A fairly brisk pace	44	35	24	18	16	11	20	14
A fast pace	6	9	2	7	2	5	2	4
Don't know	1	1		1		0	1	
Base (= 100%)	164	96	164	138	115	154	106	132
50–74								
A slow pace	27	16	15	25	26	33	47	33
A steady average pace	45	58	59	50	66	58	42	60
A fairy brisk pace	26	21	24	15	9	7	10	7
A fast pace	2	5		9		3	1	1
Don't know			2					
Base (= 100%)	94	103	39	67	25	73	24	109
All ages								
A slow pace	11	9	11	16	13	13	17	15
A steady average pace	45	49	59	53	63	62	53	62
A fairly brisk pace	38	32	26	20	19	18	24	17
A fast pace	5	11	4	11	5	8	6	7
Don't know	0	0	0	0	0	0	0	0
Base (= 100%)	378	278	336	285	291	381	300	390

Table 7.21: Do you go up and down stairs at home? (percentages of all respondents)

Response	African-Caribbean		Indian		Pakistani		Bangladeshi	
	Women	Men	Women	Men	Women	Men	Women	Men
16–29								
Yes	92	90	98	96	100	99	77	83
No	8	10	2	4	0	1	23	17
Base (= 100%)	177	114	207	129	281	235	307	211
30–49								
Yes	95	93	99	97	97	97	74	89
No	5	7	1	3	3	3	26	11
Base (= 100%)	270	140	281	227	186	268	233	182
50–74								
Yes	89	91	95	93	95	92	66	76
No	11	9	5	7	5	8	34	24
Base (= 100%)	193	174	107	106	50	124	63	170
All ages								
Yes	92	91	98	96	98	97	74	83
No	8	9	2	4	2	3	26	17
Base (= 100%)	640	428	595	462	517	627	603	563

Table 7.22: About how many times a day do you climb the stairs? (mean of all respondents who go up and down stairs)

Age group	African-Caribbean		Indian		Pakistani		Bangladeshi	
	Women	Men	Women	Men	Women	Men	Women	Men
16–29	10	11	10	10	10	11	8	9
30–49	10	10	11	9	10	8	9	7
50–74	7	8	9	7	9	6	7	7
All ages	10	10	10	9	10	9	8	8

Table 7.23: How many steps are there in your stairs? (mean of all respondents who go up and down stairs)

Age group	African-Caribbean		Indian		Pakistani		Bangladeshi	
	Women	Men	Women	Men	Women	Men	Women	Men
16–29	16	19	15	16	15	17	18	22
30–49	15	16	14	15	14	15	16	18
50–74	15	15	14	15	14	13	16	19
All ages	15	16	15	16	14	16	17	20

Table 7.24: On how many days in an average week do you climb stairs at work or elsewhere outside your home? (mean of all respondents)

Age group	African-Caribbean		Indian		Pakistani		Bangladeshi	
	Women	Men	Women	Men	Women	Men	Women	Men
16–29	9	9	9	9	10	10	5	7
30–49	9	9	10	8	9	7	6	6
50–74	6	7	8	7	8	6	4	5
All ages	8	8	9	8	9	8	6	6

Table 7.25: About how many times a day do you climb stairs at work or elsewhere? (mean of all respondents who had used stairs outside their home)

Age group	African-Caribbean		Indian		Pakistani		Bangladeshi	
	Women	Men	Women	Men	Women	Men	Women	Men
16–29	6	8	6	10	6	7	5	7
30–49	5	8	4	6	3	7	3	5
50–74	5	4	4	4	4	7	2	3
All ages	5	7	5	7	5	7	4	6

Table 7.26: And, on average, how many steps did you climb each time? (mean of all respondents who had used stairs outside their home)

Age group	African-Caribbean Women	Men	Indian Women	Men	Pakistani Women	Men	Bangladeshi Women	Men
16–29	25	24	30	25	19	31	27	25
30–49	25	23	20	28	17	21	32	17
50–74	21	27	15	22	16	13	35	15
All ages	25	24	25	26	18	25	29	21

Table 7.27: On how many days in an average week do you carry a child around? (percentages of all respondents)

Days	African-Caribbean Women	Men	Indian Women	Men	Pakistani Women	Men	Bangladeshi Women	Men
16–29								
Rarely/never	61	82	62	75	41	69	65	73
1–2 days	6	9	10	7	11	12	12	13
3–5 days	4	3	4	6	3	4	2	5
Most days	30	6	24	12	45	15	22	9
Base (= 100%)	*178*	*114*	*208*	*129*	*280*	*234*	*306*	*213*
30–49								
Rarely/never	70	67	78	68	71	68	78	52
1–2 days	6	8	5	9	6	6	11	23
3–5 days	3	4	3	4	5	6	4	9
Most days	22	21	14	19	18	20	8	16
Base (= 100%)	*269*	*140*	*283*	*226*	*184*	*267*	*228*	*182*
50–74								
Rarely/never	89	86	85	88	73	90	88	77
1–2 days	6	8	4	6	11	3	6	15
3–5 days	3	1	5	2	6	2		4
Most days	2	5	6	4	10	5	5	4
Base (= 100%)	*193*	*174*	*107*	*106*	*49*	*122*	*63*	*170*
All ages								
Rarely/never	72	79	74	75	58	73	73	68
1–2 days	6	8	6	8	9	8	11	16
3–5 days	3	3	4	4	4	4	2	6
Most days	19	10	16	14	29	15	14	9
Base (= 100%)	*640*	*428*	*598*	*461*	*513*	*623*	*597*	*565*

Table 7.28: On how many days in an average week do you push a child in a pram or pushchair? (percentages of all respondents)

Days	African-Caribbean		Indian		Pakistani		Bangladeshi	
	Women	Men	Women	Men	Women	Men	Women	Men
16–29								
Rarely/never	74	92	74	95	65	90	76	92
1–2 days	5	4	11	2	12	8	10	6
3–5 days	9	2	4	1	7	1	8	0
Most days	12	2	12	2	15	1	6	2
Base (= 100%)	*178*	*114*	*208*	*128*	*279*	*232*	*305*	*213*
30–49								
Rarely/never	82	87	87	89	81	94	77	82
1–2 days	4	3	4	6	8	3	14	10
3–5 days	4	3	3	2	4	1	4	4
Most days	9	7	6	2	7	2	5	3
Base (= 100%)	*269*	*139*	*283*	*225*	*184*	*265*	*228*	*182*
50–74								
Rarely/never	93	96	92	96	90	97	96	97
1–2 days	7	1	3	4	4	1	2	1
3–5 days		2	2				2	
Most days		1	3	3	5	3		1
Base (= 100%)	*193*	*174*	*107*	*106*	*49*	*122*	*63*	*170*
All ages								
Rarely/never	82	92	83	93	76	93	79	91
1–2 days	5	3	6	4	9	4	11	6
3–5 days	5	2	3	1	5	1	6	1
Most days	8	3	8	2	11	2	5	2
Base (=100%)	*640*	*427*	*598*	*459*	*512*	*619*	*596*	*565*

Table 7.29: Have you undertaken any of the following physical activities during the last 4 weeks? (percentages of all respondents)

Response	African-Caribbean		Indian		Pakistani		Bangladeshi	
	Women	Men	Women	Men	Women	Men	Women	Men
16–29								
Yes	74	79	61	83	49	74	33	76
No	26	21	39	17	51	26	67	24
Base (= 100%)	*177*	*112*	*205*	*129*	*281*	*232*	*305*	*209*
30–49								
Yes	63	73	27	49	19	29	5	33
No	37	27	73	51	81	71	95	67
Base (= 100%)	*267*	*139*	*280*	*224*	*185*	*267*	*232*	*180*
50–74								
Yes	29	29	7	23	9	9	0	10
No	71	71	93	77	91	91	100	90
Base (= 100%)	*192*	*174*	*107*	*106*	*50*	*123*	*63*	*168*
All ages								
Yes	58	59	35	54	31	42	18	44
No	42	41	65	46	69	58	82	56
Base (= 100%)	*636*	*425*	*592*	*459*	*516*	*622*	*600*	*557*

Table 7.30: Which of these physical activities have you engaged in during the last 4 weeks (percentages of all respondents who had engaged in physical activity during the last 4 weeks)

Activity	African-Caribbean		Indian		Pakistani		Bangladeshi	
	Women	Men	Women	Men	Women	Men	Women	Men
16–29								
Cycling/exercise bike	19	29	18	26	9	23	10	25
Exercises (press-ups, sit-ups, etc.)	39	52	37	40	52	43	46	29
Aerobics/keep fit/ gymnastics/dancing	51	19	40	8	35	4	17	7
Other types of dancing	35	19	26	4	8	2	20	4
Weight training	13	39	8	44	8	38	4	33
Swimming	14	16	29	12	14	13	11	20
Running/jogging	21	30	23	26	25	21	14	30
Football/rugby	1	44	3	56	5	44	7	71
Badminton/tennis	6	10	19	20	·26	22	20	37
Squash				4	4	4	1	4
Other sports or exercise	7	13	9	17	16	22	15	6
Base (= 100%)	*127*	*84*	*117*	*103*	*123*	*158*	*97*	*151*
30–49								
Cycling/exercise bike	13	20	26	16	30	15	31	9
Exercises (press-ups, sit-ups, etc.)	39	48	37	38	59	31	61	38
Aerobics/keep fit/ gymnastics/dancing	41	18	20	3	21	9	14	1
Other types of dancing	21	23	11	4	3		6	1
Weight training	12	28	4	18	3	16		5
Swimming	23	18	25	25	6	11	12	10
Running/jogging	18	26	5	18	6	34		15
Football/rugby	1	19	1	16	4	16		21
Badminton/tennis	3	7	3	9		21		10
Squash	0	1		4		2		
Other sports or exercise	5	19	7	15	2	18		22
Base (= 100%)	*168*	*99*	*84*	*109*	*34*	*78*	*16*	*59*
50–74								
Cycling/exercise bike	21	30	48	21		30		14
Exercises (press-ups, sit-ups, etc.)	43	47	11	54	32	38		62
Aerobics/keep fit/ gymnastics/dancing	26	12			13		100	
Other types of dancing	17	14	11	3				
Weight training	8			3				
Swimming	8	7	18	11	30			6
Running/jogging	13	9		11	25	5		
Football/rugby						5		
Badminton/tennis				19	25	2		
Squash								
Other sports or exercise	2	14	12	7		29		20
Base (= 100%)	*56*	*46*	*10*	*26*	*4*	*12*	*1*	*15*

Continued on next page

Table 7.30: *continued*

Activity	African-Caribbean		Indian		Pakistani		Bangladeshi	
	Women	Men	Women	Men	Women	Men	Women	Men
All ages								
Cycling/exercise bike	17	26	22	21	14	21	12	21
Exercises (press-ups, sit-ups, etc.)	40	50	36	40	53	40	48	33
Aerobics/keep fit/ gymnastics/dancing	44	17	31	5	31	5	17	5
Other types of dancing	27	19	20	4	6	2	18	3
Weight training	12	28	6	30	6	30	3	25
Swimming	17	15	27	17	13	12	11	17
Running/jogging	19	25	16	21	20	24	13	25
Football/rugby	1	27	2	35	5	35	6	55
Badminton/tennis	4	7	13	16	19	21	18	29
Squash	0	0	0	4	3	3	1	3
Other sports or exercise	5	15	8	15	12	21	13	11
Base (= 100%)	*351*	*229*	*211*	*238*	*161*	*248*	*114*	*225*

Table 7.31: On how many separate occasions did you engage in this activity during the last 4 weeks? (Mean no. of occasions on which all respondents had engaged in physical activity during the last 4 weeks)

Activity	African-Caribbean		Indian		Pakistani		Bangladeshi	
	Women	Men	Women	Men	Women	Men	Women	Men
16–29								
Cycling/exercise bike	8	8	4	8	17	11	11	10
Exercises (press-ups, sit-ups, etc.)	10	13	11	10	13	11	16	17
Aerobics/keep fit/ gymnastics/dancing	7	9	6	4	10	8	10	7
Other types of dancing	6	11	6	6	9	6	8	3
Weight training	4	7	6	10	4	9	4	8
Swimming	2	4	4	4	4	4	4	3
Running/jogging	7	8	6	10	10	13	10	9
Football/rugby	2	6	2	7	2	10	2	10
Badminton/tennis	3	6	3	5	5	5	5	6
Squash				7	2	5	1	3
Other sports or exercise	7	8	4	5	8	7	10	11
30–49								
Cycling/exercise bike	9	10	9	10	8	19	8	11
Exercises (press-ups, sit-ups, etc.)	12	12	14	15	15	14	18	14
Aerobics/keep fit/ gymnastics/dancing	7	7	5	14	5	11	4	28
Other types of dancing	6	6	2	2	8		13	1
Weight training	6	9	7	9	6	12		8
Swimming	3	5	3	3	2	4	4	3
Running/jogging	8	10	7	9	6	8		9
Football/rugby	3	4	2	5	1	8		4
Badminton/tennis	2	3	4	6		4		5
Squash	1	4		3		12		
Other sports or exercise	7	9	17	8	30	7		24

Continued on next page

Table 7.31: *continued*

Activity	African-Caribbean		Indian		Pakistani		Bangladeshi	
	Women	Men	Women	Men	Women	Men	Women	Men
50–74								
Cycling/exercise bike	12	12	17	7		28		29
Exercises (press-ups, sit-ups, etc.)	18	18	3	17	2	16		14
Aerobics/keep fit/ gymnastics/dancing	6	9			4		4	
Other types of dancing	4	3	4	4				
Weight training	15			30				
Swimming	2	5	4	6	4			4
Running/jogging	6	10		22	3	8		
Football/rugby						8		
Badminton/tennis				3	1	2		
Squash								
Other sports or exercise	14	15	5	20		10		29
All ages								
Cycling/exercise bike	9	9	7	9	12	14	10	11
Exercises (press-ups, sit-ups, etc.)	12	14	12	13	14	12	16	16
Aerobics/keep fit/ gymnastics/dancing	7	9	6	6	9	9	9	8
Other types of dancing	6	8	5	4	9	6	8	3
Weight training	6	8	6	10	4	9	4	8
Swimming	3	4	4	4	4	4	4	3
Running/jogging	7	9	6	10	9	11	10	9
Football/rugby	2	6	2	7	2	10	2	10
Badminton/tennis	3	5	3	5	5	5	5	6
Squash	1	4		5	2	6	1	3
Other sports or exercise	8	9	7	7	9	7	10	19

Table 7.32: How much time did you usually spend on this activity on each occasion? (Mean no. of minutes in which all respondents had engaged in physical activity during the last 4 weeks)

Activity	African-Caribbean		Indian		Pakistani		Bangladeshi	
	Women	Men	Women	Men	Women	Men	Women	Men
16–29								
Cycling/exercise bike	28	64	43	31	32	71	47	41
Exercises (press-ups, sit-ups, etc.)	30	37	25	39	22	27	22	35
Aerobics/keep fit/ gymnastics/dancing	58	56	50	72	43	53	54	114
Other types of dancing	174	191	82	179	61	60	51	25
Weight training	59	65	45	55	25	55	38	73
Swimming	76	100	73	65	72	84	52	76
Running/jogging	31	43	27	41	24	51	25	42
Football/rugby	23	89	80	98	38	95	45	91
Badminton/tennis	84	95	80	97	52	86	64	75
Squash				44	80	143	20	65
Other sports or exercise	59	73	85	203	66	174	47	66

Continued on next page

Table 7.33: *continued*

Activity	African-Caribbean		Indian		Pakistani		Bangladeshi	
	Women	Men	Women	Men	Women	Men	Women	Men
All ages								
Cycling/exercise bike	70	61	59	69	59	63	70	62
Exercises (press-ups, sit-ups, etc.)	65	68	60	61	65	62	90	78
Aerobics/keep fit/ gymnastics/dancing	87	67	77	90	89	82	93	68
Other types of dancing	59	62	68	58	81	76	57	27
Weight training	69	78	80	79	90	84	45	82
Swimming	39	47	45	47	56	44	65	60
Running/jogging	76	80	82	92	75	78	95	88
Football/rugby	86	81	47	81	78	83	70	93
Badminton/tennis	69	74	61	74	57	75	93	78
Squash	100	100		91	100	100	100	47
Other sports or exercise	58	72	55	71	60	56	76	64
All activities	*77*	*73*	*70*	*75*	*74*	*79*	*82*	*87*

Table 7.34: Do you help care for anyone who is disabled or has difficulty in walking? (percentages of all respondents)

Response	African-Caribbean		Indian		Pakistani		Bangladeshi	
	Women	Men	Women	Men	Women	Men	Women	Men
16–29								
Yes	7	6	18	10	17	14	8	12
No	93	94	82	90	83	86	92	88
Base (= 100%)	*178*	*114*	*207*	*126*	*280*	*232*	*305*	*209*
30–49								
Yes	12	3	12	9	6	4	6	5
No	88	97	88	91	94	96	94	95
Base (= 100%)	*268*	*139*	*283*	*227*	*186*	*265*	*233*	*178*
50–74								
Yes	22	6	15	12	7	7	4	5
No	78	94	85	88	93	93	96	95
Base (= 100%)	*192*	*172*	*106*	*105*	*50*	*121*	*63*	*168*
All ages								
Yes	13	5	15	10	11	9	7	8
No	87	95	85	90	89	91	93	92
Base = 100%)	*638*	*425*	*596*	*458*	*516*	*618*	*601*	*555*

Table 7.35: Average number of days on which a disabled adult is lifted or carried (percentages of all respondents)

Days	African-Caribbean Women	African-Caribbean Men	Indian Women	Indian Men	Pakistani Women	Pakistani Men	Bangladeshi Women	Bangladeshi Men
16–29								
Rarely/never	93	57	46	70	64	84	59	47
1–2 days			36	8	23	6	39	36
3–5 days		30	2	8	3	2		
Most days	7	14	16	15	10	9	3	17
Base (= 100%)	*10*	*4*	*31*	*11*	*42*	*23*	*24*	*22*
30–49								
Rarely/never	65	56	77	84	65	55	13	35
1–2 days	7		10	13	21	10	10	35
3–5 days	16	44			6	6		8
Most days	12		13	4	9	29	77	22
Base (= 100%)	*29*	*5*	*29*	*19*	*14*	*13*	*12*	*8*
50–74								
Rarely/never	52	95	80	86	42	74	12	59
1–2 days	4	5	6					
3–5 days	15							16
Most days	28		14	14	58	26	88	26
Base (= 100%)	*32*	*10*	*13*	*7*	*4*	*4*	*3*	*6*
All ages								
Rarely/never	65	77	64	79	62	77	38	47
1–2 days	4	3	21	8	20	6	25	30
3–5 days	12	17	1	3	3	2	0	4
Most days	19	3	14	10	15	15	37	19
Base (= 100%)	*71*	*19*	*73*	*37*	*60*	*40*	*39*	*36*

Table 7.36: Average number of days on which walking support is given to a disabled adult (percentages of all respondents)

Days	African-Caribbean		Indian		Pakistani		Bangladeshi	
	Women	Men	Women	Men	Women	Men	Women	Men
16–29								
Rarely/never	67	100	45	29	45	40	52	51
1–2 days	5		18	49	19	12	31	33
3–5 days	21		9	17	14	28	11	
Most days	7		28	6	22	20	6	16
Base (= 100%)	*10*	*4*	*31*	*11*	*43*	*23*	*24*	*22*
30–49								
Rarely/never	35	33	42	48	56	39	71	70
1–2 days	21		25	26	21	10		8
3–5 days	26	67	9	4	18	6	17	
Most days	17		25	22	6	45	11	22
Base (= 100%)	*29*	*5*	*29*	*19*	*14*	*13*	*12*	*8*
50–74								
Rarely/never	20	43	12	57	25		100	59
1–2 days	11	20	31	10		7		
3–5 days	31	10	21	10				16
Most days	38	28	36	23	75	93		26
Base (= 100%)	*32*	*10*	*13*	*7*	*4*	*4*	*3*	*6*
All ages								
Rarely/never	35	54	37	44	46	33	63	56
1–2 days	13	11	23	30	17	11	17	23
3–5 days	27	20	11	10	14	20	12	3
Most days	25	15	28	16	23	37	8	19
Base (= 100%)	*71*	*19*	*73*	*37*	*61*	*40*	*39*	*36*

Table 7.37: Average number of days on which a wheelchair is pushed (percentages of all respondents who help care for someone who is disabled or has difficulty in walking)

Days	African-Caribbean		Indian		Pakistani		Bangladeshi	
	Women	Men	Women	Men	Women	Men	Women	Men
16–29								
Rarely/never	51	27	79	79	95	67	81	73
1–2 days	21	43	11	8	1	8	13	16
3–5 days	21	30	2	8	3	23	6	
Most days	7		8	6	1	2		10
Base (= 100%)	*10*	*4*	*31*	*11*	*42*	*23*	*24*	*22*
30–49								
Rarely/never	53	56	91	95	79	76	80	78
1–2 days	15		4	5	15			8
3–5 days	23	44				7		
Most days	9		4		6	17	20	13
Base (= 100%)	*29*	*5*	*29*	*19*	*14*	*12*	*12*	*8*
50–74								
Rarely/never	46	82	76	76	67	74	100	59
1–2 days	24	18	6	10				16
3–5 days	12		10					
Most days	18		8	14	33	26		26
Base (= 100%)	*31*	*10*	*13*	*7*	*4*	*4*	*3*	*6*
All ages								
Rarely/never	49	63	83	85	88	70	82	72
1–2 days	20	20	8	7	4	5	7	15
3–5 days	18	17	3	3	2	17	3	0
Most days	13	0	7	6	6	8	7	14
Base (= 100%)	*70*	*19*	*73*	*37*	*60*	*39*	*39*	*36*

Table 7.38: And do any of the following stop you from getting more exercise? (percentages of all respondents)

Reason	African-Caribbean Women	Men	Indian Women	Men	Pakistani Women	Men	Bangladeshi Women	Men
16–29								
(a) My husband/wife/partner would disapprove			6	2	5	1	8	0
(b) Other members of my family would disapprove	1	2	6		15	2	16	2
(c) I don't want to go to mixed sex places	4	2	9	1	16	4	20	4
(d) I don't like to go to places where I can't speak my language			3	3	2	2	5	1
(e) I don't want to go to a place where people show parts of their bodies	1	1	9	2	15	7	24	5
(f) I have older relatives to look after	1		3	1	2	1	4	1
(g) I don't like to go out alone	17	6	24	4	15	10	29	9
(h) I would not know what to do	2	1	3		6	4	9	6
(i) I never see anyone from my culture doing these things	2		6	3	10	2	13	3
None of these	76	87	54	85	48	75	34	75
Don't know	0	0		3	2	1	7	3
Base (= 100%)	*178*	*114*	*208*	*129*	*281*	*235*	*307*	*213*
30–49								
(a) My husband/wife/partner would disapprove	1	2	4	2	17	2	10	0
(b) Other members of my family would disapprove	1		3	0	9	3	3	3
(c) I don't want to go to mixed sex places	6		10	4	28	7	18	15
(d) I don't like to go to places where I can't speak my language	1		6	3	12	2	13	9
(e) I don't want to go to a place where people show parts of their bodies	3		10	6	22	8	15	13
(f) I have older relatives to look after	1	1	6	2	4	1	4	1
(g) I don't like to go out alone	13	4	14	6	9	3	15	6
(h) I would not know what to do	2		4	3	2	1	4	7
(i) I never see anyone from my culture doing these things	2	0	6	2	7	3	6	9
None of these	77	93	60	82	46	81	43	62
Don't know	1	0	3	4	4	2	16	9
Base (= 100%)	*270*	*140*	*283*	*227*	*186*	*268*	*233*	*183*

Continued on next page

Table 7.38: *continued*

Reason	African-Caribbean		Indian		Pakistani		Bangladeshi	
	Women	Men	Women	Men	Women	Men	Women	Men
50–74								
(a) My husband/wife/ partner would disapprove	0	1	3	2	2	1	11	3
(b) Other members of my family would disapprove	1		3				5	2
(c) I don't want to go to mixed sex places	4	1	7	3	16	7	25	19
(d) I don't like to go to places where I can't speak my language	1	3	8	6	14	4	15	7
(e) I don't want to go to a place where people show parts of their bodies	4	1	8	6	14	4	21	17
(f) I have older relatives to look after	0	1	5		3		2	4
(g) 1 don't like to go out alone	23	3	16	5	9	2	12	3
(h) I would not know what to do	4		7	6	5	1	3	10
(i) I never see anyone from my culture doing these things	0		8	0		1	2	7
None of these	69	91	64	77	55	73	32	49
Don't know	3	2	7	3	12	17	24	16
Base (= 100%)	*193*	*174*	*107*	*107*	*50*	*124*	*63*	*171*
All ages								
(a) My husband/wife/ partner would disapprove	0	1	4	2	10	2	9	1
(b) Other members of my family would disapprove	1	1	4	0	10	2	9	2
(c) I don't want to go to mixed sex places	5	1	9	3	21	6	20	12
(d) I don't like to go to places where I can't speak my language	1	1	5	4	8	3	10	5
(e) I don't want to go to a place where people show parts of their bodies	3	1	9	5	18	6	20	11
(f) I have older relatives to look after	1	0	5	1	3	1	4	2
(g) I don't like to go out alone	17	4	18	5	12	6	21	6
(h) I would not know what to do	3	0	4	3	5	2	6	7
(i) I never see anyone from my culture doing these things	1	0	6	2	7	2	8	6
None of these	74	90	59	82	48	77	37	63
Don't know	1	1	3	4	4	5	13	8
Base (= 100%)	*641*	*428*	*598*	*463*	*517*	*627*	*603*	*567*

Chapter 8 Diet and nutrition

Table 8.1: How many of the meals taken at home in the last seven days included traditional foods? (percentages of all respondents)

Frequency	African-Caribbean		Indian		Pakistani		Bangladeshi	
	Women	Men	Women	Men	Women	Men	Women	Men
16–29								
All	8	15	25	25	33	46	36	45
Most	16	23	29	35	32	29	36	33
About half	21	32	27	26	24	15	19	16
Just a few	32	18	16	8	10	9	7	5
None	21	9	3	4	2	2	2	
None in last 7 days	0	1		1	1	0		
Don't know	1	2		1	0			
Base (= 100%)	*178*	*114*	*208*	*129*	*281*	*235*	*307*	*213*
30–49								
All	7	13	45	48	55	57	47	76
Most	20	18	27	26	27	29	32	15
About half	22	28	19	15	13	8	18	6
Just a few	33	24	5	9	3	5	4	3
None	16	16	3	1	1	1		
None in last 7 days	1	1	0			0		
Don't know	2	0	1	0	1	1		
Base (= 100%)	*270*	*140*	*283*	*227*	*186*	*268*	*233*	*183*
50–74								
All	16	18	70	61	81	71	57	87
Most	17	29	18	23	11	21	36	8
About half	29	21	6	12	4	5	6	4
Just a few	28	19	3	2	5			0
None	6	8	2	1		3		
None in last 7 days	2	0				0		
Don't know	1	4	1	0				
Base (= 100%)	*193*	*174*	*107*	*107*	*50*	*124*	*63*	*171*
All ages								
All	10	15	43	43	49	55	43	67
Most	18	24	26	29	26	27	35	21
About half	23	27	19	18	16	10	17	10
Just a few	31	20	9	7	6	5	5	3
None	15	11	2	2	1	2	1	0
None in last 7 days	1	1	0	0	0	0	0	0
Don't know	1	2	0	1	0	0	0	0
Base (= 100%)	*641*	*428*	*598*	*463*	*517*	*627*	*603*	*567*

Table 8.2: How many of the meals eaten away from home in the last seven days included traditional foods? (percentages of all respondents)

Frequency	African-Caribbean Women	African-Caribbean Men	Indian Women	Indian Men	Pakistani Women	Pakistani Men	Bangladeshi Women	Bangladeshi Men
16–29								
All	4	4	9	7	14	14	13	8
Most	8	6	4	3	8	6	9	11
About half	2	4	8	4	12	11	8	13
Just a few	21	28	8	21	6	16	11	18
None	47	41	39	44	31	27	25	25
None in last 7 days	16	15	30	18	28	26	32	21
Don't know	1	2	2	2	2	0	1	3
Base (= 100%)	*178*	*114*	*208*	*129*	*281*	*235*	*307*	*213*
30–49								
All	3	3	13	12	24	16	13	14
Most	1	6	9	6	11	13	11	11
About half	3	9	5	10	6	7	4	6
Just a few	15	18	5	14	2	3	1	8
None	42	40	15	21	12	16	2	4
None in last 7 days	33	23	46	37	41	44	68	51
Don't know	3	1	7	1	3	2	1	7
Base (= 100%)	*270*	*140*	*283*	*227*	*186*	*268*	*233*	*183*
50–74								
All	2	2	31	21	29	15	13	23
Most	2	4	7	7	4	14	8	6
About half	7	6	1	5	7	4	2	3
Just a few	5	11	1	4			2	0
None	25	18	2	8	5	3		1
None in last 7 days	58	53	52	55	55	63	70	63
Don't know	1	5	5	0		1	5	3
Base (= 100%)	*193*	*174*	*107*	*107*	*50*	*124*	*63*	*171*
All ages								
All	3	3	15	12	20	15	13	14
Most	4	5	7	5	9	10	9	10
About half	4	6	5	7	9	8	6	8
Just a few	14	19	5	14	3	8	6	10
None	39	33	21	26	20	18	13	12
None in last 7 days	34	31	41	35	37	41	51	42
Don't know	2	3	5	1	2	1	1	4
Base (= 100%)	*641*	*428*	*598*	*463*	*517*	*627*	*603*	*567*

Table 8.3: What kind of foods should be included in a healthy diet? (percentages of all respondents)

Item	African-Caribbean Women	African-Caribbean Men	Indian Women	Indian Men	Pakistani Women	Pakistani Men	Bangladeshi Women	Bangladeshi Men
16–29								
Well-balanced diet	2	5	5	3	3	6	1	5
Fresh fruit	69	48	66	61	68	59	55	49
Fresh vegetables/salad	85	76	80	79	82	73	72	79
High fibre/fibre/roughage/cereals	42	25	28	31	28	20	20	13
Fish	39	38	24	18	18	26	30	33
White meat/chicken/lean meat	30	26	17	17	14	21	10	18
Vitamins/minerals/trace elements	8	4	9	10	6	8	8	6
Dairy products/cheese/eggs	26	22	27	21	32	36	28	23
Low fat	7	1	8	6	6	6	6	8
Low fat spreads/margarine	2		3		4	0	1	1
Meat	24	21	21	22	26	39	19	22
Rice	19	16	9	5	15	7	15	13
Grilled foods/steamed	4	4	2	1	5	3	2	2
Fresh food (unspecified)	1		1		1		2	1
Carbohydrates/starchy foods (unspecified)	13	8	4	7	5	6	4	5
Sunflower margarine/polyunsaturates			0	1				
Varied diet/little bit of everything	1	0	2	2	1		0	1
Drink plenty of water/fluids	15	15	8	9	11	6	8	5
Moderation in everything/nothing in excess	1	3	0	0	0	1	0	1
Skimmed milk/semi-skimmed milk	3	4	5		1	1	0	1
Eat regularly/regular meals	0							
Light meals		3	0		1	1		
Concept not related to diet			0		0		0	
Other food substance	0	7	4	2	4	4	3	6
Reduce meat/little meat	4	4	2	3	2	3	2	2
No red meat	3	1	1	2	2	0	1	2
Low sugar/reduced sugar intake	4	1	5	2	4	2	3	3
Low salt/no salt	4	1	1		1	2	0	0
Avoid fatty foods/greasy foods	4	5	7	5	2	2	4	4
Avoid fried foods	3	1	1	0	4	3	1	0
Avoid chips and crisps	1				1			
Less convenience foods/refined/no additives	1	1	1	1	2		0	
Less fizzy drinks					0	1	0	
Protein	11	5	8	10	7	13	7	5
Low alcohol intake	1	1	0	2				
Limit dairy products	1		1			1	1	0
Herbs	1					0	1	1
Include small amount of fat/fat in diet	2	2	1	2	1	2	2	2
Low calorie intake/low calorie drinks	2	1	4	4	4	3	2	5
Pulses/beans/lentils	7	1	11	7	11	6	4	2
Fruit juice	4	2	7	3	5	7	7	3
Low saturated fats	0	2	1					
One main meal per day		0		1	0			
No fat/fat free			0	2		0	2	1
Watch cholesterol level					0			1
Sufficient sugar intake		1	1		2		1	1
No snacks/eating between meals				0				
Indian food (unspecified)	1	3	2		1	0	1	2
West Indian food								
Use oil/olive oil		1	1	0	0	1		
Vegetarian diet			1		1	0		1
Nuts	1	1	2	1	3	1	1	
Bread/chapatties	6	8	13	6	15	14	9	5
Curries			1	1	1	3	1	2
Noodles and pasta	13	16	6	5	4	2	2	1
Less spicy foods					1		0	1
Miscellaneous	0		2	1	1	1	0	
Don't know	1	5	7	3	3	4	14	1
Base (= 100%)	*178*	*114*	*208*	*129*	*281*	*235*	*307*	*213*

Continued on next page

Table 8.3: *continued*

Item	African-Caribbean		Indian		Pakistani		Bangladeshi	
	Women	Men	Women	Men	Women	Men	Women	Men
30–49								
Well-balanced diet	3	2	1	2	1	2	0	1
Fresh fruit	61	61	66	57	55	51	50	41
Fresh vegetables/salad	86	77	87	78	81	86	64	78
High fibre/fibre/ roughage/cereals	30	26	31	20	10	14	5	5
Fish	41	36	19	21	23	34	31	56
White meat/chicken/ lean meat	29	21	12	18	21	32	10	27
Vitamins/minerals/ trace elements	10	9	4	3	0	2		1
Dairy products/cheese/ eggs	21	15	41	26	37	25	28	25
Low fat	5	4	4	5	1	3	1	3
Low fat spreads/ margarine	2	1	2	2				0
Meat	17	22	13	14	33	40	17	28
Rice	22	16	17	6	16	7	11	16
Grilled foods/steamed	7	8	3	3	5	1	2	2
Fresh food (unspecified)	0	0	3	2	0	1		
Carbohydrates/starchy foods (unspecified)	17	14	3	3		2		
Sunflower margarine/ polyunsaturates	0			1				
Varied diet/little bit of everything		4	1	1	2	2	1	
Drink plenty of water/ fluids	14	8	5	4	4	5	4	1
Moderation in everything/nothing in excess	4	2	0	0	1		0	4
Skimmed milk/ semi-skimmed milk	2	3	2	3	3	3		1
Eat regularly/regular meals			0		0			
Light meals			1	1				
Concept not related to diet	0			0		0		
Other food substance	2	6	4	6	3	7	2	4
Reduce meat/little meat	7	2	1	3	1	3	1	8
No red meat	1	2	2	4	1	1	0	5
Low sugar/reduced sugar intake	4	2	3	2	1	1	1	1
Low salt/no salt	2		0		1		1	
Avoid fatty foods/ greasy foods	1	3	6	7	2	5	1	5
Avoid fried foods	3	1	3	3	2	1		1
Avoid chips and crisps	0					0		
Less convenience foods/ refined/no additives	2	2	0		1	2		1
Less fizzy drinks			1	0		1		1
Protein	14	8	5	4	0	4		1
Low alcohol intake	1	2	0	2				
Limit dairy products	1		0	0	0	1		
Herbs	1	4		1	1	1		2
Include small amount of fat/fat in diet	1		1	1				
Low calorie intake/low calorie drinks	2	2	4	2	1		2	1
Pulses/beans/lentils	9	4	20	14	18	16	7	13
Fruit juice	4	1	6	3	1	6	1	2
Low saturated fats	0	1		0				
One main meal per day	0		0	0				
No fat/fat free	0	1	2	1	1	1	1	1
Watch cholesterol level			0					
Sufficient sugar intake	1		0					1
No snacks/eating between meals				0				0
Indian food (unspecified)	2	4	1	5	1	2	1	3
West Indian food								
Use oil/olive oil	1	1	1		3	2	1	
Vegetarian diet		0	2	2		2		
Nuts	1	2	3	4	0			0
Bread/chapatties	7	1	17	9	26	14	8	8
Curries			2	1	1	2		2
Noodles and pasta	14	11	4	1	1			
Less spicy foods	1		1	2			0	1
Miscellaneous	0		2	2		0		1
Don't know	3	4	3	3	5	2	23	4
Base (= 100%)	270	140	283	227	186	268	233	183

Continued on next page

Table 8.3: *continued*

Item	African-Caribbean Women	African-Caribbean Men	Indian Women	Indian Men	Pakistani Women	Pakistani Men	Bangladeshi Women	Bangladeshi Men
50–74								
Well-balanced diet	1			1		3		1
Fresh fruit	53	45	48	49	50	50	29	33
Fresh vegetables/salad	87	82	86	69	68	71	51	72
High fibre/fibre/roughage/cereals	23	17	18	18	4	11	5	8
Fish	41	33	13	21	26	25	34	55
White meat/chicken/lean meat	34	27	9	24	20	23	3	25
Vitamins/minerals/trace elements	4	2	3	5	8	3		
Dairy products/cheese/eggs	13	17	34	24	21	28	24	20
Low fat	5	3	2	6	5	3		4
Low fat spreads/margarine	3	3	2	1	1	0		
Meat	13	9	14	8	11	42	9	26
Rice	19	12	21	17	6	6	0	33
Grilled foods/steamed	11	0	1		5	3	2	4
Fresh food (unspecified)	1	1	1	0	10			
Carbohydrates/starchy foods (unspecified)	6	4	1	1	5			
Sunflower margarine/polyunsaturates								0
Varied diet/little bit of everything	2	4	2	2		2		
Drink plenty of water/fluids	5	2		6	4	1		1
Moderation in everything/nothing in excess	2	2	1	1	1			1
Skimmed milk/semi-skimmed milk	1	2	1	1	1	1	8	2
Eat regularly/regular meals			1			0		1
Light meals		2	4	4	8	2		
Concept not related to diet		1						
Other food substance	6	8	11	4		6		5
Reduce meat/little meat	2	3	1	4	12	8	14	6
No red meat	3	1	2	2	8			3
Low sugar/reduced sugar intake	7	2	1	7			3	2
Low salt/no salt	1	1		2	2	1		1
Avoid fatty foods/greasy foods	7	5	6	7	10	6	0	8
Avoid fried foods	5	1	2		2	1	2	1
Avoid chips and crisps					4			
Less convenience foods/refined/no additives	1	2	3	4		6		1
Less fizzy drinks			2					
Protein	6	5	1	9	7	1		
Low alcohol intake	3							
Limit dairy products	0		1	2	6			1
Herbs	1			1				1
Include small amount of fat/fat in diet	0	0			1			
Low calorie intake/low calorie drinks	3	2	1	2				0
Pulses/beans/lentils	3	4	40	28	25	20	2	6
Fruit juice	6	4	3	2	1	8		2
Low saturated fats								
One main meal per day					1			
No fat/fat free	0	1		1	2	2		0
Watch cholesterol level								
Sufficient sugar intake		0						
No snacks/eating between meals								
Indian food (unspecified)	2	5	2	2	1			1
West Indian food								
Use oil/olive oil	2	1		2		1		1
Vegetarian diet				2		1		0
Nuts			4	2		2		
Bread/chapatties	4	3	28	19	15	19	6	8
Curries			6	1	3	2	2	4
Noodles and pasta	10	1	1					
Less spicy foods				3	4	0		
Miscellaneous	0	0	1	1	3	2		1
Don't know	4	5	1	1	11	0	35	4
Base (= 100%)	*193*	*174*	*107*	*107*	*50*	*124*	*63*	*171*

Continued on next page

Table 8.3: *continued*

Item	African-Caribbean Women	African-Caribbean Men	Indian Women	Indian Men	Pakistani Women	Pakistani Men	Bangladeshi Women	Bangladeshi Men
All ages								
Well-balanced diet	2	2	2	2	2	4	1	3
Fresh fruit	62	51	62	57	60	54	49	42
Fresh vegetables/salad	86	78	84	76	80	78	66	76
High fibre/fibre/ roughage/cereals	33	22	27	23	17	16	12	9
Fish	40	35	19	20	21	29	31	46
White meat/chicken/ lean meat	30	25	13	19	18	26	9	22
Vitamins/minerals/ trace elements	8	5	5	6	4	5	4	3
Dairy products/cheese/ eggs	21	18	35	24	32	30	27	22
Low fat	6	3	5	6	4	4	3	5
Low fat spreads/ margarine	2	1	2	1	2	0	1	0
Meat	18	17	16	15	27	40	17	25
Rice	20	15	15	8	14	7	12	20
Grilled foods/steamed	7	4	3	2	5	2	2	3
Fresh food (unspecified)	1	0	2	1	2	0	1	0
Carbohydrates/starchy foods (unspecified)	12	8	3	4	3	3	2	2
Sunflower margarine/ polyunsaturates	0	0	0	0	0	0	0	0
Varied diet/little bit of everything	1	3	1	2	1	1	0	0
Drink plenty of water/ fluids	12	8	5	6	7	5	5	2
Moderation in everything/nothing in excess	2	3	0	1	1	1	0	2
Skimmed milk/ semi-skimmed milk	2	3	3	1	2	2	1	1
Eat regularly/regular meals	0	0	0	1	0	0	0	0
Light meals	0	2	1	1	2	1	0	0
Concept not related to diet	0	0	0	0	0	0	0	0
Other food substance	2	7	5	4	3	5	2	5
Reduce meat/little meat	5	3	2	3	3	4	3	5
No red meat	2	1	2	3	2	0	1	3
Low sugar/reduced sugar intake	5	2	3	3	2	1	2	2
Low salt/no salt	2	0	1	1	1	1	0	0
Avoid fatty foods/ greasy foods	4	4	6	6	3	4	3	5
Avoid fried foods	3	1	2	1	3	2	1	1
Avoid chips and crisps	0	0	0	0	1	0	0	0
Less convenience foods/ refined/no additives	1	2	1	1	2	2	0	1
Less fizzy drinks	0	0	1	0	0	1	0	0
Protein	11	6	6	7	4	7	3	3
Low alcohol intake	1	1	0	1	0	0	0	0
Limit dairy products	1	0	1	1	1	1	0	0
Herbs	1	1	0	0	0	0	0	1
Include small amount of fat/fat in diet	1	1	1	1	1	1	1	1
Low calorie intake/low calorie drinks	2	2	3	2	2	1	2	2
Pulses/beans/lentils	6	3	21	15	16	13	5	6
Fruit juice	5	2	6	3	3	7	4	2
Low saturated fats	0	1	1	0	0	0	0	0
One main meal per day	0	0	0	0	0	0	0	0
No fat/fat free	0	1	1	1	1	1	1	1
Watch cholesterol level	0	0	0	0	0	0	0	0
Sufficient sugar intake	0	0	1	0	1	0	0	1
No snacks/eating between meals	0	0	0	0	0	0	0	0
Indian food (unspecified)	2	4	1	3	1	1	1	2
West Indian food								
Use oil/olive oil	1	1	1	1	1	1	0	0
Vegetarian diet	0	0	1	1	0	1	0	1
Nuts	1	1	3	2	1	1	0	0
Bread/chapatties	6	4	18	10	19	15	8	7
Curries	0	0	2	1	2	2	1	2
Noodles and pasta	13	9	4	2	2	1	1	0
Less spicy foods	0	0	0	2	1	0	0	1
Miscellaneous	0	0	2	2	1	1	0	0
Don't know	3	4	4	3	5	2	20	3
Base (= 100%)	641	428	598	463	517	627	603	567

Table 8.4: Understanding of terms regarding diet and nutrition (percentages of all respondents)

Term understood	African-Caribbean		Indian		Pakistani		Bangladeshi	
	Women	Men	Women	Men	Women	Men	Women	Men
16–29								
Starchy foods	90	79	70	68	58	54	39	48
Dietary fibre	79	70	72	58	55	54	40	47
Fat	99	99	98	100	98	99	99	97
Saturated fat	51	54	49	36	39	45	28	31
Base (= 100%)	*177*	*112*	*202*	*121*	*253*	*207*	*288*	*196*
30–49								
Starchy foods	98	91	65	59	38	48	5	10
Dietary fibre	84	73	57	57	48	45	7	22
Fat	96	98	98	97	97	97	100	100
Saturated fat	66	56	43	55	23	41	8	9
Base (= 100%)	*265*	*138*	*273*	*204*	*128*	*224*	*204*	*164*
50–74								
Starchy foods	97	97	61	64	45	33		8
Dietary fibre	78	64	50	52	34	22		11
Fat	97	92	94	94	100	100	100	99
Saturated fat	49	46	39	51	23	32		8
Base (= 100%)	*186*	*168*	*94*	*94*	*32*	*98*	*56*	*145*
All ages								
Starchy foods	95	89	66	63	49	47	21	26
Dietary fibre	80	69	61	56	50	44	22	29
Fat	97	96	97	98	98	99	100	99
Saturated fat	56	52	44	48	31	41	17	18
Base (= 100%)	*628*	*418*	*569*	*419*	*413*	*529*	*548*	*505*

Table 8.5: What types of food contain a lot of starch? (percentages of all those respondents who understood the meaning of the term starch)

Food	African-Caribbean Women	Men	Indian Women	Men	Pakistani Women	Men	Bangladeshi Women	Men
16–29								
Bread (including nan, chapati, puri, roti	32	13	35	13	33	26	30	23
Rice	66	41	51	33	32	29	34	30
Potatoes	73	64	64	55	65	48	39	47
Yams, plantain, sweet potatoes	20	30	10	4	2	10	4	3
Brown/wholemeal bread	4	1	3	4	9	3	2	5
Brown rice	4	4	5	3	5	2	2	3
Noodles/pasta/macaroni, etc.	28	10	22	10	10	6	10	5
Maize/sweetcorn	1		2	2	4	5	1	1
Lentils/peas/beans/dhal	2		4	4	5	4	6	1
Cooking oil/vegetable oil			1	1		2	1	
Butter	1		1	3	5	3	1	2
Ghee			0		1	2		2
Lard				1		0		
Cheese		4	2	1		2		
Meat/red meat	1		2		0	7	5	2
Eggs			1	1		2	1	2
Burgers/sausages/hot dogs		1	1					
Crisps	3	3	4	3	9	2	7	6
Fried snacks, e.g. samosa, pakora, bhaji	1	0	3		2	4	1	
Sweets: halva, kulfi, gulabjamun, etc.	1	2	4	2	3	6	3	5
Milk puddings with rice/semolina/sago/vermicelli	1	1	3		2	3	1	1
Nuts	0		0		3	2	1	
Shellfish/seafood, such as prawns	1		0		1	1	1	
Cakes/biscuits	3	2	1	3	2	2	4	5
Cereals	1	2	0	3	1	1	4	1
Vegetables	2		0	4	2	4	4	4
Fruits	1		1		1	1	2	4
Flour, cornflour, cornmeal, wheat	2	1			0	1	1	
Chips	1	3	1	2		0	1	5
Casava								
Cocoa								
(Other) wrong answers			3	4	7	5	5	1
Other	12	12	11	18	23	17	22	12
Don't know of any examples	3	2	6	8	6	5	17	11
Base (= 100%)	160	90	139	77	136	113	109	87

Continued on next page

Table 8.5: *continued*

Food	African-Caribbean		Indian		Pakistani		Bangladeshi	
	Women	Men	Women	Men	Women	Men	Women	Men
30–49								
Bread (including nan, chapati, puri, roti	31	15	26	15	29	27	17	33
Rice	73	40	75	57	57	56	42	44
Potatoes	69	69	66	60	51	52	54	34
Yams, plantain, sweet potatoes	39	47	11	6	5	10		11
Brown/wholemeal bread	3	2	1	2	3	3		4
Brown rice	4	2	3	4	7	4	7	4
Noodles/pasta/macaroni, etc.	22	10	12	9	19	6	9	
Maize/sweetcorn	0	1	3	2		4		
Lentils/peas/beans/dhal	1		7	1	6	2	7	
Cooking oil/vegetable oil			0			1		
Butter			3		1			
Ghee			2	1		1		
Lard			1					6
Cheese	1	3	1	1	2			
Meat/red meat	0	1	2	3	6	2		
Eggs	0		0	1			7	
Burgers/sausages/hot dogs	1							
Crisps	1	0	2	1		1		
Fried snacks, e.g. samosa, pakora, bhaji	1		1	1	1	3		
Sweets: halva, kulfi, gulabjamun, etc.	0	1	1	1	3	4		6
Milk puddings with rice/semolina/sago/vermicelli	0	0	2	1	6	1	7	
Nuts		1						
Shellfish/seafood, such as prawns								
Cakes/biscuits	1	1	1	2	3	2	4	
Cereals	4	1	1	1	1	1		
Vegetables	3	1	2	3	4	1	7	4
Fruits	5	8	1	3	4	1		
Flour, cornflour, cornmeal, wheat	8	5	1	4		1		
Chips	2	1	1	1				
Casava								
Cocoa								
(Other) wrong answers	0			1		2		
Other	16	16	13	17	13	10	7	
Don't know of any examples	0	4	3	7	5	5	24	41
Base (= 100%)	*257*	*128*	*175*	*117*	*49*	*91*	*13*	*16*

Continued on next page

Food	African-Caribbean		Indian		Pakistani		Bangladeshi	
	Women	Men	Women	Men	Women	Men	Women	Men
50–74								
Bread (including nan, chapati, puri, roti	21	10	37	29	26	33		24
Rice	68	48	80	56	53	15		56
Potatoes	63	51	61	40	76	29		21
Yams, plantain, sweet potatoes	65	72	4	1		10		
Brown/wholemeal bread	3	2	2	2	4			5
Brown rice	5	8	2		4			23
Noodles/pasta/ macaroni, etc	8	2	15	2	6	2		
Maize/sweetcorn	3		5			4		
Lentils/peas/beans/dhal	1	0	9		15	2		
Cooking oil/vegetable oil			0					
Butter	0		9	4		3		
Ghee			0	1		3		
Lard								
Cheese								17
Meat/red meat				3		12		
Eggs	0					1		
Burgers/sausages/ hot dogs	0	1				1		
Crisps	1			1	15			
Fried snacks, e.g. samosa, pakora, bhaji	0	1		3				
Sweets: halva, kulfi, gulabjamun, etc.	0		6		10	9		
Milk puddings with rice/ semolina/sago/vermicelli		1	8	3		9		
Nuts								
Shellfish/seafood, such as prawns								
Cakes/biscuits	0	1	3	1				
Cereals	2	2		4		14		14
Vegetables	0	1		5				8
Fruits	4	11		1		11		16
Flour, cornflour, cornmeal, wheat	5	2	2	1		14		
Chips				8				
Casava								
Cocoa								
(Other) wrong answers				1				
Other	20	16	14	12	14	21		29
Don't know of any examples	0	2	2	2	4	22		
Base (= 100%)	*180*	*161*	*55*	*51*	*12*	*29*		*10*

Continued on next page

Table 8.5: *continued*

Food	African-Caribbean Women	African-Caribbean Men	Indian Women	Indian Men	Pakistani Women	Pakistani Men	Bangladeshi Women	Bangladeshi Men
All ages								
Bread (including nan, chapati, puri, roti	29	12	32	17	31	27	29	25
Rice	69	43	67	48	41	37	34	34
Potatoes	69	60	64	54	63	47	41	43
Yams, plantain, sweet potatoes	40	51	9	4	2	10	3	3
Brown/wholemeal bread	3	2	2	3	7	3	2	5
Brown rice	4	5	4	3	5	2	3	5
Noodles/pasta/ macaroni, etc	20	7	17	8	12	6	10	4
Maize/sweetcorn	1	0	3	2	2	4	1	1
Lentils/peas/beans/dhal	1	0	6	2	6	3	6	1
Cooking oil/vegetable oil	0	0	0	1	0	1	0	0
Butter	1	0	3	2	3	2	1	2
Ghee	0	0	1	1	1	2	0	1
Lard	0	0	0	0	0	0	0	1
Cheese	0	2	2	1	0	2	0	1
Meat/red meat	1	0	2	2	2	6	5	2
Eggs	0	0	1	1	0	1	1	1
Burgers/sausages/ hot dogs	0	1	0	0	0	0	0	0
Crisps	2	1	2	2	7	1	6	5
Fried snacks, e.g. samosa, pakora, bhaji	1	0	2	1	1	3	1	0
Sweets: halva, kulfi, gulabjamun, etc.	1	1	3	1	4	6	3	5
Milk puddings with rice/ semolina/sago/vermicelli	0	1	3	1	3	3	1	1
Nuts	0	0	0	0	2	1	1	0
Shellfish/seafood, such as prawns	0	0	0	0	1	0	1	0
Cakes/biscuits	2	1	1	2	2	2	4	4
Cereals	2	2	0	2	1	3	4	2
Vegetables	2	1	1	4	3	2	4	4
Fruits	3	7	1	1	2	3	2	5
Flour, cornflour, cornmeal, wheat	5	3	1	2	0	3	1	0
Chips	1	1	1	1	1	0	0	4
Casava	0	0	0	0	0	0	0	0
Cocoa	0	0	0	0	0	0	0	0
(Other) wrong answers	0	0	1	2	4	3	4	1
Other	15	15	12	16	20	15	21	12
Don't know of any examples	1	3	4	6	6	8	17	13
Base (= 100%)	*597*	*379*	*369*	*245*	*197*	*233*	*122*	*113*

Table 8.6: What types of food contain a lot of dietary fibre? (percentages of all those respondents who understood the meaning of the term dietary fibre)

Food	African-Caribbean		Indian		Pakistani		Bangladeshi	
	Women	Men	Women	Men	Women	Men	Women	Men
16–29								
Bread (including nan, chapati, puri, roti	16	16	20	19	21	32	18	11
Rice	3	4	6	1	10	9	17	7
Potatoes	8	5	9	6	4	12	1	5
Yams, plantain, sweet potatoes	3	2	2	5	2	4	1	
Brown/wholemeal bread	55	36	51	52	42	38	41	21
Brown rice	18	3	25	17	13	13	21	11
Noodles/pasta/macaroni, etc.	6	2	10	4	3	1	4	4
Maize/sweetcorn	5	8	5	4	6	5	4	
Lentils/peas/beans/dhal	10	2	12	9	11	13	8	6
Cooking oil/vegetable oil			1		1	1	2	1
Butter	2	2			2	3	1	1
Ghee							1	1
Lard								1
Cheese	1	1	1	2	1	1	2	1
Meat/red meat	0	1	0		2	4		1
Eggs		0	2		1	3	2	3
Burgers/sausages/hot dogs			0					1
Crisps	1		1			1	1	2
Fried snacks, e.g. samosa, pakora, bhaji			2		1		1	
Sweets: halva, kulfi, gulabjamun, etc.						1		
Milk puddings with rice/semolina/sago/vermicelli	0		2			2	1	5
Nuts		1	4	4	1	3	4	2
Shellfish/seafood, such as prawns			3	1		1		
Cereals	48	41	16	17	31	26	30	29
Fruits	7	11	7	6	10	7	7	14
Vegetables	11	12	4	4	6	2	10	9
Bran	12	13	3	4	3	1	1	0
(Other) wrong answers	0				1	2	5	
Other	46	38	53	33	63	44	50	27
Don't know of any examples	1	2	5	3	7	4	8	13
Base (= 100%)	*133*	*76*	*147*	*71*	*141*	*112*	*113*	*86*

Continued on next page

Table 8.6: *continued*

Food	African-Caribbean Women	Men	Indian Women	Men	Pakistani Women	Men	Bangladeshi Women	Men
30–49								
Bread (including nan, chapati, puri, roti	13	14	26	20	19	18	14	15
Rice	3	4	1	2	13	5		5
Potatoes	5	6	6	6	11	6		3
Yams, plantain, sweet potatoes	2	7	4	3	2	3		
Brown/wholemeal bread	38	40	56	53	38	60	56	38
Brown rice	12	6	23	6	11	13	26	16
Noodles/pasta/macaroni, etc.	3	5	4	3	2	1		
Maize/sweetcorn	2	7	2	4	2	3	5	
Lentils/peas/beans/dhal	13	10	13	12	6	5	9	6
Cooking oil/vegetable oil	0		1	1	1	1		
Butter	0							
Ghee				1				
Lard				1				
Cheese		0	0	2		1	5	
Meat/red meat	1	1	0		2	2		
Eggs			0	1	1	2		
Burgers/sausages/hot dogs								
Crisps				1				
Fried snacks, e.g. samosa, pakora, bhaji				1		2		
Sweets: halva, kulfi, gulabjamun, etc.								
Milk puddings with rice/semolina/sago/vermicelli	1	1	1	2	2	1		
Nuts		3	0	1	3	1		
Shellfish/seafood, such as prawns		0	1	1		2		
Cereals	51	36	23	31	21	27	17	13
Fruits	14	10	6	11	17	9	6	9
Vegetables	17	9	6	10	21	10	12	21
Bran	10	7	1	10	1	6		
(Other) wrong answers	0	1			1			2
Other	50	49	44	41	58	37	13	29
Don't know of any examples	1	2	5	2	7	5	22	15
Base (= 100%)	*217*	*103*	*159*	*115*	*59*	*89*	*17*	*33*

Continued on next page

Table 8.6: *continued*

Food	African-Caribbean		Indian		Pakistani		Bangladeshi	
	Women	Men	Women	Men	Women	Men	Women	Men
50–74								
Bread (including nan, chapati, puri, roti)	5	15	43	8	13	36		18
Rice	2	3	4	2	13	3		8
Potatoes	8	4	3	1	14			4
Yams, plantain, sweet potatoes	3	6	2	5	8	3		
Brown/wholemeal bread	31	31	54	36	35	40		37
Brown rice	6	11	18	3	19	7		8
Noodles/pasta/macaroni, etc.	2	1	5					
Maize/sweetcorn	8	7	2	3		3		
Lentils/peas/beans/dhal	5	8	17	33	56	20		6
Cooking oil/vegetable oil								
Butter			1	3				6
Ghee			1	1	1			
Lard				1				
Cheese								6
Meat/red meat	0		2					6
Eggs			2	2				6
Burgers/sausages/hot dogs								
Crisps								
Fried snacks, e.g. samosa, pakora, bhaji			1					
Sweets: halva, kulfi, gulabjamun, etc.								12
Milk puddings with rice/semolina/sago/vermicelli			2					
Nuts		3	3	2	3			
Shellfish/seafood, such as prawns				2				
Cereals	36	39	21	22	11	22		10
Fruits		6	9	5	5		5	
Vegetables	12	13	16	12	5	2		9
Bran		4	3		3			
(Other) wrong answers				2				
Other	53	38	22	45	38	45		24
Don't know of any examples	10	6		10		6		
Base (= 100%)	*140*	*103*	*49*	*42*	*10*	*22*		*16*

Continued on next page

Table 8.6: *continued*

Food	African-Caribbean		Indian		Pakistani		Bangladeshi	
	Women	Men	Women	Men	Women	Men	Women	Men
All ages								
Bread (including nan, chapati, puri, roti	69	67	98	79	103	115	117	98
Rice	11	10	24	17	19	19	19	11
Potatoes	10	6	8	5	12	13	1	6
Yams, plantain, sweet potatoes	6	7	6	10	8	7	1	1
Brown/wholemeal bread	46	36	54	48	41	40	41	23
Brown rice	35	24	63	53	33	49	28	21
Noodles/pasta/macaroni, etc.	11	4	25	7	8	9	7	8
Maize/sweetcorn	7	9	6	6	6	5	4	0
Lentils/peas/beans/dhal	9	8	14	20	17	16	9	6
Cooking oil/vegetable oil	7	4	10	9	4	4	3	3
Butter	1	1	1	2	2	3	1	2
Ghee	0	1	0	0	0	1	1	0
Lard	0	0	0	0	0	0	0	0
Cheese	1	1	1	2	1	1	2	2
Meat/red meat	0	1	1	2	2	4	1	1
Eggs	1	2	1	2	3	3	3	1
Burgers/sausages/hot dogs	0	0	1	0	1	1	0	1
Crisps	1	0	1	0	0	1	1	2
Fried snacks, e.g. samosa, pakora, bhaji	0	0	2	0	1	0	1	0
Sweets: halva, kulfi, gulabjamun, etc.	0	0	0	1	0	2	0	2
Milk puddings with rice/semolina/sago/vermicelli	0	0	2	0	0	2	1	5
Nuts	2	4	5	4	3	4	2	0
Shellfish/seafood, such as prawns	0	1	2	2	1	1	0	0
Cereals	43	39	18	19	28	26	30	26
Fruits	36	26	23	30	19	23	9	16
Vegetables	20	16	11	15	14	8	11	11
Bran	19	12	6	12	13	7	2	6
(Other) wrong answers	6	3	1	8	2	5	5	0
Other	49	38	45	37	58	44	50	27
Don't know of any examples	34	25	35	37	35	28	10	19
Base (= 100%)	*276*	*182*	*199*	*115*	*152*	*136*	*114*	*103*

Table 8.7: What types of food contain a lot of fat? (percentages of all those respondents who understood the meaning of the term fat)

	African-Caribbean		Indian		Pakistani		Bangladeshi	
Food	Women	Men	Women	Men	Women	Men	Women	Men
16–29								
Bread (including nan, chapati, puri, roti		2	5	1	4	4	3	
Rice	0		5	1	4	2	3	4
Potatoes	7	7	11	10	9	17	7	8
Yams, plantain, sweet potatoes		2	1	1		0		2
Brown/wholemeal bread	0				0	2		0
Brown rice			1			2	0	
Noodles/pasta/ macaroni, etc.	1			1		1	0	0
Maize/sweetcorn						0		
Lentils/peas/beans/dhal	0		0	1		4	1	2
Cooking oil/vegetable oil	18	8	19	18	21	20	20	12
Butter	42	24	46	30	41	38	51	41
Ghee	1	2	16	14	11	20	25	21
Lard	11	1	7	8	6	11	7	1
Cheese	16	16	25	7	14	16	16	18
Meat/red meat	37	44	32	26	35	28	53	47
Eggs	3	3	4	2	4	3	7	5
Burgers/sausages/ hot dogs	23	19	23	10	7	10	8	7
Crisps	14	10	27	9	11	11	13	9
Fried snacks, e.g. samosa, pakora, bhaji	19	15	30	23	25	27	14	14
Sweets: halva, kulfi, gulabjamun, etc.	12	8	19	12	11	7	7	5
Milk puddings with rice/ semolina/sago/vermicelli	5	8	13	6	7	4	5	9
Nuts	3	8	8	1	1	1	2	1
Shellfish/seafood, such as prawns			1			2	1	
Cakes/biscuits/pastries	8	9	7	3	9	3	8	5
Fried foods, including chips, fish in batter	13	19	6	15	15	20	8	13
Chocolate	6	1	4	5	8	5	6	3
Cream/ice-cream	3	2	4	1	4	2	2	2
Milk, yoghurt, dairy products	9	4	2	2	7	8	4	2
Margarine	5	2	1		3	3	2	1
Fish	2	1			0	2	4	1
Bacon	4	2	1			0		
Curry/curries			0	3	1	3	1	1
(Other) wrong answer	2	4	3	2	3	6	5	1
Other	32	28	39	25	42	29	26	15
Don't know of any examples	1		0	3	3	2	2	4
Base (= 100%)	*174*	*111*	*198*	*121*	*250*	*205*	*285*	*191*

Continued on next page

Table 8.7: *continued*

Food	African-Caribbean		Indian		Pakistani		Bangladeshi	
	Women	Men	Women	Men	Women	Men	Women	Men
30–49								
Bread (including nan, chapati, puri, roti	0		6	3	6	4	5	2
Rice	1	2	5	4	7	2	5	5
Potatoes	9	5	11	12	8	8	12	6
Yams, plantain, sweet potatoes	0	2	0	1		0	0	
Brown/wholemeal bread					1		0	
Brown rice		1		0		0		
Noodles/pasta/macaroni, etc.			0	1		0		
Maize/sweetcorn								
Lentils/peas/beans/dhal	0		0	1	1	2	0	
Cooking oil/vegetable oil	20	15	15	14	22	18	16	18
Butter	44	24	57	40	55	54	59	52
Ghee	2	4	32	21	28	33	43	45
Lard	10	5	6	4	4	11	4	2
Cheese	22	13	23	23	12	17	7	16
Meat/red meat	54	50	33	45	54	48	90	74
Eggs	2	4	5	5	5	2	6	6
Burgers/sausages/hot dogs	23	21	8	11	4	3	2	2
Crisps	9	8	14	5	7	4	2	2
Fried snacks, e.g. samosa, pakora, bhaji	11	12	34	19	28	25	3	5
Sweets: halva, kulfi, gulabjamun, etc.	2	5	20	8	12	6	4	8
Milk puddings with rice/semolina/sago/vermicelli	3	8	13	6	7	6	6	6
Nuts	3		7	1	2	2		1
Shellfish/seafood, such as prawns	1		0	1	2	1	13	1
Cakes/biscuits/pastries	13	8	2	3	3	2		1
Fried foods, including chips, fish in batter	13	10	3	10	3	4	0	3
Chocolate	2	1	0	1		1		1
Cream/ice-cream	2	1	1	2	4	3		1
Milk, yoghurt, dairy products	8	4	2	10	1	5	1	1
Margarine	5	2	4	2	2	1		
Fish	4			0	1	0	5	2
Bacon	7	6	1	2			0	
Curry/curries	0		1	1		2		
(Other) wrong answer	2	2	1	1	1	0	1	
Other	27	26	22	20	21	16	4	6
Don't know of any examples	1	4	2	3	2	1	1	4
Base (= 100%)	*255*	*134*	*269*	*198*	*123*	*220*	*204*	*164*

Continued on next page

Table 8.7: *continued*

Food	African-Caribbean Women	Men	Indian Women	Men	Pakistani Women	Men	Bangladeshi Women	Men
50–74								
Bread (including nan, chapati, puri, roti	1	1	8	1	7	4	5	
Rice	1	2	5	4	5	7	2	
Potatoes	14	8	8	11	7	8	14	5
Yams, plantain, sweet potatoes	1	1		1				
Brown/wholemeal bread	0							
Brown rice								
Noodles/pasta/ macaroni, etc.								
Maize/sweetcorn	1							
Lentils/peas/beans/dhal		0	2			3		
Cooking oil/vegetable oil	10	13	19	13	10	14	18	13
Butter	27	24	56	49	36	54	45	56
Ghee	1	1	38	22	32	37	32	45
Lard	11	9	4	7	3	7		4
Cheese	14	13	13	13	6	9	4	16
Meat/red meat	66	58	31	46	39	49	97	76
Eggs	2	3	3	4		3	4	4
Burgers/sausages/ hotdogs	20	11	6	12		2	1	1
Crisps	3	4	11	3	5	2	4	0
Fried snacks, e.g. samosa, pakora, bhaji	7	5	28	6	35	15	2	3
Sweets: halve, kulfi, gulabjamun, etc.	1		25	10	10	9		1
Milk puddings with rice/ semolina/sago/vermicelli	1	4	13	6	5	9	3	8
Nuts	1	2	6	3		2		0
Shellfish/seafood, such as prawns	2			1			6	1
Cakes/biscuits/pastries	4		4	3		2		
Fried foods, including chips, fish in batter	1	7	3	5		4		1
Chocolate	1	2				2	2	1
Cream/ice-cream		2	4	1	7			
Milk, yoghurt, dairy products	2	4	5	4		1		
Margarine	1		1	3		1		
Fish	6			1			7	4
Bacon	4	3		2				
Curry/curries	0				3			
(Other) wrong answer	0	2	5			1		1
Other	20	11	12	17	23	8		3
Don't know of any examples	5	9	2	1	11	2	1	2
Base (= 100%)	*179*	*153*	*88*	*88*	*32*	*98*	*56*	*144*

Continued on next page

Table 8.7: *continued*

Food	African-Caribbean Women	African-Caribbean Men	Indian Women	Indian Men	Pakistani Women	Pakistani Men	Bangladeshi Women	Bangladeshi Men
All ages								
Bread (including nan, chapati, puri, roti	0	1	6	2	5	4	4	0
Rice	1	2	5	3	5	3	3	3
Potatoes	9	7	11	11	8	12	10	7
Yams, plantain, sweet potatoes	0	1	1	1	0	0	0	1
Brown/wholemeal bread	0	0	0	0	0	1	0	0
Brown rice	0	0	0	0	0	1	0	0
Noodles/pasta/ macaroni, etc.	0	0	0	1	0	1	0	0
Maize/sweetcorn	0	0	0	0	0	0	0	0
Lentils/peas/beans/dhal	0	0	1	1	0	3	0	1
Cooking oil/vegetable oil	17	12	17	15	20	18	18	14
Butter	39	24	53	38	45	47	53	48
Ghee	1	2	27	19	20	29	33	35
Lard	10	5	6	6	5	10	5	2
Cheese	18	14	22	16	12	15	11	17
Meat/red meat	51	51	32	38	42	40	73	63
Eggs	2	3	4	4	4	3	6	5
Burgers/sausages/ hot dogs	22	17	13	11	5	6	5	4
Crisps	9	7	18	6	9	6	8	4
Fried snacks, e.g. samosa, pakora, bhaji	13	11	32	18	27	24	8	8
Sweets: halva, kulfi, gulabjamun, etc.	6	5	20	10	11	7	5	5
Milk puddings with rice/ semolina/sago/vermicelli	3	7	13	6	6	6	5	8
Nuts	3	3	8	2	1	1	1	1
Shellfish/seafood, such as prawns	1	0	1	1	1	1	6	0
Cakes/biscuits/pastries	9	5	4	3	6	2	4	3
Fried foods, including chips, fish in batter	10	12	4	11	9	10	4	7
Chocolate	3	2	1	2	4	3	3	2
Cream/ice-cream	2	2	3	1	4	2	1	1
Milk, yoghurt, dairy products	7	4	3	6	4	5	2	1
Margarine	4	2	2	2	2	2	1	1
Fish	4	0	0	0	1	1	5	2
Bacon	5	4	1	2	0	0	0	0
Curry/curries	0	0	1	1	1	2	0	0
(Other) wrong answer	2	3	2	1	2	3	3	1
Other	27	22	26	21	32	20	14	9
Don't know of any examples	2	4	1	2	3	2	2	4
Base (= 100%)	*608*	*398*	*555*	*407*	*405*	*523*	*545*	*499*

Table 8.8: What types of food contain a lot of saturated fat? (percentages of all respondents who understood the meaning of the term saturated fat)

Food	African-Caribbean		Indian		Pakistani		Bangladeshi	
	Women	Men	Women	Men	Women	Men	Women	Men
16–29								
Bread (including nan, chapati, puri, roti			1	2		5		
Rice			1		2	2	3	
Potatoes	2		2			2	7	
Yams, plantain, sweet potatoes	0			1		1		
Brown/wholemeal bread								
Brown rice						1	2	
Noodles/pasta/ macaroni, etc.			2			0	3	
Maize/sweetcorn			1		1	2		
Lentils/peas/beans/dhal	1		2			2		
Cooking oil/vegetable oil	10	13	16	8	20	10	5	8
Butter	32	24	31	27	33	22	27	24
Ghee	2	5	13	4	4	15	9	6
Lard	7	5	13	8	9	7	8	
Cheese	10	7	8	8	6	21	9	4
Meat/red meat	19	11	16	3	6	6	12	6
Eggs		1	6	7	3	3	2	
Burgers/sausages/ hot dogs	3	7	5	6	1	1	4	
Crisps	4	5	9	8	6	4	5	3
Fried snacks, e.g. samosa, pakora, bhaji	5	12	9	9	7	24	11	2
Sweets: halva, kulfi, gulabjamun, etc.	1		7	2	3	7	7	3
Milk puddings with rice/ semolina/sago/vermicelli	4	1	6	7	5	4	6	5
Nuts			4			0	1	
Shellfish/seafood, such as prawns			6		1		2	
Cakes/biscuits/pastries	7	2			4	2	2	
Fried foods, including chips, fish in batter	6	6	2		5	2	6	5
Chocolate	3						3	3
Cream/ice-cream		2					3	
Milk, yoghurt, dairy products	6	3		9	3	11	5	8
Margarine	10	1	4	4	6	9	7	16
Fish	4			4	1	2		
Bacon	2	1	2					
(Other) wrong answers						1	5	1
Other	21	9	27	19	28	19	26	9
Don't know of any examples	18	22	15	12	19	10	21	30
Base (= 100%)	84	62	94	40	97	82	77	57

Continued on next page

Table 8.8: *continued*

Food	African-Caribbean		Indian		Pakistani		Bangladeshi	
	Women	Men	Women	Men	Women	Men	Women	Men
30–49								
Bread (including nan, chapati, puri, roti			7	8		3		
Rice	1		3	2	2			
Potatoes		1	1	1	2	1		
Yams, plantain, sweet potatoes								
Brown/wholemeal bread	1				2			
Brown rice			1					
Noodles/pasta/macaroni, etc.		2						
Maize/sweetcorn	1		2	1				
Lentils/peas/beans/dhal				1		1		
Cooking oil/vegetable oil	15	19	28	16	21	22	5	
Butter	26	22	31	26	14	22	9	24
Ghee	2	2	13	21	8	5	17	25
Lard	13	10	10	7	1	4	4	
Cheese	8	11	3	8	1	4	6	
Meat/red meat	19	12	10	15	6	19	16	
Eggs	1	1	4	1		3	12	
Burgers/sausages/hotdogs	16	5	2	3	10	8	6	
Crisps	6	6	6	4	6	10	17	
Fried snacks, e.g. samosa, pakora, bhaji	7	9	16	21	5	13		15
Sweets: halva, kulfi, gulabjamun, etc.	0	1	6	3	2	2	8	7
Milk puddings with rice/semolina/sago/vermicelli	1	8	5	2		5		5
Nuts	1		6	3	3	1		
Shellfish/seafood, such as prawns	1		1			4	14	
Cakes/biscuits/pastries	3		5	1	2			7
Fried foods, including chips, fish in batter	5	7	1	2	2			
Chocolate	1							
Cream/ice-cream	2		2	1				
Milk, yoghurt, dairy products	8	6	3	5	2	5	5	5
Margarine	12	9	5	6	3	2	4	7
Fish	2		1	1	2			
Bacon	5	1		1	5			
(Other) wrong answers		1	4	1				
Other	25	17	25	18	31	19	6	22
Don't know of any examples	18	20	15	17	21	10	26	36
Base (= 100%)	*164*	*80*	*119*	*112*	*27*	*77*	*19*	*15*

Continued on next page

Food	African-Caribbean Women	African-Caribbean Men	Indian Women	Indian Men	Pakistani Women	Pakistani Men	Bangladeshi Women	Bangladeshi Men
50–74								
Bread (including nan, chapati, puri, roti			2			4		
Rice					12			
Potatoes	1		2	3		3		
Yams, plantain, sweet potatoes								
Brown/wholemeal bread								5
Brown rice								
Noodles/pasta/macaroni, etc.								
Maize/sweetcorn	2		2					
Lentils/peas/beans/dhal				3				
Cooking oil/vegetable oil	19	17	24	11	24	21		
Butter	36	22	20	24	19	21		29
Ghee		2	33	12		24		10
Lard	13	1	9	4		2		
Cheese	11	12	9	3	12	15		32
Meat/red meat	26	23	18	20		19		10
Eggs	0	4				19		
Burgers/sausages/hot dogs	9	12	5	2				
Crisps	2	4	16		12			
Fried snacks, e.g. samosa, pakora, bhaji	3	6	38	21		4		
Sweets: halva, kulfi, gulabjamun, etc.		1	17	8	12	5		
Milk puddings with rice/semolina/sago/vermicelli	2	4	4	1		6		
Nuts		4	5					
Shellfish/seafood, such as prawns	1	1						
Cakes/biscuits/pastries	2		3					
Fried foods, including chips, fish in batter	2	5		2				
Chocolate			3					
Cream/ice-cream								
Milk, yoghurt, dairy products	3	7	4	2		3		
Margarine	8					2		
Fish	3							
Bacon	3		2					
(Other) wrong answers			3					
Other	26	14	16	17	4	6		
Don't know of any examples	18	18	7	27	53	6		47
Base (= 100%)	*86*	*75*	*35*	*45*	*7*	*25*		*12*

Continued on next page

Table 8.8: *continued*

Food	African-Caribbean		Indian		Pakistani		Bangladeshi	
	Women	Men	Women	Men	Women	Men	Women	Men
All ages								
Bread (including nan, chapati, puri, roti	0	0	3	4	0	4	0	0
Rice	0	0	2	1	3	1	3	0
Potatoes	1	0	2	1	1	2	6	0
Yams, plantain, sweet potatoes	0	0	0	0	0	1	0	0
Brown/wholemeal bread	0	0	0	0	1	0	0	1
Brown rice	0	0	0	0	0	0	1	0
Noodles/pasta/macaroni, etc.	0	1	1	0	0	0	2	0
Maize/sweetcorn	1	0	2	0	1	1	0	0
Lentils/peas/beans/dhal	0	0	1	1	0	1	0	0
Cooking oil/vegetable oil	14	16	23	13	20	16	5	6
Butter	31	23	29	26	27	22	24	24
Ghee	1	3	16	15	5	13	10	9
Lard	11	5	11	7	6	5	8	0
Cheese	9	10	6	7	6	14	9	7
Meat/red meat	21	15	13	13	6	13	12	6
Eggs	1	2	4	2	2	6	4	0
Burgers/sausages/hot dogs	10	8	4	3	3	4	5	0
Crisps	5	5	9	4	6	6	7	2
Fned snacks, e.g. samosa, pakora, bhaji	5	9	17	18	6	17	9	3
Sweets: halva, kulfi, gulabjamun, etc.	0	1	8	4	4	5	7	3
Milk puddings with rice/semolina/sago/vermicelli	2	4	5	3	3	5	5	5
Nuts	0	1	5	1	1	1	1	0
Shellfish/seafood, such as prawns	0	0	3	0	1	2	4	0
Cakes/biscuits/pastries	4	1	2	0	3	1	2	5
Friedfoods, including chips, fish in batter	5	6	1	1	4	1	5	3
Chocolate	1	0	0	0	0	0	3	2
Cream/ice-cream	1	1	1	1	0	0	2	0
Milk, yoghurt, dairy products	6	5	2	5	3	8	5	7
Margarine	10	3	4	4	5	5	6	13
Fish	3	0	0	1	1	1	0	0
Bacon	4	1	1	0	1	0	0	0
(Other) wrong answers	0	0	2	1	0	0	4	1
Other	24	13	24	18	27	17	23	10
Don't know of any examples	18	20	14	18	23	9	22	33
Base(= 100%)	*334*	*217*	*248*	*197*	*131*	*184*	*96*	*84*

Table 8.9: What types of food should be cut down in order to reduce the amount of salt in your diet? (percentages of all respondents)

Type of food	African-Caribbean		Indian		Pakistani		Bangladeshi	
	Women	Men	Women	Men	Women	Men	Women	Men
16–29								
Processed foods/tinned foods in general	6	5	7	3	4	6	1	1
Ready prepared meals	2	5	6	1	1	3	2	1
Salt cod/salt mackerel/ salt beef	18	10	4	1	2	4	2	4
Bacon	10	11	8	5	1	1	2	1
Crisps, roasted peanuts, salty snacks	22	10	23	21	22	29	22	14
Other	22	12	15	21	19	13	13	17
No, would not avoid or cut down	13	11	14	15	19	22	15	16
Just use less salt in cooking/put less salt	33	22	36	24	39	29	34	28
Don't know	11	25	17	21	13	12	25	27
Base (= 100%)	*178*	*114*	*208*	*129*	*281*	*235*	*307*	*213*
30–49								
Processed foods/tinned foods in general	11	12	10	5	3	7	1	3
Ready prepared meals	3	4	5	3	3	5	1	
Salt cod/salt mackerel/ salt beef	17	12	3	4	2	6	2	1
Bacon	13	6	7	8		2	0	
Crisps, roasted peanuts, salty snacks	21	12	22	18	10	17	8	4
Other	22	12	13	12	7	8	6	6
No, would not avoid or cut down	11	17	7	10	9	15	27	14
Just use less salt in cooking/put less salt	41	37	54	42	62	39	47	44
Don't know	6	16	13	23	18	19	17	32
Base (= 100%)	*270*	*140*	*283*	*227*	*186*	*268*	*233*	*183*
50–74								
Processed foods/tinned foods in general	8	5	6	14		4		2
Ready prepared meals	2	4	3	1		3		2
Salt cod/salt mackerel/ salt beef	17	12		8		4	0	1
Bacon	17	7	2	4	1	2		0
Crisps, roasted peanuts, salty snacks	14	8	12	15	9	13	5	5
Other	20	10	7	8	8	10		9
No, would not avoid or cut down	8	17	12	10	3	15	18	16
Just use less salt in cooking/put less salt	56	44	64	42	67	47	54	46
Don't know	8	13	12	19	20	14	27	24
Base (= 100%)	*193*	*174*	*107*	*107*	*50*	*124*	*63*	*171*
All ages								
Processed foods/tinned foods in general	8	7	8	7	3	6	1	2
Ready prepared meals	2	4	5	2	2	4	2	1
Salt cod/salt mackerel/ salt beef	17	11	3	4	2	5	2	2
Bacon	13	8	6	6	1	1	1	0
Crisps, roasted peanuts, salty snacks	20	10	20	19	15	21	15	9
Other	22	11	12	14	12	10	8	11
No, would not avoid or cut down	11	15	10	12	13	18	20	15
Just use less salt in cooking/put less salt	42	34	50	36	52	37	42	38
Don't know	9	18	14	22	16	15	22	27
Base (= 100%)	*641*	*428*	*598*	*463*	*517*	*627*	*603*	*567*

Table 8.10: Are there any foods that you would not consider eating, or any dietary restrictions you keep, for religious or cultural reasons (percentages of all respondents)

Type of food	African-Caribbean		Indian		Pakistani		Bangladeshi	
	Women	Men	Women	Men	Women	Men	Women	Men
16–29								
Pork, pork products	13	19	31	27	71	84	84	89
Beef	3	2	43	44	19	13	13	12
Meat which isn't halal	1	1	18	17	65	73	73	51
Meat of any kind	2	1	22	8	5	3	5	2
Animal fat of unknown origin (e.g. in manufactured foods such as biscuits)	0		11	4	17	31	35	9
Onions/garlic/tomatoes	0			1	1	1	2	0
Don't drink alcohol	1		13	15	22	36	49	46
Other	7	13	9	3	6	4	4	11
No dietary restrictions	77	74	23	29	4	5	3	2
Base(= 100%)	*178*	*114*	*208*	*129*	*281*	*235*	*307*	*213*
30–49								
Pork, pork products	16	13	29	33	83	89	78	90
Beef	2	1	39	41	16	15	4	8
Meat which isn't halal	0	1	19	22	73	75	86	64
Meat of any kind	1	1	41	19	4	3	8	1
Animal fat of unknown origin (e.g. in manufactured foods such as biscuits)	1	1	11	10	22	33	60	22
Onions/garlic/tomatoes		1	1	0	2	2	2	
Don't drink alcohol	0		12	15	26	45	59	52
Other	9	13	6	5	3	3	3	4
No dietary restrictions	77	72	11	23	4	1	5	2
Base (= 100%)	*270*	*140*	*283*	*227*	*186*	*268*	*233*	*183*
50–74								
Pork, pork products	14	5	28	28	71	94	81	91
Beef	4	2	42	50	18	13		9
Meat which isn't halal	1		15	18	67	82	92	59
Meat of any kind	1	0	60	16	9	2	4	1
Animal fat of unknown origin (e.g. in manufactured foods such as biscuits)			17	9	12	39	56	25
Onions/garlic/tomatoes	1		5	0	2	1	1	1
Don't drink alcohol	3	0	10	8	15	50	71	61
Other	7	5	13	1	3	1	1	5
No dietary restrictions	80	88	6	24	6	1	1	
Base (= 100%)	*193*	*174*	*107*	*107*	*50*	*124*	*63*	*171*
All ages								
Pork, pork products	14	13	30	30	76	88	81	90
Beef	3	2	41	44	17	14	8	10
Meat which isn't halal	1	0	18	20	68	75	81	57
Meat of any kind	2	1	38	14	6	3	6	1
Animal fat of unknown origin (e.g. in manufactured foods such as biscuits)	0	0	12	8	18	34	48	18
Onions/garlic/tomatoes	0	0	1	0	2	2	2	1
Don't drink alcohol	2	0	12	13	23	43	56	52
Other	8	10	8	3	4	3	3	7
No dietary restrictions	78	78	14	25	4	2	4	1
Base (= 100%)	*641*	*428*	*598*	*463*	*517*	*627*	*603*	*567*

Table 8.11: Do you ever eat lamb/mutton or chicken/turkey? (percentages of all respondents who eat meat)

Type of food	African-Caribbean		Indian		Pakistani		Bangladeshi	
	Women	Men	Women	Men	Women	Men	Women	Men
16–29								
Eat lamb or mutton	91	93	81	79	91	96	86	98
Will not eat lamb or mutton	9	7	19	21	9	4	14	2
Base (= 100%)	163	110	148	108	260	184	263	206
Eat chicken or turkey	98	99	88	94	95	99	99	97
Will not eat chicken or turkey	2	1	12	6	5	1	1	3
Base(= 100%)	161	110	151	110	259	184	263	206
30–49								
Eat lamb or mutton	95	95	81	86	95	98	93	93
Will not eat lamb or mutton	5	5	19	14	5	2	7	7
Base (= 100%)	243	131	167	175	171	210	208	179
Eat chicken or turkey	98	95	94	92	99	100	93	98
Will not eat chicken or turkey	2	5	6	8	1	0	7	2
Base (= 100%)	244	131	167	174	173	210	208	179
50–74								
Eat lamb or mutton	90	92	79	70	95	93	89	93
Will not eat lamb or mutton	10	8	21	30	5	7	11	7
Base (= 100%)	181	150	41	84	43	108	60	167
Eat chicken or turkey	96	99	86	90	96	96	89	99
Will not eat chicken or turkey	4	1	14	10	4	4	11	1
Base (= 100%)	178	151	41	85	44	108	60	167
All ages								
Eat lamb or mutton	92	93	81	80	93	96	89	95
Will not eat lamb or mutton	8	7	19	20	7	4	11	5
Base (= 100%)	587	391	356	367	474	502	531	552
Eat chicken or turkey	97	98	90	93	97	98	95	98
Will not eat chicken or turkey	3	2	10	7	3	2	5	2
Base (= 100%)	583	392	359	369	476	502	531	552

Table 8.12: Do you ever eat fish, eggs or dairy products?
(percentages of all respondents)

Type of food	African-Caribbean		Indian		Pakistani		Bangladeshi	
	Women	Men	Women	Men	Women	Men	Women	Men
16–29								
Fish								
Yes	94	96	74	88	94	95	97	99
No	6	4	26	12	6	5	3	1
Base (= 100%)	*174*	*114*	*201*	*128*	*277*	*234*	*303*	*213*
Egg								
Yes	92	93	81	92	92	98	94	93
No	8	7	19	8	8	2	6	7
Base (= 100%)	*174*	*114*	*201*	*128*	*277*	*234*	*303*	*213*
Milk or yoghurt								
Yes	93	100	99	100	98	97	95	98
No	7	0	1		2	3	5	2
Base (= 100%)	*174*	*114*	*201*	*128*	*276*	*234*	*302*	*213*
Cheese								
Yes	92	90	93	97	83	85	57	74
No	8	10	7	3	17	15	43	26
Base (= 100%)	*174*	*114*	*201*	*128*	*277*	*233*	*303*	*213*
30–49								
Fish								
Yes	98	100	56	80	94	96	100	100
No	2	0	44	20	6	4		
Base (= 100%)	*257*	*140*	*274*	*221*	*185*	*266*	*233*	*183*
Eggs								
Yes	89	94	65	81	94	96	80	97
No	11	6	35	19	6	4	20	3
Base (= 100%)	*256*	*140*	*275*	*223*	*185*	*266*	*233*	*183*
Milk or yoghurt								
Yes	95	96	98	97	96	97	89	98
No	5	4	2	3	4	3	11	2
Base (= 100%)	*255*	*140*	*275*	*222*	*185*	*266*	*233*	*183*
Cheese								
Yes	91	93	86	93	67	80	22	52
No	9	7	14	7	33	20	78	48
Base (= 100%)	*256*	*140*	*275*	*222*	*185*	*266*	*233*	*181*

Continued on next page

Table 8.12: *continued*

Type of food	African-Caribbean		Indian		Pakistani		Bangladeshi	
	Women	Men	Women	Men	Women	Men	Women	Men
50–74								
Fish								
Yes	99	99	37	74	93	89	99	100
No	1	1	63	26	7	11	1	
Base (= 100%)	*188*	*173*	*100*	*106*	*50*	*124*	*63*	*169*
Eggs								
Yes	87	94	41	84	93	89	85	91
No	13	6	59	16	7	11	15	9
Base (= 100%)	*188*	*173*	*100*	*105*	*50*	*124*	*63*	*169*
Milk or yoghurt								
Yes	96	94	90	99	93	88	93	94
No	4	6	10	1	7	12	7	6
Base (= 100%)	*187*	*173*	*100*	*106*	*50*	*124*	*63*	*168*
Cheese								
Yes	87	85	80	83	63	61	16	30
No	13	15	20	17	37	39	84	70
Base (= 100%)	*188*	*173*	*100*	*104*	*49*	*121*	*63*	*169*
All ages								
Fish								
Yes	97	98	59	81	94	94	99	100
No	3	2	41	19	6	6	1	0
Base (= 100%)	*619*	*427*	*575*	*455*	*512*	*624*	*599*	*565*
Eggs								
Yes	90	94	66	86	93	95	87	93
No	10	6	34	14	7	5	13	7
Base (= 100%)	*618*	*427*	*576*	*456*	*512*	*624*	*599*	*565*
Milk or yoghurt								
Yes	95	97	97	98	97	95	92	97
No	5	3	3	2	3	5	8	3
Base (= 100%)	*616*	*427*	*576*	*456*	*511*	*624*	*598*	*564*
Cheese								
Yes	90	89	87	92	73	78	38	54
No	10	11	13	8	27	22	62	46
Base (= 100%)	*618*	*427*	*576*	*454*	*511*	*620*	*599*	*563*

Table 8.13: Do you consider yourself to be a vegetarian, a vegan or neither? (percentages of all respondents who do not eat meat)

Type of diet	African-Caribbean		Indian		Pakistani		Bangladeshi	
	Women	Men	Women	Men	Women	Men	Women	Men
16–29								
Vegetarian	72		71	100	44	19	18	
Vegan			7		12			
Neither	11	33	13		8	35	31	47
Don't know	17	67	8		37	46	52	53
Base(= 100%)	4	2	47	10	14	8	15	4
30–49								
Vegetarian	27	100	92	88				
Vegan			5				3	
Neither	55		2	3	8	42	25	100
Don't know	18		1	9	92	58	72	
Base (= 100%)	3	1	105	40	9	10	21	1
50–74								
Vegetarian	75		82	83	13			
Vegan			9					
Neither	25	100	8	10	19	50	33	55
Don't know				8	69	50	67	45
Base (= 100%)	3	1	62	19	5	4	3	2
All ages								
Vegetarian	59	36	85	89	22	8	6	0
Vegan	0	0	7	0	5	0	2	0
Neither	28	32	6	4	11	40	28	57
Don't know	13	32	2	7	63	52	64	43
Base (= 100%)	10	4	214	69	28	22	39	7

Table 8.14: Attitudes to traditional foods (percentages of all respondents)

Statement and attitudes	African-Caribbean		Indian		Pakistani		Bangladeshi	
	Women	Men	Women	Men	Women	Men	Women	Men
16–29								
Traditional foods are healthier								
Agree	45	58	39	28	37	53	47	39
Neither agree nor disagree	16	21	19	14	17	11	14	21
Disagree	30	17	37	45	41	33	32	34
Don't know	8	4	6	12	5	3	7	5
Base (= 100%)	178	114	208	128	281	234	306	213
Too much trouble to cook traditional foods								
Agree	39	43	44	38	38	29	49	61
Neither agree nor disagree	5	2	9	8	6	11	7	7
Disagree	55	52	46	48	54	58	42	30
Don't know	1	3	1	4	1	1	1	1
Base (= 100%)	178	114	207	127	280	232	306	212
Difficult to get traditional foods away from home								
Agree	57	52	37	30	36	32	51	47
Neither agree nor disagree	7	9	6	7	7	10	6	13
Disagree	33	39	54	62	56	56	40	39
Don't know	2	0	4	1	1	2	2	0
Base (= 100%)	178	114	207	129	281	233	306	212
Prefer to eat British or European food								
Agree	13	10	17	21	16	13	14	10
Neither agree nor disagree	24	17	29	23	20	16	22	22
Disagree	61	70	52	55	65	70	63	65
Don't know	2	2	1			1	1	2
Base (= 100%)	178	114	206	129	281	234	306	212
30–49								
Traditional foods are healthier								
Agree	41	60	54	51	55	57	68	52
Neither agree nor disagree	23	11	21	19	21	13	11	21
Disagree	27	20	19	23	21	27	18	19
Don't know	9	9	6	6	3	3	2	7
Base (= 100%)	270	140	282	226	186	267	232	182
Too much trouble to cook traditional foods								
Agree	36	34	37	38	24	46	74	65
Neither agree nor disagree	4	7	10	10	6	7	6	6
Disagree	59	59	52	48	69	46	19	27
Don't know	2	0	1	4	0	1	0	1
Base (= 100%)	270	140	283	227	186	266	232	182
Difficult to get traditional foods away from home								
Agree	54	59	37	25	20	26	47	39
Neither agree nor disagree	7	8	13	11	8	9	11	20
Disagree	36	30	47	63	67	63	31	40
Don't know	2	2	3	1	6	2	11	1
Base (= 100%)	270	139	283	227	185	266	232	182
Prefer to eat British or European food								
Agree	11	12	16	15	12	13	10	8
Neither agree nor disagree	26	24	24	27	16	15	15	24
Disagree	63	63	59	58	71	71	72	65
Don't know	0	0	1	0	2	1	3	2
Base (= 100%)	270	140	283	227	186	267	232	181

Continued on next page

Table 8.14: *continued*

Statement and attitudes	African-Caribbean		Indian		Pakistani		Bangladeshi	
	Women	Men	Women	Men	Women	Men	Women	Men
50–74								
Traditional foods are healthier								
Agree	51	51	70	44	61	74	78	58
Neither agree nor disagree	24	20	15	28	17	10	12	21
Disagree	17	18	11	24	18	15	8	13
Don't know	7	11	4	5	5	1	3	7
Base (= 100%)	*193*	*174*	*107*	*107*	*50*	*124*	*63*	*171*
Too much trouble to cook traditional foods								
Agree	27	22	33	39	22	42	69	63
Neither agree nor disagree	8	11	9	9	8	5	17	12
Disagree	65	66	56	50	66	52	11	24
Don't know	0	1	2	1	5	1	3	1
Base (= 100%)	*193*	*173*	*107*	*106*	*50*	*124*	*63*	*171*
Difficult to get traditional foods away from home								
Agree	43	50	19	22	14	25	53	33
Neither agree nor disagree	10	13	21	15	12	9	14	34
Disagree	40	33	53	58	62	58	26	31
Don't know	7	4	8	5	12	8	8	3
Base (= 100%)	*193*	*173*	*106*	*107*	*50*	*124*	*63*	*170*
Prefer to eat British or European food								
Agree	17	15	19	10	7	16	15	7
Neither agree nor disagree	33	25	12	22	14	10	14	18
Disagree	49	59	63	64	73	70	68	72
Don't know	0	1	5	3	6	4	3	3
Base (= 100%)	*193*	*173*	*106*	*107*	*50*	*124*	*63*	*171*
All ages								
Traditional foods are healthier								
Agree	45	56	52	42	48	59	60	49
Neither agree nor disagree	21	18	19	20	19	12	12	21
Disagree	26	18	24	31	30	27	23	24
Don't know	8	8	5	8	4	3	4	7
Base (= 100%)	*641*	*428*	*597*	*461*	*517*	*625*	*601*	*566*
Too much trouble to cook traditional foods								
Agree	35	33	39	39	30	39	62	63
Neither agree nor disagree	5	7	10	9	6	8	8	8
Disagree	59	59	51	49	62	52	29	28
Don't know	1	1	1	3	1	1	1	1
Base (= 100%)	*641*	*427*	*597*	*460*	*516*	*622*	*601*	*565*
Difficult to get traditional foods away from home								
Agree	52	53	33	26	26	28	50	40
Neither agree nor disagree	8	10	12	10	8	9	9	21
Disagree	36	34	51	62	61	59	35	37
Don't know	3	2	4	2	5	3	6	1
Base (= 100%)	*641*	*426*	*596*	*463*	*516*	*623*	*601*	*564*
Prefer to eat British or European food								
Agree	14	12	17	16	13	14	12	9
Neither agree nor disagree	27	22	24	25	17	14	18	21
Disagree	58	64	58	59	68	70	68	67
Don't know	1	1	2	1	2	2	2	2
Base (= 100%)	*641*	*427*	*595*	*463*	*517*	*625*	*601*	*564*

Black and minority ethnic groups in England

Chapter 9 Body image and body shape

Table 9.1: Perception of bodyweight (percentages of all respondents)

Respondents' views about their weight	African-Caribbean		Indian		Pakistani		Bangladeshi	
	Women	Men	Women	Men	Women	Men	Women	Men
16–29								
I weigh a lot less than I would wish to	2	5	1	4	6	6	4	8
I weigh a little less than I would wish to	9	20	10	20	9	23	10	22
I feel my weight is about right	30	52	41	38	37	44	45	48
I weigh a little more than I would wish to	31	17	30	31	33	22	29	16
I weigh a lot more than I would wish to	27	6	17	7	16	4	12	3
Don't know		2	0			1	1	3
Base (= 100%)	*165*	*114*	*188*	*126*	*253*	*235*	*266*	*211*
30–49								
I weigh a lot less than I would wish to	0	4	1		1	2	2	2
I weigh a little less than I would wish to	3	16	5	10	3	7	6	8
I feel my weight is about right	21	47	31	57	34	42	52	60
I weigh a little more than I would wish to	37	25	42	28	35	41	25	22
I weigh a lot more than I would wish to	38	7	20	6	25	7	10	5
Don't know	0	0	1	0	3	1	4	3
Base (= 100%)	*263*	*139*	*272*	*227*	*175*	*263*	*228*	*180*
50–74								
I weigh a lot less than I would wish to		1	1	3		4	0	3
I weigh a little less than I would wish to	2	3	2	9	2	6	2	15
I feel my weight is about right	22	56	45	53	40	48	53	50
I weigh a little more than I would wish to	42	29	36	27	29	24	25	24
I weigh a lot more than I would wish to	33	7	15	8	23	17	6	2
Don't know	2	4	1		6	0	13	6
Base (= 100%)	*193*	*173*	*107*	*106*	*48*	*121*	*62*	*170*
All ages								
I weigh a lot less than I would wish to	1	3	1	2	3	4	3	5
I weigh a little less than I would wish to	5	13	6	13	5	13	7	16
I feel my weight is about right	25	52	37	50	36	44	49	52
I weigh a little more than I would wish to	36	24	37	29	33	30	27	20
I weigh a lot more than I would wish to	33	6	18	7	21	8	10	3
Don't know	1	2	1	0	2	1	4	4
Base (= 100%)	*621*	*426*	*567*	*459*	*476*	*619*	*556*	*561*

Table 9.2: Knowledge of ability to put on weight (percentages of all respondents, except pregnant women, weighing less than they would wish to)

Can people do anything to add weight	African-Caribbean		Indian		Pakistani		Bangladeshi	
	Women	Men	Women	Men	Women	Men	Women	Men
16–29								
Yes	39	92	61	72	67	81	62	71
No	43	8	19	14	23	11	13	15
Don't know	17		20	14	10	9	25	14
Base (= 100%)	20	28	23	28	28	56	40	64
30–49								
Yes	45	85	59	60	28	53	21	80
No	31	10	33	37	39	39	30	14
Don't know	25	5	8	3	33	8	49	6
Base (= 100%)	8	29	22	22	9	25	19	22
50–74								
Yes	72	73	28	56		55	50	46
No	28	27	9	40		45	33	25
Don't know			63	4	100		17	29
Base (= 100%)	4	7	4	13	1	12	3	30
All ages								
Yes	43	88	57	66	58	72	47	66
No	39	11	24	25	25	21	20	17
Don't know	17	2	19	9	17	8	34	17
Base (= 100%)	32	64	49	63	38	93	62	116

Table 9.3: Actions taken to put on weight (percentages of all respondents, except pregnant women, weighing less than they would wish to, and who know it is possible to put on weight)

Action	African-Caribbean Women	Men	Indian Women	Men	Pakistani Women	Men	Bangladeshi Women	Men
16–29								
Exercising/weight training	10	20		13		14	10	23
Trying to eat more generally	10	22	35	39	32	41	47	28
Meat/protein foods		3		6	5	5	13	11
Fatty/oily foods	38	5		7		6	12	2
Fried foods						1		
Starchy foods (e.g. rice, bread, potatoes, etc.)			21				7	1
Sweet things/chocolate	38		5		6		13	2
Drinking more milk	38			10	2	12	3	2
Trying to eat more often	48	2	5		3	7	21	2
Taking food supplements, e.g. high calorie drinks		7				1		2
Other		7	14	8	3	7	4	9
No, nothing	43	50	35	46	54	38	27	55
Base (= 100%)	*7*	*26*	*13*	*19*	*18*	*42*	*24*	*44*
30–49								
Exercising/weight training		14	21	7		16		27
Trying to eat more generally	82	12	43	40	80	18	23	71
Meat/protein foods		8		22		13		
Fatty/oily foods			21	16		8		
Fried foods			21			8		
Starchy foods (e.g. rice, bread, potatoes, etc.)		15		8		8		
Sweet things/chocolate			5	8				
Drinking more milk			7	7				8
Trying to eat more often		6		23				
Taking food supplements, e.g. high calorie drinks				8				
Other	55	8	7	5		16		5
No, nothing	18	57	45	37	20	61	77	29
Base (= 100%)	*3*	*24*	*12*	*13*	*3*	*15*	*4*	*18*
50–74								
Exercising/weight training		9		7				7
Trying to eat more generally		28		7		64	100	22
Meat/protein foods				7		36		7
Fatty/oily foods		28						
Fried foods	0	0	0	0		0	0	0
Starchy foods (e.g. rice, bread, potatoes, etc.)				23				
Sweet things/chocolate	0	0	0	0		0	0	0
Drinking more milk				15		56		
Trying to eat more often		20		15				5
Taking food supplements, e.g. high calorie drinks				15		8		
Other		9		7		8		7
No, nothing	100	52	100	63		28		69
Base (= 100%)	*2*	*5*	*1*	*7*		*6*	*1*	*12*

Continued on next page

Table 9.3: *continued*

Action	African-Caribbean		Indian		Pakistani		Bangladeshi	
	Women	Men	Women	Men	Women	Men	Women	Men
All ages								
Exercising/weight training	6	17	8	10		13	8	21
Trying to eat more generally	25	18	37	35	36	40	45	34
Meat/protein foods		5		11	4	9	10	8
Fatty/oily foods	24	5	8	8		5	9	1
Fried foods			8			2		
Starchy foods (e.g. rice, bread, potatoes, etc.)		6	12	6		1	6	1
Sweet things/chocolate	24		5	2	5		10	1
Drinking more milk	24		3	10	2	14	2	3
Trying to eat more often	30	5	3	9	3	5	17	2
Taking food supplements, e.g. high calorie drinks		4		4		1		1
Other	13	8	10	7	3	8	4	8
No, nothing	45	53	42	46	51	40	34	53
Base (= 100%)	12	55	26	39	21	63	29	74

Table 9.4: Main reasons for trying to put on weight (percentages of all respondents, except pregnant women, weighing less than their ideal who know it is possible to and are actively trying to to put on weight)

Reason	African-Caribbean		Indian		Pakistani		Bangladeshi	
	Women	Men	Women	Men	Women	Men	Women	Men
16–29								
For the good of my health generally	17	31	7	39	30	18	42	70
To reduce my risk of specific health problems							18	
To have more energy/ feel less tired		15		4	8	3	47	4
To feel better about myself generally	33	57	54	23	35	41	15	23
To feel more attractive	67	18	4	15	35	16	31	5
To be able wear attractive/fashionable clothes		7	21	8	8	3		
Other	67	10	43	15	20	36	6	10
Don't know								5
Base (= 100%)	3	12	9	9	10	22	18	20
30–49								
For the good of my health generally		22	62	32	100	53		39
To reduce my risk of specific health problems		9		13				
To have more energy/ feel less tired			12	34	50			23
To feel better about myself generally	33	58				13		
To feel more attractive	67	14		13		13	100	7
To be able wear attractive/fashionable clothes						13		
Other		11		11			100	
Don't know				23		20		25
Base (= 100%)	*2*	*10*	*6*	*9*	*2*	*6*	*1*	*12*
50–74								
For the good of my health generally		100		19		73		44
To reduce my risk of specific health problems		19		39				56
To have more energy/ feel less tired				61		51	100	
To feel better about myself generally								
To feel more attractive								
To be able wear attractive/fashionable clothes								
Other								
Don't know								
Base (= 100%)		*3*		*4*		*4*	*1*	*5*

Continued on next page

Table 9.4: *continued*

Reason	African-Caribbean		Indian		Pakistani		Bangladeshi	
	Women	Men	Women	Men	Women	Men	Women	Men
All ages								
For the good of my health generally	11	34	28	35	40	28	37	59
To reduce my risk of specific health problems		5		8			15	7
To have more energy/feel less tired		9	5	19	13	9	48	9
To feel better about myself generally	33	53	33	13	30	34	13	14
To feel more attractive	67	15	2	13	30	14	33	5
To be able wear attractive/fashionable clothes		4	13	5	6	4		
Other	44	10	27	12	17	28	11	6
Don't know				7		2		10
			19			3	4	2
Base (=100%)	*5*	*25*	*15*	*22*	*12*	*32*	*20*	*37*

Table 9.5: Can people control or maintain their weight when they want to?
(percentages of all respondents, except pregnant women, weighing
about as much as they want to)

Response	African-Caribbean		Indian		Pakistani		Bangladeshi	
	Women	Men	Women	Men	Women	Men	Women	Men
16–29								
Yes	86	83	90	87	88	91	78	83
No	12	6	3	3	4	7	9	1
Don't know	2	10	7	10	8	2	13	16
Base (= 100%)	*52*	*58*	*77*	*52*	*99*	*107*	*111*	*97*
30–49								
Yes	91	83	81	86	72	86	52	79
No	4	10	2	9	9	11	27	5
Don't know	4	7	17	5	20	3	21	16
Base (= 100%)	*60*	*65*	*79*	*128*	*56*	*113*	*119*	*105*
50–74								
Yes	87	72	73	75	43	84	54	66
No	9	14	11	13	25	7	20	10
Don't know	5	15	17	12	32	10	26	24
Base (= 100%)	*46*	*94*	*45*	*55*	*18*	*62*	*32*	*83*
All ages								
Yes	88	79	82	83	74	88	63	77
No	9	10	4	9	10	8	19	5
Don't know	4	11	13	8	16	4	18	18
Base (= 100%)	*158*	*217*	*201*	*235*	*173*	*282*	*262*	*285*

Table 9.6: Actions taken to control or maintain weight (percentages of all respondents, except pregnant women, weighing about as much as they want to, and aware of ability to control their weight)

Action taken	African-Caribbean Women	African-Caribbean Men	Indian Women	Indian Men	Pakistani Women	Pakistani Men	Bangladeshi Women	Bangladeshi Men
16–29								
Take exercise	39	52	53	63	23	58	29	59
Limit total amount of food eaten	9	6	28	33	17	17	18	25
Avoid/cut down								
Meat/protein foods	7	8	11	5	3	6	12	3
Fatty/oily foods	19	16	24	23	18	20	25	13
Fried foods	6	5	14	10	8	4	4	3
Starchy foods		4	4	2	1	1	4	1
Sweet things/chocolate	3	8	12	9	4	7	15	2
Other foods	6		4	2		5	0	3
Alcoholic drinks	1	2	1	4	3	9	2	1
Sweet drinks			4	18	4	1	4	
Eat special foods for people on a diet	7	2	2		1	1	1	
Eat more								
Starchy or high-fibre foods	3	10	9			1	2	1
Lower-fat or reduced fat foods		2	6	2	1		1	1
Lean meat/white meat (e.g. chicken)		2	6			1	3	
Vegetables or fruit	11	2	12	14	8	3	12	8
Other foods	4		6	7	5	3	2	
Adopt a calorie controlled diet	5	2	2		5	5	1	
Do anything else to control/maintain weight	9	8	7	3	1	1	1	3
No, nothing	49	40	33	25	54	33	45	35
Base (= 100%)	*43*	*46*	*66*	*42*	*86*	*95*	*85*	*84*
30–49								
Take exercise	24	51	34	55	28	30	18	37
Limit total amount of food eaten	22	24	37	37	26	28	30	45
Avoid/cut down								
Meat/protein foods	4	1	3	3	6	2	20	14
Fatty/oily foods	18	13	28	13	20	16	14	17
Fried foods	8	5	15	4	8	8	2	3
Starchy foods	10	7	9	4			5	
Sweet things/chocolate	5	3	12	2	7	5	10	
Other foods	3	8	3	4		9		6
Alcoholic drinks	1	15	1	8		3	2	
Sweet drinks	2	3	13	4	2	1	2	2
Eat special foods for people on a diet			2			2		
Eat more								
Starchy or high-fibre foods	1	4	3	4	2		3	2
Lower-fat or reduced fat foods		5	4	2	2	2		
Lean meat/white meat (e.g. chicken)	4	1	1	2				
Vegetables or fruit	10	9	10	6	4	4	9	6
Other foods	12	1	1	2	4	1		
Adopt a calorie controlled diet	1	5	1	1				3
Do anything else to control/maintain weight	3	10	9	6		6	4	5
No, nothing	46	30	33	27	52	39	43	29
Base (= 100%)	*55*	*52*	*64*	*108*	*40*	*94*	*61*	*80*

Continued on next page

Table 9.6: *continued*

Action taken	African-Caribbean Women	Men	Indian Women	Men	Pakistani Women	Men	Bangladeshi Women	Men
50–74								
Take exercise	26	30	20	47	22	28	6	18
Limit total amount of food eaten	22	31	30	40	26	39	38	56
Avoid/cut down								
Meat/protein foods	6	7	2	10	19	13	39	8
Fatty/oily foods	20	8	18	20	19	20	36	8
Fried foods	11	1	8	16	11	9		1
Starchy foods	17		7	4	19	4	5	4
Sweet things/chocolate	16	2	18	10	19	11	16	3
Other foods	3	11	1	9	11			4
Alcoholic drinks	11	5		10		3	2	
Sweet drinks	1	1	2			9	2	6
Eat special foods for people on a diet	2	6	2			3		3
Eat more								
Starchy or high-fibre foods	16	3		1				2
Lower-fat or reduced fat foods	3	1	8			3		
Lean meat/white meat (e.g. chicken)	7	2				3		
Vegetables or fruit	15	4	8	10		5		3
Other foods	8		10	2			3	
Adopt a calorie controlled diet	3		4				2	
Do anything else to control/maintain weight	9	4	8	16		8		4
No, nothing	30	38	41	22	52	41	33	23
Base (= 100%)	*38*	*68*	*30*	*42*	*9*	*51*	*16*	*55*
All ages								
Take exercise	31	44	39	55	25	42	22	41
Limit total amount of food eaten	17	20	32	37	22	26	25	39
Avoid/cut down								
Meat/protein foods	6	6	6	5	6	6	18	8
Fatty/oily foods	19	12	24	17	19	19	23	13
Fried foods	8	4	14	8	8	7	3	3
Starchy foods	8	3	6	3	2	1	4	1
Sweet things/chocolate	7	5	13	5	7	7	13	2
Other foods	4	6	3	5	1	5	0	4
Alcoholic drinks	4	7	1	7	2	6	2	0
Sweet drinks	1	1	7	6	2	3	3	2
Eat special foods for people on a diet	3	3	2		0	2	0	1
Eat more								
Starchy or high-fibre foods	6	6	5	2	1	1	2	2
Lower-fat or reduced fat foods	1	3	6	1	1	1	1	1
Lean meat/white meat (e.g. chicken)	3	2	3	1		1	1	
Vegetables or fruit	12	5	11	9	6	4	9	6
Other foods	8	0	5	3	4	1	1	
Adopt a calorie controlled diet	3	2	2	0	2	2	1	1
Do anything else to control/maintain weight	7	7	8	7	0	4	2	4
No, nothing	43	37	35	25	53	37	43	30
Base (= 100%)	*136*	*166*	*160*	*192*	*135*	*240*	*162*	*219*

Table 9.7: Main reasons for controlling or maintaining weight (percentages of all respondents, except pregnant women, weighing about as much as they want to, aware of abilty to control their weight and taking action to do so)

Reason	African-Caribbean		Indian		Pakistani		Bangladeshi	
	Women	Men	Women	Men	Women	Men	Women	Men
16–29								
To reduce my risk of specific health problems	4	2	4	3	5	9	5	18
For the good of my health generally	60	41	54	55	54	48	51	66
To feel better about myself generally	24	28	19	23	9	10	29	12
Just don't want to be any fatter	12	12	9		21	7	16	6
To avoid putting on weight in specific places			11		3	12	7	13
To feel attractive	4	5	26	7	11	12	18	12
To be able to wear attractive/fashionable clothes	6		9		10	2	7	2
Pressure from family and/or friends					5	1		
Other	17	15	4	12	15	13	6	5
Don't know	14	32	23	41	22	29	16	13
Base (= 100%)	*23*	*26*	*43*	*31*	*44*	*60*	*47*	*53*
30–49								
To reduce my risk of specific health problems	5	4	5	14	3	20	19	24
For the good of my health generally	62	45	61	68	64	64	75	63
To feel better about myself generally	16	18	7	7	12	8	39	15
Just don't want to be any fatter (generally	18	13	8	6		6	14	4
To avoid putting on weight in specific places		4	8	5		5		6
To feel attractive	2	2	7	4		1		4
To be able to wear attractive/fashionable clothes	8	7	2	2		1		4
Pressure from family and/or friends				1		1		
Other	20	21	9	7	3	1	2	11
Don't know	10	14	23	17	29	15	7	13
Base (= 100%)	*31*	*34*	*41*	*80*	*21*	*55*	*35*	*56*

Continued on next page

Table 9.7: *continued*

Reason	African-Caribbean		Indian		Pakistani		Bangladeshi	
	Women	Men	Women	Men	Women	Men	Women	Men
50–74								
To reduce my risk of specific health problems	24	14	9	31	22	34	21	30
For the good of my health generally	55	52	59	70	44	64	77	57
To feel better about myself generally	11	11	3	14		16	14	8
Just don't want to be any fatter	14	3		14		5	7	2
To avoid putting on weight in specific places	2	3		5		18	7	2
To feel attractive						6		
To be able to wear attractive/fashionable clothes								
Pressure from family and/or friends	5							2
Other	6	14	21	10	33	6		
Don't know	18	23	21	14		11	9	24
Base (= 100%)	*27*	*41*	*17*	*33*	*4*	*28*	*11*	*43*
All ages								
To reduce my risk of specific health problems	11	7	5	15	6	18	13	23
For the good of my health generally	59	46	57	65	57	57	64	63
To feel better about myself generally	18	19	11	13	9	10	30	12
Just don't want to be any fatter	14	9	7	6	11	6	14	4
To avoid putting on weight in specific places	1	2	8	4	2	11	5	8
To feel attractive	2	2	14	4	6	8	9	6
To be able to wear attractive/fashionable clothes	5	2	5	1	5	1	3	2
Pressure from family and/or friends	2			1	3	1		1
Other	15	16	9	9	12	7	4	6
Don't know	14	23	23	23	23	20	12	16
Base (= 100%)	*81*	*101*	*101*	*144*	*69*	*143*	*93*	*152*

Table 9.8: Is there anything people can do to lose weight when they want to? (percentages of all respondents, except pregnant women, weighing more than they would wish to)

Reason	African-Caribbean		Indian		Pakistani		Bangladeshi	
	Women	Men	Women	Men	Women	Men	Women	Men
16–29								
Yes	96	98	99	93	93	100	87	86
No	3			5	2		7	4
Don't know	1	2	1	2	5		5	10
Base (= 100%)	*91*	*21*	*82*	*44*	*120*	*64*	*99*	*36*
30–49								
Yes	99	91	86	87	89	84	70	72
No	1	2	8	7	5	9	21	4
Don't know		7	6	6	6	7	10	24
Base (= 100%)	*190*	*43*	*162*	*69*	*91*	*111*	*70*	*40*
50–74								
Yes	95	90	85	90	89	90	46	72
No	3	4	5	10	5	6	9	10
Don't know	2	7	10		5	4	44	18
Base (= 100%)	*137*	*57*	*53*	*38*	*21*	*39*	*13*	*34*
All ages								
Yes	97	92	90	90	91	90	76	77
No	2	2	5	7	4	6	13	6
Don't know	1	6	5	3	6	4	11	17
Base (= 100%)	*418*	*121*	*297*	*151*	*232*	*214*	*182*	*110*

Table 9.9: Actions taken to lose weight (percentages of all respondents, except pregnant women, weighing more than they would wish to, aware of ability to reduce their weight)

Action taken	African-Caribbean		Indian		Pakistani		Bangladeshi	
	Women	Men	Women	Men	Women	Men	Women	Men
16–29								
Take more exercise	55	57	48	47	39	51	53	58
Eating less generally	34	35	35	21	34	16	31	35
Avoid/cut down								
Meat/protein foods			7	9	3	1	11	
Fatty/oily foods	23	14	25	9	23	10	28	11
Fried foods	6		13	7	8	4		
Starchy foods	2		3	4	7	3	6	
Sweet things/chocolate	15	7	16	3	19	8	19	
Other foods	7	3	4			4	1	
Alcoholic drinks	3		2	2	1	1		
Sweet drinks	5		4	6	4	7	5	2
Eat special foods for people on a diet	1				0		2	
Eat more								
Starchy or high-fibre foods	5		5	2	3	3	9	
Lower-fat or reduced fat foods	3		5	3	4	3	6	5
Lean meat/white meat (e.g. chicken)			1		1			
Vegetables or fruit	12	3	10	2	10	3	15	
Other foods			6	3	1		3	
Adopt a calorie-controlled or special diet	7	8	4	4	4		1	
Do anything else to lose weight	4	7	13		9	7	6	6
No, nothing	24	28	26	34	34	39	23	35
Base (= 100%)	*86*	*20*	*80*	*39*	*112*	*64*	*83*	*32*
30–49								
Take more exercise	41	43	43	50	38	41	43	20
Eating less generally	40	38	32	39	40	51	76	59
Avoid/cut down								
Meat/protein foods	6		1	3	3	8	20	11
Fatty/oily foods	26	18	28	23	28	25	20	12
Fried foods	6	5	12	5	13	7		
Starchy foods	6		4	2	5	3	7	
Sweet things/chocolate	18	4	14	7	10	13	16	2
Other foods	6	3	4	3	7			4
Alcoholic drinks	4	2		2				
Sweet drinks	5		5		2	2	3	
Eat special foods for people on a diet	0		2		2			
Eat more								
Starchy or high-fibre foods	3		4	5	4	7	7	
Lower-fat or reduced fat foods	5		5		2	3	3	
Lean meat/white meat (e.g. chicken)	3		0	2		1	4	
Vegetables or fruit	17	3	10	10	5	2	6	2
Other foods	3		2		2		3	
Adopt a calorie-controlled or special diet	6	3	5		1	2	2	3
Do anything else to lose weight	6		10	7	3	6	2	4
No, nothing	26	41	29	27	28	28	13	32
Base (= 100%)	*186*	*39*	*145*	*60*	*81*	*96*	*48*	*32*

Continued on next page

Table 9.9: *continued*

Action taken	African-Caribbean		Indian		Pakistani		Bangladeshi	
	Women	Men	Women	Men	Women	Men	Women	Men
50–74								
Take more exercise	28	45	26	47	23	52		25
Eating less generally	45	43	46	36	49	63	84	55
Avoid/cut down								
Meat/protein foods	4	9	6	1	5	1		6
Fatty/oily foods	21	23	19	3	9	21		27
Fried foods	7	3	7	4	9	1		10
Starchy foods	14	5	7	1	5			4
Sweet things/chocolate	12	11	9	6	5	6		
Other foods	5	1	2	2		2		5
Alcoholic drinks	2	9	1					
Sweet drinks	6		6		5	5		
Eat special foods for people on a diet	3	2	3		5			2
Eat more								
Starchy or high-fibre foods			4	3				
Lower-fat or reduced fat foods	4	4	1	6				
Lean meat/white meat (e.g. chicken)	2		2					
Vegetables or fruit	19	10	13	2	23	1		12
Other foods	4				18			
Adopt a calorie-controlled or special diet	2	1	2	3	11	3		
Do anything else to lose weight	8	6	8	4	6	16		2
No, nothing	24	26	31	38	28	22	16	29
Base (= 100%)	*128*	*51*	*44*	*35*	*17*	*35*	*3*	*25*
All ages								
Take more exercise	41	48	41	48	36	47	46	36
Eating less generally	40	39	35	32	39	43	51	49
Avoid/cut down								
Meat/protein foods	4	4	4	5	3	4	13	5
Fatty/oily foods	23	19	25	13	23	19	23	16
Fried foods	6	3	11	6	11	5		3
Starchy foods	8	2	4	2	6	2	6	1
Sweet things/chocolate	15	8	14	6	13	10	16	1
Other foods	6	2	4	2	3	2	1	3
Alcoholic drinks	3	4	1	2	1	0		
Sweet drinks	5		5	2	3	4	4	1
Eat special foods for people on a diet	1	1	1		1		1	1
Eat more								
Starchy or high-fibre foods	3		4	3	3	4	8	
Lower-fat or reduced fat foods	4	2	4	2	3	3	5	2
Lean meat/white meat (e.g. chicken)	2		1	1	0	0	1	
Vegetables or fruit	16	6	11	5	9	2	11	4
Eat more of other foods	2		3	1	4		3	
Adopt a calorie-controlled or special diet	5	4	4	2	4	1	1	1
Do anything else to lose weight	6	4	10	4	6	9	4	4
No, nothing	25	31	28	32	30	30	19	33
Base (= 100%)	*400*	*110*	*269*	*134*	*210*	*195*	*134*	*89*

Table 9.10: Main reasons for trying to lose weight (percentages of all respondents, except pregnant women, weighing more than they would wish to, aware of ability to reduce their weight, and taking action to lose weight)

Reason	African-Caribbean		Indian		Pakistani		Bangladeshi	
	Women	Men	Women	Men	Women	Men	Women	Men
16–29								
For the good of my health generally	32	33	38	57	56	65	41	40
To reduce my risk of specific health problems	2		7	4	8	7	13	10
To feel better about myself generally	31	29	26	31	23	18	35	17
I would like to be thinner all over	8	10	12	6	6	4	20	5
Want to lose weight from particular areas			11		8	3	10	4
To feel more attractive	23	5	13	3	11	7	16	12
To look better/more attractive	28	18	24	7	30	19	17	9
To be able to wear attractive/fashionable clothes	23	5	13		15		3	
Pressure from family and/or friends			3	3	1		3	
Other	13	3	10	3	11	24	8	9
Don't know			7	6		4		
Base (= 100%)	*63*	*15*	*55*	*25*	*73*	*40*	*62*	*20*
30–49								
For the good of my health generally	56	44	61	66	61	51	55	56
To reduce my risk of specific health problems	5		10	9	9	21	35	14
To feel better about myself generally	25	13	19	23	12	21	45	
I would like to be thinner all over	4	3	6	4	6	8	10	3
Want to lose weight from particular areas	4	12	8		11	2	10	
To feel more attractive	10	4	7	2	13	5	5	
To look better/more attractive	6	15	15	3	13	10	2	5
To be able to wear attractive/fashionable clothes	14	4	5	4	8	1	2	
Pressure from family and/or friends	0	6	2	2				
Other	19	19	8	23	2		2	15
Don't know		6	2		3		2	
Base (= 100%)	*132*	*23*	*103*	*43*	*58*	*64*	*40*	*22*

Continued on next page

Table 9.10: *continued*

Reason	African-Caribbean		Indian		Pakistani		Bangladeshi	
	Women	Men	Women	Men	Women	Men	Women	Men
50–74								
For the good of my health generally	65	45	63	70	74	46	100	60
To reduce my risk of specific health problems	16	26	16	28	17	25	14	20
To feel better about myself generally	11	17	12		15	2		17
I would like to be thinner all over	5		8	8		2		10
Want to lose weight from particular areas	1	4	8	2		19		
To feel more attractive	1	1	9			3		6
To look better/more attractive	2		12		2			
To be able to wear attractive/fashionable clothes	6	3						
Pressure from family and/or friends	0		9		6			
Other	16	12	7	16		15		3
Don't know				2		19		
Base(= 100%)	*98*	*38*	*31*	*22*	*13*	*25*	*2*	*18*
All ages								
For the good of my health generally	52	41	54	64	61	53	51	51
To reduce my risk of specific health problems	8	11	10	11	9	18	22	14
To feel better about myself generally	22	20	20	21	16	15	37	12
I would like to be thinner all over	5	4	8	5	5	5	15	6
Want to lose weight from particular areas	2	5	9	1	8	7	9	2
To feel more attractive	11	3	9	2	11	5	10	6
To look better/more attractive	11	9	18	4	18	10	10	5
To be able to wear attractive/fashionable clothes	14	4	7	2	9	1	2	
Pressure from family and/or friends	0	2	4	2	1	2		
Other	16	11	8	14	6	10	5	9
Don't know		2	3	3	1	6	1	
Base (= 100%)	*293*	*76*	*189*	*90*	*144*	*129*	*104*	*60*

Table 9.11: Ever received advice from a doctor, nurse or other health professional to gain or lose weight (percentages of all respondents)

Advice	African-Caribbean Women	African-Caribbean Men	Indian Women	Indian Men	Pakistani Women	Pakistani Men	Bangladeshi Women	Bangladeshi Men
16–29								
To lose weight	14	3	10	7	13	5	7	4
To put weight on	9	1	7	6	7	3	8	3
No, neither	76	96	81	86	80	91	83	91
Don't know	1		1	1	0	0	2	1
Base (= 100%)	*178*	*114*	*208*	*129*	*281*	*235*	*307*	*213*
30–49								
To lose weight	23	10	25	11	22	16	20	14
To put weight on	2	2	3	1	1	1	4	3
No, neither	75	88	70	87	76	83	74	83
Don't know	1		2	0	1	0	1	
Base (= 100%)	*270*	*140*	*283*	*227*	*186*	*268*	*233*	*183*
50–74								
To lose weight	57	26	36	27	30	27	8	19
To put weight on	0		1	1		3	3	4
No, neither	42	74	82	71	70	70	89	76
Don't know	1		1				1	2
Base (= 100%)	*193*	*174*	*107*	*107*	*50*	*124*	*63*	*171*
All ages								
To lose weight	29	13	22	14	19	14	13	11
To put weight on	4	1	4	3	4	2	6	3
No, neither	66	86	72	83	77	83	80	84
Don't know	1		1	0	0	0	1	1
Base (= 100%)	*641*	*428*	*598*	*463*	*517*	*627*	*603*	*567*

Table 9.12: Specific advice from health professionals on how to lose weight (percentages of all respondents advised by a health professional to lose weight)

Advice	African-Caribbean Women	African-Caribbean Men	Indian Women	Indian Men	Pakistani Women	Pakistani Men	Bangladeshi Women	Bangladeshi Men
16–29								
Take more exercise	21	58	32	36	37	54	37	52
Eat less generally	21		5		19	34	22	22
Avoid/cut down								
Meat			8	19	13	6	8	
Fatty/oily foods	19		23	54	28	23	27	33
Fried foods	10		4	10	11	6	9	12
Starchy foods			11		7	6		
Sweet things/chocolate	18		20		6	4	7	15
Other foods						10		17
Alcoholic drinks				18				
Sweet drinks	5		4		6	4	10	15
Eat special foods for								
people on a diet	3		3		1			
Eat more								
Starchy foods	2	23	2		7		6	
Lower-fat or reduced								
fat foods	3		3		3		10	3
Lean meat/white meat								
(e.g. chicken)			4					
Vegetables or fruit	19		9		13	4	24	
Other foods	8		3		6		5	
Do anything else to								
lose weight	11	35	9		6			
No, nothing			42	41	24	2	14	10
Don't know/								
can't remember	43	42	3	5	6	23	14	
Base (= 100%)	*26*	*4*	*23*	*9*	*38*	*17*	*24*	*10*
30–49								
Take more exercise	30	23	32	58	27	27	39	57
Eat less generally	20	20	29	27	29	33	63	83
Avoid/cut down								
Meat	2	10	3	7	7	15	30	14
Fatty/oily foods	28	22	32	34	27	45	34	26
Fried foods	7	12	10	4	13	5	10	3
Starchy foods	2		7	8	5	2	1	4
Sweet things/chocolate	8	3	19	8	21	6	18	9
Other foods	7	5	1	10		2		3
Alcoholic drinks	3	15		8		2		
Sweet drinks			2	9	4	6		4
Eat special foods for								
people on a diet				8	2	2	4	
Eat more								
Starchy foods	6		4	4	2			3
Lower-fat or reduced								
fat foods	5	19	6	8	11		6	
Lean meat/white meat								
(e.g. chicken)	2					5		
Vegetables or fruit	8		25	11	6	12	11	4
Other foods	2		3	3				
Do anything else to								
lose weight	9		7	8	10	15		16
No, nothing	13		19	13	16	7		3
Don't know/								
can't remember	30	41	16	4	26	20	9	1
Base (= 100%)	*66*	*13*	*62*	*24*	*46*	*40*	*47*	*25*

Continued on next page

Table 9.12: *continued*

Advice	African-Caribbean Women	African-Caribbean Men	Indian Women	Indian Men	Pakistani Women	Pakistani Men	Bangladeshi Women	Bangladeshi Men
50–74								
Take more exercise	9	37	23	39	56	34	44	34
Eat less generally	36	26	54	48	44	46	94	74
Avoid/cut down								
Meat	6	14	7	3	8	13	6	20
Fatty/oily foods	21	34	22	19	44	24	22	24
Fried foods	9	8	16	4	22	11		9
Starchy foods	19	12	9	2	16	1	6	7
Sweet things/chocolate	23	17	7	6	10	11	22	10
Other foods	5	3	4					
Alcoholic drinks	2	7				5		2
Sweet drinks	10	4	2			2	17	
Eat special foods for								
people on a diet	4	3	7				6	
Eat more								
Starchy foods	6	3		4				
Lower-fat or reduced								
fat foods	5	1	10		18			
Lean meat/white meat								
(e.g. chicken)	5	1						
Vegetables or fruit	23	7	1	4	8	26	6	6
Other foods	6		3	3	6		11	
Do anything else to								
lose weight	9	7	6	6	6		6	
No, nothing	6	3	8	22		11		
Don't know/								
can't remember	23	20	19	7		24		10
Base (= 100%)	*111*	*43*	*39*	*29*	*13*	*28*	*7*	*32*
All ages								
Take more exercise	17	36	29	45	36	34	39	45
Eat less generally	29	22	33	32	30	39	54	70
Avoid/cut down								
Meat	4	12	5	7	9	13	22	15
Fatty/oily foods	23	29	27	31	32	32	31	26
Fried foods	9	8	11	5	15	7	9	7
Starchyfoods	11	8	8	4	8	2	3	5
Sweet things/chocolate	18	13	15	6	14	8	15	10
Other foods	5	3	2	4		2		3
Alcoholic drinks	2	8		6		3		1
Sweet drinks	6	3	3	3	4	4	4	4
Eat special foods for								
people on a diet	2	2	3	3	1	1	3	
Eat more								
Starchy foods	5	4	2	3	3		2	1
Lower-fat or reduced								
fat foods	4	5	7	3	10		6	1
Lean meat/white meat								
(e.g. chicken)	3	1	1			2		
Vegetables or fruit	18	5	15	6	9	17	14	4
Other foods	5		3	2	3		2	
Do anything else to								
lose weight	10	8	7	5	8	6	0	6
No, nothing	7	2	19	22	15	8	4	2
Don't know/								
can't remember	28	27	15	6	14	23	10	5
Base (= 100%)	*203*	*60*	*124*	*62*	*97*	*85*	*78*	*67*

Table 9.13: Specific advice from health professionals on how put on weight (percentages of all respondents advised by a health professional to put on weight)

Advice	African-Caribbean Women	Men	Indian Women	Men	Pakistani Women	Men	Bangladeshi Women	Men
16–29								
Exercise/weight training			2				11	
Try to eat more								
Generally	14	52	26	12	15	15	52	36
Meat/protein foods	12		4	12	13	21	38	38
Fatty/oily foods			12	12	3		22	12
Fried foods							8	
Starchy foods	8		6				21	
Sweet things/chocolate								
Drink more milk	2		12		4	33	15	
Try to eat more often	16	52	6		3			8
Take food supplements (e.g. high calorie)					17		12	
Other	12	48	23	33	17	91	32	28
No, no specific advice given	21		34	48	35	9	14	34
Base (= 100%)	*14*	*2*	*15*	*6*	*21*	*7*	*21*	*8*
30–49								
Exercise/weight training	10		7				7	
Try to eat more								
Generally	10	33	36		33	80	54	39
Meat/protein foods			20		33	20	37	
Fatty/oily foods						20	10	20
Fried foods						20	10	
Starchy foods						20		
Sweet things/chocolate						20		
Drink more milk						20	34	20
Try to eat more often			23				20	
Take food supplements (e.g. high calorie)	13		10			20	14	
Other	13		15	32			17	54
No, no specifc advice given	58	50	20	68	33		`9	
Base (= 100%)	*6*	*3*	*12*	*3*	*3*	*5*	*10*	*5*
50–74								
Exercise/weight training				33				41
Try to eat more								
Generally			100	33		65		62
Meat/protein foods						35		24
Fatty/oily foods								
Fried foods								
Starchy foods								
Sweet things/chocolate								
Drink more milk						65		
Try to eat more often								
Take food supplements (e.g. high calorie)						65		
Other								41
No, no specific advice given	100			33			100	9
Base (= 100%)	*1*		*1*	*3*		*2*	*2*	*7*

Continued on next page

Advice	African-Caribbean Women	African-Caribbean Men	Indian Women	Indian Men	Pakistani Women	Pakistani Men	Bangladeshi Women	Bangladeshi Men
All ages								
Exercise/weight training	2		4	4			9	13
Try to eat more								
Generally	13	39	34	12	18	41	49	45
Meat/protein foods	10		9	9	15	25	36	24
Fatty/oily foods			7	9	2	4	17	10
Fried foods						4	8	
Starchy foods	6		3			4	14	
Sweet things/chocolate						4		
Drink more milk	2		7		4	39	19	5
Try to eat more often	13	16	12		2		6	3
Take food supplements								
(e.g. high calorie)	2		4		15	21	12	
Other	12	15	19	30	15	50	25	39
No, no specific advice								
given	29	35	27	51	35	5	18	17
Base (= 100%)	*21*	*5*	*28*	*12*	*24*	*14*	*33*	*20*

Table 9.14: Wish to lose weight from or alter the shape of any particular part of the body (percentages of all respondents)

Response	African-Caribbean Women	African-Caribbean Men	Indian Women	Indian Men	Pakistani Women	Pakistani Men	Bangladeshi Women	Bangladeshi Men
16–29								
Yes	64	29	58	33	53	32	41	23
No	36	71	42	67	47	68	59	77
Base (= 100%)	*177*	*114*	*208*	*127*	*280*	*234*	*303*	*210*
30–49								
Yes	68	31	60	34	64	42	22	30
No	32	69	40	66	36	58	78	70
Base (= 100%)	*265*	*140*	*279*	*224*	*186*	*265*	*232*	*181*
50–74								
Yes	60	31	55	24	55	28	9	21
No	40	69	45	76	45	72	91	79
Base (= 100%)	*187*	*171*	*107*	*106*	*49*	*123*	*63*	*168*
All ages								
Yes	64	30	58	31	58	35	29	25
No	36	70	42	69	42	65	71	75
Base (= 100%)	*629*	*425*	*594*	*457*	*515*	*622*	*598*	*559*

Table 9.15: Parts of the body from which to lose weight or alter the shape of (percentages of all respondents who would like to lose weight from a particular part of their body)

Area of the body	African-Caribbean Women	Men	Indian Women	Men	Pakistani Women	Men	Bangladeshi Women	Men
16–29								
Legs/thighs	30	18	24	8	17	6	17	14
Hips/bottom	22	4	33	6	28	6	23	13
Stomach/tummy/belly	36	53	37	67	49	60	51	57
Other	12	25	6	19	6	28	9	16
Don't know							0	
Base (= 100%)	*203*	*34*	*170*	*52*	*227*	*82*	*164*	*59*
30–49								
Legs/thighs	23	8	14	3	6	2	9	
Hips/bottom	22	7	27	2	33	5	27	4
Stomach/tummy/belly	42	71	48	88	56	92	64	96
Other	12	14	11	7	5	1	1	
Don't know								
Base (= 100%)	*280*	*48*	*228*	*81*	*164*	*108*	*68*	*52*
50–74								
Legs/thighs	11		10	2	6	1		
Hips/bottom	19	2	36	7	14	10	30	8
Stomach/tummy/belly	54	95	49	72	47	76	60	85
Other	15	3	5	10	29	12	10	
Don't know	0			10	4	1		7
Base (= 100%)	*153*	*50*	*87*	*32*	*35*	*36*	*5*	*35*
All ages								
Legs/thighs	24	9	17	5	11	3	14	6
Hips/bottom	22	4	31	4	28	6	24	9
Stomach/tummy/belly	42	72	44	77	52	77	55	76
Other	13	14	8	12	8	13	7	7
Don't know	0			2	1	0	0	2
Base (= 100%)	*636*	*132*	*485*	*165*	*426*	*226*	*237*	*146*

Table 9.16: Views about controlling weight (percentages of all respondents)

Questions and responses	African-Caribbean		Indian		Pakistani		Bangladeshi	
	Women	Men	Women	Men	Women	Men	Women	Men
16–29								
It doesn't matter how much you weigh, as long as you feel well								
Agree	50	41	52	43	57	54	55	57
Neither agree nor disagree	4	2	11	8	6	4	8	9
Disagree	45	57	37	49	35	41	34	32
Don't know	2		0	1	2	2	2	2
Controlling your weight is an important part of looking after your health								
Agree	89	92	91	89	93	89	91	90
Neither agree nor disagree	5	3	4	4	3	2	5	5
Disagree	6	4	5	6	2	6	4	3
Don't know	0	1	0		1	3	0	2
Base (= 100%)	*178*	*114*	*208*	*129*	*281*	*235*	*307*	*213*
30–49								
It doesn't matter how much you weigh, as long as you feel well								
Agree	44	37	52	53	46	47	54	52
Neither agree nor disagree	5	7	11	10	14	10	12	11
Disagree	51	54	35	37	39	43	32	35
Don't know	1	2	2	1	1	0	2	2
Controlling your weight is an important part of looking after your health								
Agree	91	91	91	89	88	94	93	89
Neither agree nor disagree	3	3	6	6	4	4	3	8
Disagree	5	4	1	4	7	2	2	2
Don't know	0	1	2	1	1	0	2	0
Base (= 100%)	*270*	*140*	*283*	*227*	*186*	*268*	*233*	*183*
50–74								
It doesn't matter how much you weigh, as long as you feel well								
Agree	57	59	53	60	36	62	52	58
Neither agree nor disagree	8	10	13	8	10	4	14	17
Disagree	34	30	29	31	50	31	25	23
Don't know	1	2	5	0	4	2	9	3
Controlling your weight is an important part of looking after your health								
Agree	93	92	91	92	87	95	76	80
Neither agree nor disagree	5	4	6	1	2	1	16	15
Disagree	0	2	2	3	2	1		3
Don't know	1	3	2	3	8	3	8	2
Base (= 100%)	*193*	*174*	*107*	*107*	*50*	*124*	*63*	*171*
All ages								
It doesn't matter how much you weigh, as long as you feel well								
Agree	50	46	52	51	49	53	55	56
Neither agree nor disagree	5	6	12	9	10	6	10	12
Disagree	44	46	35	39	39	40	32	30
Don't know	1	1	2	1	2	1	3	2
Controlling your weight is an important part of looking after your health								
Agree	91	92	91	90	90	92	90	87
Neither agree nor disagree	5	3	5	5	3	3	6	9
Disagree	4	3	3	5	4	3	2	3
Don't know	1	2	1	1	2	2	2	2
Base (= 100%)	*641*	*428*	*598*	*463*	*517*	*627*	*603*	*567*

Table 9.17: Average Body Mass Index (means of all respondents)

Age group	African-Caribbean		Indian		Pakistani		Bangladeshi	
	Women	Men	Women	Men	Women	Men	Women	Men
16–29	24.9	23.7	22.9	23.5	23.5	22.9	22.3	22.1
30–49	27.8	25.6	26.6	25.2	27.5	26.0	25.3	24.3
50–74	30.5	27.2	28.2	24.9	29.3	26.5	24.7	24.4
All ages	*27.5*	*25.5*	*25.6*	*24.6*	*26.1*	*24.9*	*23.9*	*23.4*

Table 9.18: Average waist hip ratio (means of all respondents)

Age group	African-Caribbean		Indian		Pakistani		Bangladeshi	
	Women	Men	Women	Men	Women	Men	Women	Men
16–29	0.8	0.9	0.8	0.9	0.8	0.9	0.8	0.9
30–49	0.8	0.9	0.8	0.9	0.8	0.9	0.9	0.9
50–74	0.9	0.9	0.8	1.0	0.9	1.0	0.9	1.0
All ages	*0.8*	*0.9*	*0.8*	*0.9*	*0.8*	*0.9*	*0.9*	*0.9*

Table 9.19: Average waist measurement (mean [centimetres] of all respondents)

Age group	African-Caribbean		Indian		Pakistani		Bangladeshi	
	Women	Men	Women	Men	Women	Men	Women	Men
16–29	76.6	80.7	72.7	81.9	75.7	82.5	74.0	78.3
30–49	83.3	84.9	82.9	87.8	88.2	89.6	85.1	86.9
50–74	95.2	92.5	88.9	93.5	96.9	92.0	87.1	91.4
All ages	*84.2*	*86.0*	*80.6*	*87.0*	*84.3*	*87.3*	*80.6*	*84.7*

Table 9.20: Average hip measurement (mean [centimetres] of all respondents)

Age group	African-Caribbean		Indian		Pakistani		Bangladeshi	
	Women	Men	Women	Men	Women	Men	Women	Men
16–29	99.2	94.7	95.0	96.1	96.0	93.4	92.1	90.6
30–49	104.3	97.7	103.0	96.4	103.7	97.2	97.0	92.9
50–74	111.4	98.6	106.1	98.1	108.7	96.4	95.4	94.1
All ages	*104.5*	*96.9*	*100.9*	*96.7*	*101.2*	*95.5*	*94.7*	*92.3*

Table 9.21: Average height (mean [centimetres] of all respondents)

Age group	African-Caribbean		Indian		Pakistani		Bangladeshi	
	Women	Men	Women	Men	Women	Men	Women	Men
16–29	164.2	176.4	158.0	172.5	158.4	172.5	154.0	166.8
30–49	162.3	175.2	155.9	169.3	158.0	170.4	151.5	165.1
50–74	161.3	169.7	154.4	168.1	156.4	168.9	151.0	163.5
All ages	*162.7*	*173.8*	*156.4*	*170.1*	*157.9*	*170.9*	*152.6*	*165.3*

Table 9.22: Average weight (mean [kilograms] of all respondents)

Age group	African-Caribbean		Indian		Pakistani		Bangladeshi	
	Women	Men	Women	Men	Women	Men	Women	Men
16–29	67.0	73.8	57.2	70.4	58.9	68.3	53.0	61.4
30–49	73.1	78.7	64.6	72.6	68.8	75.5	58.1	66.2
50–74	79.2	78.7	67.0	70.4	71.0	75.2	56.7	65.4
All ages	*72.6*	*76.9*	*62.6*	*71.4*	*65.0*	*72.6*	*55.7*	*64.0*

MORI/7296   AFRICAN-CARIBBEAN VERSION   21.3.94

BLACK AND MINORITY ETHNIC GROUPS

HEALTH AND LIFESTYLE SURVEY 1994

Good morning, etc. I'm ... from MORI. We are carrying out a survey on behalf of the Health Education Authority, about the health and lifestyle of people living in Britain today. I would like to start by asking you some questions about your health in general. Everything you tell me is totally confidential.

STICK ADDRESS NUMBER LABEL IN THIS SPACE

(11-16)

CODE DAY OF WEEK OF INTERVIEW

                                                   (17)

Monday 1
Tuesday 2
Wednesday 3
Thursday 4
Friday 5
Saturday 6
Sunday 7   (17)

INTERVIEWER DECLARATION

I confirm that I have conducted this interview face-to-face with the person named on the contact sheet for this address and that I asked all the relevant questions and recorded the answers in conformance with the survey specifications and within the MRS Code of Conduct.

DATE OF INTERVIEW . . . .

INTERVIEWER NAME . . . .

SIGNATURE . . . .

INTERVIEWER NUMBER   ☐☐☐☐/☐

                 (18)   (19)   (20)   (21)   (22)   (18-22)

Q1 **First I would like to ask you some questions about your health in general. How do you feel about your health? Would you say that for your age your health is . . .**

READ OUT. ALTERNATE ORDER. TICK START

0

☐ **Very good** 1

Fairly good 2

Fairly poor 3

☐ **Very poor** 4

Don't know 5   (37)

Q2 **As far as you know, is there anything people can do to improve their health, or to help themselves stay in good health?**

0

Yes 1   ASK Q3
No 2   GO TO
Don't know 3   Q6

ASK IF YES AT Q2 (OTHERS GO TO Q6)
Q3 **What are the most important things which people can do to improve their health, or to help themselves stay in good health?**

DO NOT PROMPT. MULTICODE OK

0

Eat a healthy diet 1
Take (regular) exercise 2
Not to smoke 3
Not to drink (too much) alcohol 4
Not to work too hard 5
Not to worry (too much) 6
Get a good night's sleep/plenty of rest 7
Avoid getting overweight 8
Avoid fatty foods 9
Other comments about diet/food (WRITE IN
  & CODE 0)

. . . .

. . . . 0

Other (WRITE IN & CODE X)

. . . .

. . . . X

Don't know . . . . Y

Q4   **And do you do anything yourself, on a regular basis, to improve your health, or to help yourself stay in good health?**

0

Yes 1   ASK Q5
No 2   GO TO
Don't know 3   Q6

ASK IF YES AT Q4 (OTHERS GO TO Q6)
Q5   **What do you do (to improve your health, or to help yourself stay in good health)?**

DO NOT PROMPT. MULTICODE OK

0

Eat a healthy diet 1
Take (regular) exercise 2
Not to smoke 3
Not to drink (too much) alcohol 4
Not to work too hard 5
Not to worry (too much) 6
Get a good night's sleep/plenty of rest 7
Avoid getting overweight 8
Avoid fatty foods 9
Other comments about diet/food (WRITE IN
   & CODE 0)

   . . . .

   0
Other (WRITE IN & CODE X)

   . . . .

   X
Don't know . . . . Y

Q6 **Which serious illnesses or health problems, if any, are linked to people's diet and the food they eat?**

DO NOT PROMPT. MULTICODE OK

Q7 **Which serious illnesses or health problems, if any, are linked to smoking?**

DO NOT PROMPT. MULTICODE OK

Q8 **Which serious illnesses or health problems, if any, are linked to not taking enough exercise?**

DO NOT PROMPT. MULTICODE OK

Q9 **Which serious illnesses or health problems, if any, are linked to drinking too much alcohol?**

DO NOT PROMPT. MULTICODE OK

	Q6 Diet	Q7 Smoking	Q8 Exercise	Q9 Alcohol
	0	0	0	0
Heart trouble/disease/attack	1	1	1	1
Diabetes	2	2	2	2
Stroke	3	3	3	3
Overweight/obesity	4	4	4	4
High blood pressure	5	5	5	5
Constipation	6	6	6	6
Bowel cancer	7	7	7	7
Lung cancer	8	8	8	8
Breast cancer	9	9	9	9
Cancer in general/ unspecified type of cancer	0	0	0	0
Liver disease/cirrhosis of the liver	X	X	X	X
Kidney disease	Y	Y	Y	Y
	0	0	0	0
Arthritis/rheumatism/ problems with joints	1	1	1	1

Other (WRITE IN & CODE 2)

Q6   2

Q7   2

Q8   2

Q9   2

None (no serious illnesses are linked to this)	3	3	3	3
Don't know	4	4	4	4

Q10   **What kinds of health problems, if any, are people who are overweight more likely to suffer from?**

DO NOT PROMPT. CODE BELOW

```
                                                                    ( )
Heart disease  . . . . . . . . . . . . . . . . . . . . . . . . . . . . . . . . . . . . . 1
Heart attack  . . . . . . . . . . . . . . . . . . . . . . . . . . . . . . . . . . . . . . 2
Stroke  . . . . . . . . . . . . . . . . . . . . . . . . . . . . . . . . . . . . . . . . . . 3
High blood pressure . . . . . . . . . . . . . . . . . . . . . . . . . . . . . . . . 4
Diabetes . . . . . . . . . . . . . . . . . . . . . . . . . . . . . . . . . . . . . . . . . 5
Other (WRITE IN AND CODE 6)
        . . . . . . . . . . . . . . . . . . . . . . . . . . . . . . . . . . . . . . .

        . . . . . . . . . . . . . . . . . . . . . . . . . . . . . . . . . . . . . . .

        . . . . . . . . . . . . . . . . . . . . . . . . . . . . . . . . . . . . . . . 6
None   . . . . . . . . . . . . . . . . . . . . . . . . . . . . . . . . . . . . . . . . . 7
Don't know . . . . . . . . . . . . . . . . . . . . . . . . . . . . . . . . . . . . . . 8
```

Q11   **As far as you know, is there anything people can do to reduce their risk of getting serious illnesses (such as heart disease or cancer), or not?**

```
                                                                    0
Yes   . . . . . . . . . . . . . . . . . . . . . . . . . . . . . . . . . . . . . . . . . 1
No    . . . . . . . . . . . . . . . . . . . . . . . . . . . . . . . . . . . . . . . . . 2
Don't know . . . . . . . . . . . . . . . . . . . . . . . . . . . . . . . . . . . . . . 3
```

Q12 Do you have any long-standing illness, disability or infirmity? By long standing I mean anything that has troubled you over a period of time or that is likely to affect you over a period of time.

```
                                                            0
Yes ......................................... 1    ASK Q13
No .......................................... 2    GO TO Q15    (38)
```

ASK IF YES AT Q12 (IF NO, GO TO Q15)

Q13 **What is the matter with you?** PROBE IN DETAIL **What else?** IF UNCLEAR ASK: **What do you mean by that?** WRITE IN

```
...........................................................    0

...........................................................    0

...........................................................    0

...........................................................    0

...........................................................    0

...........................................................    0

...........................................................    0

...........................................................    0
```

Q14 **Does this illness or disability (Do any of these illnesses or disabilities) limit your activities in any way?**

```
                                                       0
Yes ..................................... 1
No ...................................... 2             (55)
```

Q15 **Have you ever been told by a doctor or a nurse that you had...READ OUT CONDITIONS LISTED BELOW ?**

ROTATE ORDER. TICK START.

		Yes	No	Don't know
☐ a)	**Diabetes**	1	2	3
b)	**High blood pressure**	1	2	3
c)	**Angina**	1	2	3
☐ d)	**Heart attack (including myocardial infarction or coronary thrombosis)**	1	2	3
e)	**Any other kind of heart trouble**	1	2	3
☐ f)	**Stroke**	1	2	3

ASK WOMEN WHO HAVE BEEN TOLD THEY HAD DIABETES (OTHER WOMEN SEE Q18.)
(MEN GO TO Q21, P7)

Q16 **Can I just check, were you pregnant when you were told that you had diabetes?**

```
                                              (  )
Yes ........................................... 1   ASK Q17
No ............................................ 2   SEE Q18
```

ASK IF YES AT Q16 (OTHER WOMEN SEE Q18)

Q17 **Have you ever had diabetes apart from when you were pregnant?**

```
                                              (  )
Yes ........................................... 1
No ............................................ 2
```

ASK WOMEN WHO SAY THEY HAVE EVER HAD HIGH BLOOD PRESSURE (YES AT Q15B).
(OTHER WOMEN GO TO Q20)

Q18 **Can I just check, were you pregnant when you were told that you had high blood pressure?**

```
                                              (  )
Yes ........................................... 1   ASK Q19
No ............................................ 2   GO TO Q20
```

ASK IF YES AT Q18 (OTHER WOMEN GO TO Q20)

Q19   **Have you <u>ever</u> had high blood pressure apart from when you were pregnant?**

                                                        ( )

Yes 1
No 2

ASK WOMEN AGED 16-49 (DO NOT ASK IF LIKELY TO GIVE OFFENCE, EG UNMARRIED WOMEN)

Q20   **(May I just check) Are you pregnant now?**

                                                       (63)

Yes   1   <u>GO TO Q32, P12</u>
No   2   ASK Q21
Not sure 3
Question not asked 4

ASK ALL EXCEPT PREGNANT WOMEN (PREGNANT WOMEN GO TO Q32, P12)

Q21   **And how much do you weigh at the moment?**   TAKE RESPONDENT'S ESTIMATE IF NECESSARY

   ☐☐   stone   ☐☐   pounds   OR   ☐☐☐   kilogrammes

   (70) (71)   (72) (73)   (74) (75) (76)

Don't know at all . . . . Y

Q22   **Which of these best describes you?** READ OUT a) TO e)

                                                     0

a)   **I weigh a lot less than I would wish to** 1

b)   **I weigh a little less than I would wish to** 2   <u>ASK Q23</u>

c)   **I feel my weight is about right** 3   <u>GO TO Q26,P8</u>

d)   **I weigh a little more than I would wish to** 4   GO TO Q29,P10

e)   **I weigh a lot more than I would wish to** . . . . <u>5</u>

Don't know 6   GO TO Q32, P12

ASK IF a) OR b) AT Q22 (WEIGH A LITTLE/LOT LESS)

Q23   **As far as you know, is there anything people can do to put on weight, when they want to?**

                                                       0

Yes   1   ASK Q24
No   2   GO TO Q32, P12
Don't know 3

ASK IF YES AT Q23
Q24   **Are <u>you</u> doing anything at the moment to put weight on? IF YES: What are you doing?**

DO NOT PROMPT. CODE BELOW. MULTICODE OK

                                                   0

Yes:

       Exercising/weight training 1
       Trying to eat more generally 2
       Trying to eat more of specific foods:
          meat/protein foods 3
          fatty foods 4
          fried foods 5
          starchy foods (eg rice, bread, potatoes, sweet
            potatoes, yams) 6   **ASK**
          sweet things/chocolate 7   **Q25**
       Drinking more milk 8
       Trying to eat more often 9
       Taking food supplements eg high calorie drinks 0
       Other (WRITE IN AND CODE X)

        X
No,nothing . . . . Y   **GO TO Q32,P12**

ASK IF DOING SOMETHING TO PUT WEIGHT ON AT Q24 (OTHERS GO TO Q32, P12)
Q25   **What would you say are your main reasons for trying to put on weight?**

DO NOT PROMPT. MULTICODE OK

                                                    0

For the good of my health generally 1
To reduce my risk of specific health
 problems 2
To have more energy/feel less tired 3
To feel better about myself generally/more confident 4
To feel more attractive 5
To be able to wear attractive/fashionable clothes 6
Other (WRITE IN AND CODE 7)

        . . . .

        7
Don't know 8   **NOW GO TO Q32, P12**

ASK IF c) AT Q22 (ABOUT THE RIGHT WEIGHT)
Q26   **As far as you know, is there anything people can do to control or maintain their weight, when they want to?**

                                                    0

Yes   1   **ASK Q27**
No   2   **GO TO Q32,P12**
Don't know 3

ASK IF YES AT Q 26
Q27 **Do <u>you</u> do anything at the moment to control or maintain your weight, or not? IF YES: What do you do? What else?**

DO NOT PROMPT. CODE BELOW. MULTICODE OK

0

<u>Yes:</u>
Take exercise 1
Limit total amount of food eaten 2
Avoid or cut down on particular foods:
      meat 3
      fatty/oily foods 4
      fried foods 5
      starchy foods (rice, bread, potatoes, sweet
       potatoes, yams etc) 6
      sweet things/chocolate 7
      avoid or cut down on other foods
       (WRITE IN AND CODE 8)

    . . . .

    8   ASK
Avoid or cut down on alcoholic drinks 9   Q28
Avoid or cut down on sweet drinks 0
Eat special foods for people on a diet X
Eat more of particular foods:
      starchy or high-fibre foods (eg rice, bread,
       potatoes, sweet potatoes, yams etc) . . . . Y   ASK Q

0
      lower-fat or reduced fat foods (skimmed or semi-
       skimmed milk, low-fat cheese, low-fat spread etc) . . . 1
      lean meat/white meat such as chicken or turkey 2
      vegetables or fruit 3
      eat more of other foods (WRITE IN AND CODE 4)

    . . . .

    4
Do anything else to control/maintain weight (WRITE IN AND CODE 5)
    . . . .

    . . . . <u>5</u>

<u>No, nothing</u> 6   GO TO Q32, P12

ASK IF DOING SOMETHING TO CONTROL WEIGHT AT Q27 (IF NOT, GO TO Q32)

Q28 **What would you say are your main reasons for controlling/maintaining your weight?**

DO NOT PROMPT. CODE BELOW. MULTICODE OK

0

For the good of my health generally 1
To reduce my risk of specific health
  problems (eg diabetes, heart disease) 2
To feel better about myself generally/more confident 3
Just don't want to be any fatter (generally) 4
To avoid putting on weight in specific
  places eg stomach, hips, thighs 5
To feel attractive 6
To be able to wear attractive/fashionable clothes 7
Pressure from family and/or friends 8
Other (WRITE IN AND CODE 9)

. . . . 9
Don't know 0   NOW GO TO Q32, P12

ASK IF d) OR e) AT Q22 (WEIGH A LOT/LITTLE MORE)

Q29 **As far as you know, is there anything people can do to lose weight when they want to?**

0

Yes   1   ASK Q30
No   2   GO TO
Don't know 3   Q32,P12

Q30 **Are you doing anything at the moment to lose weight? IF YES: What are you doing? What else?**

DO NOT PROMPT. CODE BELOW. MULTICODE OK

0

<u>Yes:</u>
Taking more exercise 1
Eating less generally 2
Avoiding or cutting down on particular foods:
      meat 3
      fatty/oily foods 4
      fried foods 5
      starchy foods (rice, bread, potatoes, sweet
        potatoes, yams etc) 6
      sweet things/chocolate 7
      avoiding or cutting down on other foods
        (WRITE IN AND CODE 8)

      . . . .

      8
Avoiding or cutting down on alcoholic drinks 9
Avoiding or cutting down on sweet drinks 0
Eating special foods for people on a diet X   ASK
Eating more of particular foods:
      starchy or high-fibre foods (eg rice, bread, potatoes,
        sweet potatoes, yams etc) . . . . Y   Q31

0

      lower-fat or reduced fat foods (skimmed or
      semi-skimmed milk, low-fat cheese, low-fat spread etc) 1
      lean meat/white meat such as chicken or turkey 2
      vegetables or fruit 3
      eating more of other foods (WRITE IN AND CODE 4)

      . . . .

      4
Calorie controlled diet/special diet 5
Doing anything else to lose weight (WRITE IN AND CODE 5)

      . . . .

      . . . . 5 _____
<u>No, nothing</u> 6   GO TO Q32, P12

ASK THOSE WHO ARE TRYING TO LOSE WEIGHT AT Q30 (OTHERS GO TO Q32, P12)

Q31   **What would you say are your main reasons for trying to lose weight?**

DO NOT PROMPT. CODE BELOW. MULTICODE OK

                                                                          0
For the good of my health generally 1
To reduce my risk of specific health problems
   (eg diabetes, heart disease) 2
To feel better about myself generally/more confident 3
I would like to be thinner all over 4
I would like to be a different shape/lose weight from
   particular parts of me, eg stomach, hips, thighs 5
To feel more attractive 6
To look better/more attractive 7
To be able to wear attractive/fashionable clothes 8
Pressure from family and/or friends 9
Other (WRITE IN AND CODE 0)

   0
Don't know X

ASK ALL

Q32   **Have you ever been advised by a doctor or nurse or any other health professional to lose weight or to put on weight?**

                                                                          0
Yes:

        To lose weight 1   <u>ASK Q33</u>
        To put on weight 2   <u>GO TO Q34</u>
No, neither 3   GO TO Q35
Don't know 4

ASK IF ADVISED TO LOSE WEIGHT AT Q32
Q33   **Did they give you any specific advice about how to lose weight, or not? IF YES What was that advice?**

DO NOT PROMPT. CODE BELOW. MULTICODE OK

                                                    0

Yes:

Take more exercise 1
Eat less generally 2
Avoid or cut down on particular foods:
  meat 3
  fatty/oily foods 4
  fried foods 5
  starchy foods (rice, bread, potatoes,
    sweet potatoes, yams etc) 6
  sugar/sweet things/chocolate 7
  avoid or cut down on other foods
    (WRITE IN AND CODE 8)

  . . . .
  8
Avoid or cut down on alcoholic drinks 9
Avoid or cut down on sweet drinks 0
Eat special foods for people on a diet X
Eat more of particular foods:
  starchy or high-fibre foods (eg rice, bread, potatoes,
  sweet potatoes, yams etc) . . . . Y

                                                    0
  lower-fat or reduced fat foods (skimmed or semi-
    skimmed milk, low-fat cheese, low-fat spread etc) . . . 1
  lean meat/white meat such as chicken or turkey 2
  vegetables or fruit 3
  eat more of other foods: (WRITE IN AND CODE 4)

  . . . .
  4
Do anything else to lose weight
  (WRITE IN AND CODE 5)

  . . . .
  5
No, no advice given 6
Don't know/can't remember 7   **NOW GO TO Q35**

ASK IF ADVISED TO PUT ON WEIGHT AT Q32
Q34 **Did they give you any specific advice about how to put on weight, or not? IF YES What was that advice?**

DO NOT PROMPT. CODE BELOW. MULTICODE OK

0

Yes:
```
        Exercise/weight training . . . . . . . . . . . . . . . . . . . . . . 1
        Try to eat more generally . . . . . . . . . . . . . . . . . . . . . 2
        Try to eat more of specific foods:
            meat/protein foods . . . . . . . . . . . . . . . . . . . . . . . 3
            fatty foods . . . . . . . . . . . . . . . . . . . . . . . . . . . . 4
            fried foods . . . . . . . . . . . . . . . . . . . . . . . . . . . . 5
            starchy foods (eg rice, bread, potatoes,
                sweet potatoes, yams) . . . . . . . . . . . . . . . . . . . 6
            sweet things/chocolate . . . . . . . . . . . . . . . . . . . . 7
        Drink more milk . . . . . . . . . . . . . . . . . . . . . . . . . . 8
        Try to eat more often . . . . . . . . . . . . . . . . . . . . . . . 9
        Take food supplements eg high calorie
        drinks . . . . . . . . . . . . . . . . . . . . . . . . . . . . . . . . . 0
        Other (WRITE IN AND CODE X)
```

. . . .

. . . . X

No, no specific advice given . . . . Y

ASK ALL
Q35 **Would you like to lose weight from, or alter the shape of, any particular part of your body?**

0

Yes   1   ASK Q36
No   2   GO TO Q37

ASK IF YES AT Q35 (OTHERS GO TO Q37)
Q36 **Which parts would you like to lose weight from or alter the shape of?**

DO NOT PROMPT. MULTICODE OK

0

Legs/thighs 1
Hips/bottom 2
Stomach/tummy/belly 3
Other (WRITE IN AND CODE 4)

. . . . 4

Don't know 5

Q37 I am going to read out some statements about people's weight and I would like you to tell me whether you agree or disagree with each one

READ OUT STATEMENTS. ALTERNATE ORDER. TICK START.

		Agree	Neither agree nor disagree	Disagree	Don't know
☐ a)	It doesn't matter how much you weigh as long as you feel well	1	2	3	4
☐ b)	Controlling your weight is an important part of looking after your health	1	2	3	4

SMOKING

ASK ALL
Q38 I would now like to ask you a few questions about smoking. Have you ever smoked a cigarette, a cigar or a pipe?

			0		
Yes	....	1	ASK Q39	
No	....	2	GO TO Q47	(46)

ASK ALL WHO EVER SMOKED. OTHERS GO TO Q47, P17
Q39 Do you smoke cigarettes at all nowadays?

			0		
Yes	....	1	GO TO Q43, P16	
No	....	2	ASK Q40	(47)

ASK IF NO AT Q39
Q40 Have you ever smoked cigarettes regularly?

			0		
Yes	....	1	ASK Q41	
No	....	2	GO TO Q42	0

ASK IF EVER SMOKED CIGARETTES REGULARLY (YES AT Q40)

Q41 **About how many cigarettes did you smoke in a day when you smoked them regularly?** PROBE WHETHER HAND-ROLLED OR MANUFACTURED CIGARETTES

☐☐☐ cigarettes a day

(53) (54) (55)

Don't know . . . . . Y

NB. IF HAND-ROLLED CIGARETTES SMOKED, GIVE AMOUNT OF TOBACCO, NOT NUMBER OF CIGARETTES
1 oz = 28 gr, ½ = 14 gr, ¼ = 7 gr

☐☐ GRAMMES

(56) (57)

Don't know . . . . Y

ASK ALL EX-CIGARETTE SMOKERS (NO AT Q39)

Q42 **How long ago did you give up smoking - the last time, if you have given up more than once?**

WRITE IN BOXES BELOW. USING LEADING ZEROES IF NECESSARY

☐☐ years ☐☐ months

Don't know . . . . Y NOW GO TO Q 47, P17

ASK IF YES AT Q39

Q43 **Do you smoke cigarettes regularly nowadays?**

0

Yes 1
No 2

Q44 **About how many cigarettes a day do you usually smoke on weekdays?** PROBE WHETHER HAND-ROLLED OR MANUFACTURED CIGARETTES

☐☐☐ cigarettes

(78) (79) (80)

Don't know . . . . Y

NB. IF HAND-ROLLED CIGARETTES SMOKED, GIVE AMOUNT OF TOBACCO, NOT NUMBER OF CIGARETTES
1 oz = 28 gr, ½ = 14 gr, ¼ = 7 gr

☐☐ GRAMMES

(11) (12)   (11-12)

Don't know . . . . Y

Q45 **About how many cigarettes a day do you usually smoke at weekends?** PROBE WHETHER HAND-ROLLED OR MANUFACTURED CIGARETTES

☐☐☐ cigarettes

(78) (79) (80)

Don't know .... Y

NB. IF HAND-ROLLED CIGARETTES SMOKED, GIVE AMOUNT OF TOBACCO, NOT NUMBER OF CIGARETTES

1 oz = 28 gr, ½ = 14 gr, ¼ = 7 gr

☐☐ GRAMMES

(11) (12)   (11-12)

Don't know .... Y

Q46 **Have you ever tried to give up smoking?**

0

Yes 1

No 2

(SKIP QQ47-48)

NUTRITION

ASK ALL
Q49   SHOWCARD   Thinking now of all the meals or snacks you have eaten at home in the last seven days, which of the statements on this card do you think best describes them?

                                                                    ()

They all included traditional West Indian foods of some kind . . 1
Most of them included traditional West Indian foods 2
About half of them included traditional West Indian foods 3
Just a few of them included traditional West Indian foods 4
None of them included traditional West Indian foods 5

Haven't eaten any meals/snacks at home in last seven days . . 6
Don't know/can't remember 7

Q50   SHOWCARD   AGAIN And thinking now of any meals or snacks you have eaten away from home in the last seven days, which of the statements on this card do you think best describes them?

                                                                    ()

They all included traditional West Indian foods of some kind . . 1
Most of them included traditional West Indian foods 2
About half of them included traditional West Indian foods 3
Just a few of them included traditional West Indian foods 4
None of them included traditional West Indian foods 5

Haven't eaten any meals/snacks away from home in last
    seven days 6
Don't know/can't remember 7

Q51 **What kind of foods do you think a person should include in a healthy diet?**

PROBE FOR DETAILS. WRITE IN

. . . .

. . . .

. . . .

. . . .

. . . .

Q52   **I'm going to read out some words relating to diet and nutrition and I'd like you to tell me for each one whether you feel you understand what this term means, or not. IF NECESSARY, ADD: (I don't just want to know whether you have heard of this, I want to know whether you feel you understand what it means.)**

READ OUT EACH TERM. ROTATE ORDER. TICK START

		Under-stand	Don't under-stand	Never heard of it	Don't know/not sure
☐ a)	**Starchy foods**	1	2	3	4
☐ b)	**Dietary fibre**	1	2	3	4
☐ c)	**Fat**	1	2	3	4
☐ d)	**Saturated fat**	1	2	3	4

IF NONE OF THE ABOVE TERMS UNDERSTOOD - GO TO Q57, P22.
IF 'STARCHY FOODS' UNDERSTOOD - ASK Q53
IF 'DIETARY FIBRE' UNDERSTOOD - ASK Q54
IF 'FAT' UNDERSTOOD - ASK Q55
IF 'SATURATED FAT' UNDERSTOOD - ASK Q56

ASK IF 'STARCHY FOODS' UNDERSTOOD
Q53 Could you give me some examples of foods which contain a lot of starch?

(DO NOT PROMPT. CODE BELOW)

ASK IF 'DIETARY FIBRE' UNDERSTOOD
Q54 Could you give me some examples of foods which contain a lot of dietary fibre?

(DO NOT PROMPT. CODE BELOW)

ASK IF 'FAT' UNDERSTOOD
Q55 Could you give me some examples of foods which contain a lot of fat?

(DO NOT PROMPT. CODE BELOW)

ASK IF 'SATURATED FAT' UNDERSTOOD
Q56 Could you give me some examples of foods which contain a lot of saturated fat?

(DO NOT PROMPT. CODE BELOW)

	Q53	Q54	Q55	Q56
	0	0	0	0
Bread (including nan, chapati, puri, roti, poppodum)	1	1	1	1
Rice	2	2	2	2
Potatoes	3	3	3	3
Yams, plantain, sweet potatoes	4	4	4	4
Brown/wholemeal bread	5	5	5	5
Brown rice	6	6	6	6
Noodles/pasta/macaroni etc	7	7	7	7
Maize/sweetcorn	8	8	8	8
Lentils/peas/beans/dhal	9	9	9	9
Cooking oil/vegetable oil	0	0	0	0
Butter	X	X	X	X
Ghee	Y	Y	Y	Y
	0	0	0	0
Lard	1	1	1	1
Cheese	2	2	2	2
Meat/red meat	3	3	3	3
Eggs	4	4	4	4
Burgers/sausages/hot dogs	5	5	5	5
Crisps	6	6	6	6
Fried snacks eg samosa, pakora, bhaji, dokra, chevro, gartia, bombay mix	7	7	7	7
Sweets: halva, kulfi, gulabjamun etc	8	8	8	8
Milk puddings with rice/semolina/sago/vermicelli	9	9	9	9
Nuts	0	0	0	0
Shellfish/seafood such as prawns	X	X	X	X

Other (WRITE IN & CODE Y)

Q53 . . . . Y

Q54 . . . . Y

Q55 . . . . Y

Q56 . . . . Y

	Q53	Q54	Q55	Q56
	0	0	0	0
Don't know	1	1	1	1

ASK ALL

Q57 **If you wanted to reduce the amount of salt in your diet, are there any particular foods you would avoid or cut down on? IF YES Which ones?**

DO NOT PROMPT. MULTICODE OK

( )

Yes:
Processed foods/tinned foods in general 1
Ready prepared meals 2
Salt cod/salt mackerel/salt beef 3
Bacon 4
Crisps, roasted peanuts, salty snacks 5
Other (WRITE IN AND CODE 6)

. . . .

. . . . 6
No, would not avoid or cut down on any particular foods 7
Just use less salt in cooking/put less salt on food 8
Don't know 9

Q58 **Are there any foods that you would not consider eating, or any dietary restrictions that you keep, for religious or cultural reasons? IF YES What foods are these?**

DO NOT PROMPT. MULTICODE OK

( )

Yes:
Pork, pork products 1
Beef 2
Meat which isn't halal 3
Meat of any kind 4
Animal fat of unknown origin (eg in
  manufactured foods such as biscuits) 5
Onions/garlic/tomatoes 6
Don't drink alcohol 7
Other (WRITE IN AND CODE 8)

. . . .

. . . . 8
No dietary restrictions 9

ASK ALL EXCEPT THOSE WHO SAID THEY DON'T EAT MEAT AT Q58

Q59 **(Can I just check,) do you ever eat.. READ OUT**

		Yes	No
a)	**Meat such as lamb/mutton or beef**	1	2
b)	**Chicken or turkey**	1	2

Q60   Can I just check, do you ever eat...   READ OUT

		Yes	No
a)	Fish	1	2
b)	Eggs	1	2
c)	Milk or yoghurt	1	2
d)	Cheese	1	2

ASK IF MEAT NOT EATEN (AT Q58 OR Q59)
Q61   Do you consider yourself to be a vegetarian, or a vegan, or neither?

0

Vegetarian 1
Vegan 2
Neither 3
Don't know 4

Q62   Do you agree or disagree with the following statements?

READ OUT .ROTATE ORDER. TICK START.

		Agree	Neither agree nor disagree	Disagree	Don't know
☐ a)	The traditional foods eaten by people of West Indian origin are healthier than the foods eaten by most people in this country	1	2	3	4
☐ b)	It's too much trouble to try to cook traditional West Indian foods all the time	1	2	3	4
☐ c)	It can be very difficult to get traditional West Indian foods if you have to eat away from home	1	2	3	4
☐ d)	I prefer to eat British or European style food rather than traditional West Indian food	1	2	3	4

HYPERTENSION

ASK ALL
Q63   Do you know what is meant by the term 'high blood pressure'?

                                                                    0
Yes   1   ASK Q64
No   2   GO TO
Don't know 3   Q67, P25

ASK IF YES AT Q63 (OTHERS GO TO Q67)
Q64   **What do you think are the health risks, if any, of having high blood pressure?**

DO NOT PROMPT MULTICODE OK

                                                                    0
Increased risk of:
Overweight/obesity 1
Diabetes 2
Coronary heart disease 3
Heart attack 4
Stroke 5
Headaches or migraines 6
Other (WRITE IN & CODE '7')

        7
No health risks 8
Don't know 9

Q65   **What, if anything, do you think causes high blood pressure?**

DO NOT PROMPT. CODE BELOW. MULTICODE OK

                                                                    ( )
Eating too much salt 1
Drinking too much alcohol 2
Being overweight/obese 3
Stress/worry/pressure 4
Runs in families/genetic/hereditary 5
Hardened arteries/clogged up arteries 6
Other (WRITE IN AND CODE 7)

        . . . .

        7
Nothing in particular 8
Don't know 9

Q66   SHOWCARD AGAIN **If somebody you knew wanted to reduce their risk of having high blood pressure, which of these pieces of advice would you give them?**

MULTICODE OK

	0
Lose weight/avoid becoming overweight	1
Avoid fatty/oily foods and drinks	2
Avoid sugary/sweet foods and drinks	3
Avoid drinking alcohol/cut down	4
Don't smoke/give up smoking	5
Avoid salty foods	6
Eat more of foods such as bread, rice, potatoes and yams	7
Eat plenty of fresh fruit and vegetables	8
Take (regular) exercise	9
Other (WRITE IN & CODE 0)	
....	0
None of these	X
There is nothing you can do to reduce risk of high blood pressure	Y
	0
Don't know	1

CHECK BACK TO Q15B. ASK THOSE WHO DID <u>NOT</u> SAY THEY HAVE BEEN TOLD BY DOCTOR/NURSE THAT THEY HAD HIGH BLOOD PRESSURE. OTHERS GO TO Q70)

Q67   **Have you ever had your blood pressure measured by a doctor or nurse?**

	(66)	
Yes	1	ASK Q68
No	2	GO TO
Don't know	3	Q70 (66)

ASK IF YES AT Q67 (OTHERS GO TO Q70)

Q68   **Thinking about the last time your blood pressure was measured, were you told it was...**
READ OUT

	( )
Alright/fine/normal	1
Higher than normal	2
Lower than normal	3
or not told anything?	4
Don't know/can't remember	5

Q69   **Can I just check, were you pregnant at the time of the test?**

                                                              ( )
Yes   1
No   2

PHYSICAL ACTIVITY

Q70   **I'd now like to ask you some questions about exercise and physical activity, including walking, cycling, dancing, swimming, running, doing exercises, playing energetic sports, and other kinds of physical activity.**

First of all, if a person is taking any of these kinds of exercise or doing other physical activities in order to keep fit, do they need to do it a certain number of times each week or each month, or not?

                                                             0
Yes, has to be done a number of times a week 1   ASK Q71
No   2   GO TO Q72
Don't know 3

ASK IF YES AT Q70 (OTHERS GO TO Q72)
Q71   **And how many times a week do you think a person has to take exercise or do physical activities, in order to keep fit?**

DO NOT PROMPT. SINGLE CODE ONLY

                                                             0
1   1
2   2
3   3
4 or 5 4
Most days/6 or 7 times a week 5
More than seven times a week 6
Don't know 7

ASK ALL
Q72   **And does a person have to take exercise or do physical activities for at least a certain length of time, on each occasion, for it to help them keep physically fit, or not?**

                                                             0
Yes, have to do it for a certain length of time 1   ASK Q73
No, don't have to do it for a certain length of time 2   GO TO
Don't know 3   Q74

ASK IF YES AT Q72

Q73   How long does a person need to spend taking exercise or doing physical activities, on each occasion, for it to help them to keep physically fit?

DO NOT PROMPT. SINGLE CODE ONLY

0

Up to 5 minutes 1
6 to 10 minutes 2
11 to 15 minutes 3
16 to 20 minutes 4
21 to 25 minutes 5
26 to 30 minutes 6
31 to 45 minutes 7
46 to 60 minutes 8
Over an hour 9
Don't know 0

ASK ALL

Q74   If a person is taking exercise or doing other physical activities in order to keep physically fit, which of the following statements best describes how much effort they need to put into it? Please tell me the first statement you think applies.

READ OUT . SINGLE CODE ONLY

0

It should leave you feeling exhausted 1

It should leave you feeling out of breath and sweaty 2

It should make your heart beat a bit faster than normal and make you feel slightly warmer 3

It should <u>not</u> make your heart beat any faster than normal . . 4

Don't know 5

Black and minority ethnic groups in England

Q75 What health effects, if any, is it likely to have, if a person does not take enough exercise or do enough physical activities?

DO NOT PROMPT. MULTICODE OK

Get fat/overweight 1
Diabetes 2
Heart disease/heart attack 3
Stroke 4
Stiff joints/ arthritis 5
Backache 6
Get out of breath easily 7
Less able to cope with worries/stress 8
Minor ailments such as colds, coughs 9
Other (WRITE IN & CODE 0)

. . . .

. . . . 0
None X
Don't know . . . . Y

READ OUT:
Now I'd like to ask you about some of the things you have done at work or in your free time that involve physical activity <u>in the past 4 weeks</u> that is from . . . . . up to yesterday.

A - ACTIVITY AT WORK AND AROUND THE HOUSE

Q76 (Can I just check) were you in paid employment or self employment in the past 4 weeks?

	( )	
Yes (paid employment or self employed)	1	<u>ASK Q77</u>
No	2	GO TO Q78, P29

ASK IF YES AT Q76 (OTHERS GO TO Q78)
Q77 Thinking about your job in general would you say that you are . . . READ OUT

( )

very physically active 1

fairly physically active 2

not very physically active 3

or not at all physically active in your job? 4

Don't know 5

IF YES AT Q76, READ OUT:
I'd like you to think about the physical activities you have done when you were <u>not</u> doing your paid job.

ASK ALL

Q78   Have you done any housework in the past 4 weeks?

( )

Yes 1   ASK Q79
No 2   GO TO Q82

ASK IF YES AT Q78 (OTHERS GO TO Q82)

Q79   SHOWCARD   Some kinds of housework are heavier than others. This card gives examples of heavy housework, it does not include everything. These are just examples. Was any of the housework you did in the past 4 weeks this kind of heavy housework?

0

Yes 1   ASK Q80
No 2   GO TO Q82

ASK IF YES AT Q80 (OTHERS GO TO Q82)

Q80   During the past 4 weeks on how many days have you done that kind of heavy housework? WRITE IN

No of days   [ ] [ ]
              ( ) ( )

Don't know . . . . Y

Q81   On the day you most recently did some heavy housework, how long in total did you spend doing it? Please don't include any time you spent on lighter housework, or any breaks you took. We want to know the actual time you spent on heavy housework.

RECORD ANSWER IN HOURS AND MINUTES, IN BOXES BELOW

HOURS   [ ] [ ]   MINUTES   [ ] [ ]
         0   0   0   0

Don't know . . . . Y

ASK ALL

Q82   Have you done any gardening, DIY or building work in the past 4 weeks? (Again, I am asking about physical activities you have done when you were not doing your paid job.)

( )

Yes 1   ASK Q83
No 2   GO TO Q86, P31

ASK IF YES AT Q82 (OTHERS GO TO Q86)
Q83   SHOWCARD   **Could you have a good look at this card which gives examples of heavy manual gardening and DIY work. Was the gardening or DIY you did in the past 4 weeks of the <u>heavy manual</u> kind?**

                                                                           0
         Yes 1   ASK Q84
         No 2   GO TO Q86

ASK IF YES AT Q83 (OTHERS GO TO Q86)
Q84   **During the past 4 weeks, on how many days in total did you do this kind of heavy manual gardening or DIY?**

         WRITE IN

         No of days   ☐☐
                             ( ) ( )
         Don't know . . . . Y

Q85   **On the day you most recently did some heavy gardening, how long in total did you spend doing it? Please don't include any time you spent on lighter gardening, or any breaks you took. We want to know the actual time you spent on heavy gardening.**

         RECORD ANSWER IN HOURS AND MINUTES, IN BOXES BELOW

         HOURS   ☐☐   MINUTES   ☐☐
                 ( ) ( )   ( ) ( )
         Don't know . . . . Y

Q86 **Have you done any walks of a quarter of a mile or more in the past 4 weeks? That would usually be _continuous_ walking lasting 5 to 10 minutes.**

                                                              0
        Yes 1   ASK Q87
        No 2   GO TO
        Can't walk at all 3   Q91, P32

ASK IF YES AT Q86 (OTHERS GO TO Q91,P32)
Q87 **I'd like you to think about _all_ the walking you have done in the past 4 weeks either locally or away from here. Please include any country walks, walking in the course of your work, walking to and from work and any other walks that you have done.**

Did you do any walks of 1 mile or more in the past 4 weeks? That would usually be _continuous_ walking for at least 20 minutes.

                                                              0
        Yes 1   ASK Q88
        No 2   GO TO Q91, P32

ASK IF YES AT Q87 (OTHERS GO TO Q91)
Q88 **During the past 4 weeks, how many times did you do any walks of 1 mile or more? WRITE IN**

        No of times   ☐☐
                           ( ) ( )
        Don't know .... Y

Q89 **And how many of these walks were 2 miles or more? WRITE IN**

        No of walks   ☐☐
                           ( ) ( )
        Don't know .... Y

Q90 **Which of the following best describes your usual walking pace ... READ OUT**

                                                              0
        a slow pace 1

        a steady average pace 2

        a fairly brisk pace 3

        or a fast pace - at least 4 mph? 4

        Don't know 5

B - SPORTS AND EXERCISE

ASK ALL

Q91 SHOWCARD   **Can you tell me if you have done any of the activities on this card during the last 4 weeks?**

(READ OUT SHOWCARD ITEMS IF NECESSARY)

<pre>
                                                            0
        Yes 1   ASK Q92
        No 2   GO TO Q96
</pre>

ASK IF YES AT Q91 (OTHERS GO TO Q96)

Q92 **Which ones? CODE BELOW**

Q93 **Can you tell me on how many separate occasions did you (ACTIVITY) during the past 4 weeks?**

Q94 **How much time did you usually spend (ACTIVITY) on each occasion?**

Q95 **During the past 4 weeks was the effort of (ACTIVITY) usually enough to make you out of breath or sweaty?**

	Q92 Activities done ( )	Q93 No of occasions	Q94 Time spent per occasion HRS MINS	Q95 Effort YES NO
Cycling/exercise bike 1				1 2 0
Exercises (press ups, sit ups etc) 2				1 2 0
Aerobics/keep fit/gymnastics/ dance for fitness 3				1 2 ( )
Other types of dancing ... 4				1 2 ( )
Weight training 5				1 2 ( )
Swimming 6				1 2 ( )
Running/jogging 7				1 2 ( )
Football/rugby 8				1 2 ( )
Badminton/tennis 9				1 2 ( )
Squash 0				1 2 ( )
Other sports or exercise . X				1 2 ( )

C - OTHER PHYSICAL ACTIVITIES

ASK ALL
Finally in this section on activities I'd like to talk briefly about other things that may involve you in physical activity.

Q96   **First, stairs. Do you go up and down stairs at home?** INCLUDE STAIRS FROM STREET LEVEL TO FRONT DOOR, EG IN FLAT OR MAISONETTE

                                                                0

Yes 1   ASK Q97

No 2   GO TO Q99

ASK IF YES AT Q96 (OTHERS GO TO Q99)
Q97   **About how many times a day do you climb the stairs?** WRITE IN

No of times   ☐☐
              ( ) ( )

Don't know . . . . Y

Q98   **And how many steps are there in your stairs?**

No of steps   ☐☐
              ( ) ( )

Don't know . . . . Y

ASK ALL
Q99   **In an average week on how many days, if any, do you usually climb stairs at work or elsewhere other than your home?** WRITE IN OR CODE

No of days_____ ☐☐   ASK Q100

None 0   GO TO Q102

Don't know . . . . Y

ASK IF SOME AT Q99 (IF NONE, GO TO Q102)
Q100   **About how many times a day do you climb up stairs at work or elsewhere?** WRITE IN

No of times   ☐☐
              ( ) ( )

Don't know . . . . Y

Q101   **And, on average, how many steps do you go up each time?**

No of steps   ☐☐
              ( ) ( )

Don't know . . . . Y

Q102 And now, caring for others. In an average week on how many days, if any, do you carry a child around? Would you say rarely or never, 1-2 days, 3-5 days or most days? CODE BELOW

Q103 And in an average week, on how many days, if any, do you push a child in a pram or pushchair? Would you say rarely or never, 1-2 days, 3-5 days or most days? CODE BELOW

Q104 And in an average week, on how many days, if any, do you play games with a young child that involve you in physical effort? Would you say rarely or never, 1-2 days, 3-5 days or most days? CODE BELOW

	Q102 Carry child ( )	Q103 Push child ( )	Q104 Play games ( )
Rarely/never	1	1	1
1-2 days	2	2	2
3-5 days	3	3	3
Most days	4	4	4

Q105 Do you help care for anyone who is disabled or has difficulty walking?

	( )	
Yes	1	ASK Q106
No	2	GO TO Q109

ASK IF YES AT Q105 (OTHERS GO TO Q109)

Q106 In an average week on how many days, if any, do you lift or carry a disabled adult? Would you say rarely or never, 1 to 2 days, 3 to 5 days or most days? CODE BELOW

Q107 In an average week on how many days, if any, do you give walking support to a disabled adult? Would you say rarely or never, 1 to 2 days, 3 to 5 days or most days? CODE BELOW

Q108 In an average week on how many days, if any, do you push a wheel chair? Would you say rarely or never, 1 to 2 days, 3 to 5 days or most days? CODE BELOW

	Q106 Lift/ carry ( )	Q107 Support ( )	Q108 Push chair ( )
Rarely/never	1	1	1
1-2 days	2	2	2
3-5 days	3	3	3
Most days	4	4	4

D - ATTITUDES TO ACTIVITY AND HEALTH

ASK ALL
Q109   Compared to other people of your age would you describe yourself as . . . . . READ OUT

( )
very physically active 1

fairly physically active 2

not very physically active 3

or not at all physically active? 4

Don't know 5

Q110   Compared to other people of your age would you say you are . . . .   READ OUT

( )
very fit 1

fairly fit 2

not very fit 3

or not at all fit? 4

Don't know 5

Q111   Do you think you get enough exercise at present to keep you fit?

( )
Yes 1
No 2
Don't know 3

Q112   Do you think most people get enough exercise in everyday life to keep themselves fit?

( )
Yes 1
No 2
Don't know 3

Q113 SHOWCARD   I'm going to show you a list of things that people say stop them getting more exercise and I'd like you to tell me which, if any, apply to you.   PROBE AS NECESSARY: What others?

(READ OUT SHOWCARD ITEMS IF NECESSARY)   CODE ALL ITEMS THAT APPLY TO RESPONDENT - MULTICODE OK

( )
I'm not the sporty type 1
I haven't got the time 2
I've got young children to look after 3
I'm too shy or embarrassed 4
There's no-one to do it with 5
I'm too old 6
I have an injury or disability that stops me 7
My health is not good enough 8
There's no suitable facilities nearby 9
I need to rest and relax in my spare time 0
I don't have time because of my work X
I might get injured or damage my health . . . . Y
( )
I haven't got the right clothes or equipment 1
I'd never keep it up 2
I'm too fat 3
I haven't got the energy 4
I can't afford it 5
I don't enjoy physical activity 6
None of these 7
Don't know 8

Q114 SHOWCARD   And do any of the following stop you from getting more exercise?

(READ OUT SHOWCARD ITEMS IF NECESSARY)   CODE ALL ITEMS THAT APPLY TO RESPONDENT - MULTICODE OK

( )
My husband/wife/partner would disapprove 1
Other members of my family would disapprove 2
I don't want to go to 'mixed sex' places 3
I don't like to go to places where I
    can't speak my language 4
I don't want to go to a place where people
    show parts of their bodies 5
I have older relatives to look after 6
I don't like to go out alone 7
I would not know what to do 8
I never see anyone from my culture
    doing these things 9
None of these 0
Don't know X

Q115 When people talk about vigorous exercise they often mean different things. I'd like you to thing about vigorous exercise as something which makes you out of breath or sweaty. Do you do this kind of vigorous exercise three times a week or more for at least 20 minutes per occasion?

		( )	
Yes	....	1	GO TO Q117
No	....	2	ASK Q116

ASK IF NO AT Q115 (OTHERS GO TO Q117)
Q116 Do you do this kind of vigorous exercise at least once a week?

		( )
Yes	....	1
No	....	2

ASK ALL
Q117 I'm going to read out advice that people often give to those who want to be healthy. I'd like you to tell me how important you think each one is, for a person of your age who wants to be healthy

READ OUT. ROTATE ORDER. TICK START

		Very important	Fairly important	Not very important	Not at all important	Don't know
☐ a)	to get out and about	1	2	3	4	5
b)	to get a good night's sleep	1	2	3	4	5
☐ c)	to avoid getting overweight	1	2	3	4	5
d)	to avoid worrying too much	1	2	3	4	5
☐ e)	not to smoke	1	2	3	4	5
f)	to exercise regularly	1	2	3	4	5
☐ g)	not to drink much alcohol	1	2	3	4	5
h)	to avoid fatty foods	1	2	3	4	5

DEMOGRAPHICS

Q118   RECORD RESPONDENT'S GENDER

```
                                                           0
Female  . . . . . . . . . . . . . . . . . . . . . . . . . . . . . . . . . . . . . . . 1
Male    . . . . . . . . . . . . . . . . . . . . . . . . . . . . . . . . . . . . . 2
```

Q119   **Now I'd like to ask some more general questions about yourself and your household. May I just check your age?**

GET ESTIMATE IF NECESSARY. WRITE IN BOXES BELOW.

□□ YEARS

(23)(24)

Q120   **How many people are there usually living here in this household - that includes yourself, any other adults and children?**

WRITE NUMBER IN BOXES. USE LEADING ZERO IF NECESSARY

NB INCLUDE THOSE 75+   □□ people

(23)(24)   (23-24)

Q121   **How many of the people in your household are aged 16 or over?**

WRITE NUMBER IN BOXES. USE LEADING ZERO IF NECESSARY

□□ people

(23)(24)

Q122   **And how many of those people are aged between 16 and 74 (inclusive)?**

WRITE NUMBER IN BOXES. USE LEADING ZERO IF NECESSARY

□□ people

(23)(24)

ASK OR RECORD IF ALREADY KNOWN

Q123   SHOWCARD   **Which of the statements on this card best describes you? Reading from the top of the list, please call out the first one which applies to you.** SINGLE CODE ONLY

```
                                                           (20)
1       Married  . . . . . . . . . . . . . . . . . . . . . . . . . . . . . . . . . . 1
2       Living with partner  . . . . . . . . . . . . . . . . . . . . . . . . . . 2
3       Regular partner but not living with him/her  . . . . . . . . 3
4       Single  . . . . . . . . . . . . . . . . . . . . . . . . . . . . . . . . . . . . 4
5       Separated  . . . . . . . . . . . . . . . . . . . . . . . . . . . . . . . . 5
6       Divorced  . . . . . . . . . . . . . . . . . . . . . . . . . . . . . . . . . 6
7       Widowed  . . . . . . . . . . . . . . . . . . . . . . . . . . . . . . . . . 7              (20)
```

Q124 **Are there any children or young people aged 15 or under, living in the household?**

```
                                                    0
Yes      . . . . . . . . . . . . . . . . . . . . . . . . . . . . . . . . . . . . . . 1    ASK Q125 or Q126
No       . . . . . . . . . . . . . . . . . . . . . . . . . . . . . . . . . . . . . . 2    GO TO Q129
```

ASK IF CHILDREN IN HH AND RESPONDENT IS NOT SINGLE AT Q123
Q125 **Do you have any children of your own, or any step-children, aged 15 or under and living in the household?**

INCLUDE CHILDREN OF PARTNER EVEN IF NOT MARRIED TO HIM/HER. INCLUDE ADOPTED CHILDREN. CODE BELOW

ASK IF CHILDREN IN HH AND RESPONDENT IS SINGLE AT Q123
Q126 **Can I just check, do you have any children of your own aged 15 or under and living in the household?**

INCLUDE ADOPTED OR STEP-CHILDREN

```
                                                 Q125/126
                                                    0
Yes      . . . . . . . . . . . . . . . . . . . . . . . . . . . . . . . . . . . . . 1      ASK Q127
No       . . . . . . . . . . . . . . . . . . . . . . . . . . . . . . . . . . . . . 2      GO TO Q129
```

ASK IF YES AT Q125/126
Q127 How many?

☐☐   children
0 0

Q128 What are their ages, starting with the youngest?

RECORD AGES IN BOXES BELOW, USING LEADING ZERO IF NECESSARY. BABIES UNDER 1 YEAR OLD SHOULD BE RECORDED AS '00'.

Child 1 ☐☐ years   Child 2 ☐☐ years
         0   0   0   0

Child 3 ☐☐ years   Child 4 ☐☐ years
         0   0   0   0

Child 5 ☐☐ years   Child 6 ☐☐ years
         0   0   0   0

Child 7 ☐☐ years   Child 8 ☐☐ years
         0   0   0   0

Q129 **May I just check, were you in paid employment or self-employed in the week ending last Saturday?**

PROBE TO FIND OUT WHICH. CODE YES IF EMPLOYED/SELF-EMPLOYED FOR ANY NUMBER OF HOURS.

PAID EMPLOYMENT INCLUDES: SATURDAY JOBS; CASUAL WORK EG BABYSITTING; PEOPLE BEING PAID BY THEIR EMPLOYER TO ATTEND AN EDUCATIONAL ESTABLISHMENT; WIVES/HUSBANDS WORKING UNPAID IN A BUSINESS BELONGING TO THEIR SPOUSE, PROVIDED THEY WORK FOR 15 HRS OR MORE A WEEK; PEOPLE WORKING IN A FRIEND'S OR RELATIVE'S BUSINESS AS LONG AS THEY RECEIVE PAY OR A SHARE OF THE PROFITS; PEOPLE WORKING FOR EMPLOYERS ON GOVERNMENT TRAINING SCHEMES; PEOPLE ABSENT BECAUSE OF MATERNITY LEAVE, HOLIDAY, STRIKE, SICKNESS, TEMPORARY LAY-OFF OR ANY SIMILAR REASON PROVIDED THE HAVE A JOB TO RETURN TO WITH THE SAME EMPLOYER.

0

Yes:		
Employed	1	ASK
Self-employed	2	Q130
Government training scheme	3	
No	4	GO TO Q138, P42

ASK IF YES AT Q129 (OTHERS GO TO Q138, P42)
Q130 **Were you working full-time or part-time?**

FULL-TIME = MORE THAN 30 HRS PER WEEK; PART-TIME = 30 HOURS OR LESS

0

Full-time 1
Part-time 2

Q131 **What is the name or title of your job?**

PROBE FOR GRADE IF NECESSARY

. . . .

Q132 **What industry do you work in?**

. . . .

Q133 **What kind of work do you do most of the time?**

. . . .

Q134 **Do you have any special training or qualifications for that job, or do you use any machinery or special skills?** IF YES: **What are these?** WRITE IN

. . . .

. . . .

ASK IF EMPLOYED OR ON GOVT TRAINING AT Q129 (SELF-EMPLOYED GO TO Q147)

Q135 **Are you a manager or a foreman or supervisor, or not?**

	0	
Manager	1	
Foreman/supervisor	2	ASK Q136
Other type of employee	3	GO TO Q158, P46

ASK IF MANAGER/FOREMAN

Q136 **How many employees work in the establishment?**

	0
1-2	4
3-24	5
25-99	6
100-999	7
1000 or more	8
Don't know	9

IF RESPONDENT IS EMPLOYEE OR GOVT TRAINING, NOW GO TO Q158 ON P46

ASK IF SELF-EMPLOYED (CODE 2 AT Q129)

Q137 **Do you employ any other people? How many?**

	0	
1-5 employees	1	
6-24 employees	2	
25 or more employees	3	
No employees	4	NOW GO TO Q158, P46

Q138 **Last week were you...** READ OUT. CODE FIRST THAT APPLIES

0
Waiting to take up a job that you had already obtained? . . . 1   GO TO Q139,P43

THIS MEANS PEOPLE WHO HAVE A JOB FIXED UP BUT HAVEN'T STARTED WORK IN IT

Looking for work? 2   GO TO Q140,P43

THIS MEANS PEOPLE OUT OF EMPLOYMENT BUT ACTIVELY SEEKING WORK; INCLUDE PEOPLE DOING VOLUNTARY WORK IF THEY ARE ALSO SEEKING PAID WORK

Intending to look for work but prevented by temporary
sickness or injury? 3   GO TO Q140,P43

EXCLUDE ANYONE WHOSE TEMPORARY SICKNESS/INJURY HAS ALREADY LASTED LONGER THAN 28 DAYS (IE 4 WEEKS) - THESE PEOPLE SHOULD BE CODED AS 'DOING SOMETHING ELSE', CODE 8

Going to school or college full-time? 4   GO TO Q140,P43

THIS APPLIES ONLY TO STUDENTS, NOT TEACHERS/LECTURERS. USE THIS CODE ONLY FOR PEOPLE AGED 16-49 - OLDER PEOPLE WHO ARE STUDENTS SHOULD BE CODED 8, BELOW

Permanently unable to work because of long-term
sickness or disability? 5   GO TO Q140, P43

USE THIS CODE ONLY FOR MEN AGED 16-64 OR WOMEN AGED 16-59 - IF OUTSIDE THIS AE RANGE, CODE 8 BELOW

Retired? 6   GO TO Q150, P44

FOR WOMEN, CHECK THE AGE AT WHICH THEY STOPPED WORK - ONLY USE THIS CODE IF THEY STOPPED.WORK AT AGE 50 OR OLDER

Looking after the home or family? 7   GO TO Q140, P43

THIS INCLUDES WOMEN WHO STOPPED PAID WORK BEFORE AGE 50

Or were you doing something else?

THIS CODE COVERS ALL THOSE WHO COULD NOT BE CODED ABOVE
  (WRITE IN AND CODE 8) . . . .

. . . . 8   GO TO Q140, P43

ASK IF WAITING TO TAKE UP A JOB (CODE 1 AT Q138)
Q139 Apart from the job you are waiting to take up, have you ever been in paid employment?

0

Yes 1   GO TO Q141 BELOW

No 2   GO TO Q158, P46

ASK IF CODES 2-5 OR 7,8 AT Q138 (NOT CURRENTLY WORKING BUT NOT RETIRED)
Q140 Have you ever been in paid employment?

0

Yes 1   ASK Q141

No 2   GO TO Q158, P46

ASK IF YES AT Q139 OR Q140
Q141 In your last paid job or paid work, what was the name or title of your job?

(PROBE GRADE IF NECESSARY)

. . . .

Q142 What industry did you work in?

. . . .

Q143 What kind of work did you do most of the time?

. . . .

Q144 Did you have any special training or qualifications for that job, or did you use any machinery or special skills? IF YES: What were these? WRITE IN

. . . .

. . . .

Q145 Were you an employee or self-employed?

0

Employee 1   ASK Q146

Self-employed 2   GOTO Q148

ASK IF EMPLOYEE AT Q145
Q146 **Were you a manager or a foreman or supervisor, or not?**

		0		
Manager	. . . .	1		
Foreman/supervisor	. . . .	2	ASK Q147	
Other type of employee	. . . .	3	SEE Q149, BELOW	0

ASK IF MANAGER/FOREMAN
Q147 **How many employees worked in the establishment?**

	0
1-2	1
3-24	2
25-99	3
100-999	4
1000 or more	5
Don't know	6

IF RESPONDENT WAS EMPLOYEE, NOW SEE Q149 BELOW

ASK IF SELF-EMPLOYED AT Q145
Q148 **Did you employ any other people? How many?**

	(11)
1-5 employees	1
6-24 employees	2
25 or more employees	3
No employees	4

NOW CHECK Q138:

ASK Q149 IF RESPONDENT CODED 1, 2 OR 3 AT Q138 ON P42.
IF RESPONDENT CODED 4,5,7 OR 8, GO TO Q158 ON P46.
(IF RESPONDENT CODED 6 - RETIRED - GO TO Q150 BELOW)

ASK IF RESPONDENT UNEMPLOYED LAST WEEK (CODE 1, 2 OR 3 AT Q138)
Q149 **How long altogether have you been out of employment but wanting work, in this current period of unemployment?**

READ OUT IF NECESSARY

		0	
Less than 6 months	. . . .	1	
6 months but less than 12 months	. . . .	2	
12 months but less than 2 years	. . . .	3	
2 years or more	. . . .	4	NOW GO TO Q158, P46

ASK IF RETIRED (CODE 6 AT Q138)
Q150 **In the main job you did before you retired, what was the name or title of your job?**

(PROBE GRADE IF NECESSARY) WRITE IN

. . . .

Q151 **What industry did you work in?** WRITE IN

. . . .

Q152 **What kind of work did you do most of the time?** WRITE IN

. . . .

Q153 **Did you have any special training or qualifications for that job, or did you use any machinery or special skills?** IF YES: **What were these?** WRITE IN DESCRIPTION OF TRAIN

. . . .

. . . .

Q154 **Were you an employee or self-employed?**

                                                                0

Employee 1   ASK Q155
Self-employed 2   GOTO Q157

ASK IF EMPLOYEE AT Q154
Q155 **Were you a manager or a foreman or supervisor, or not?**

                                                                 0

Manager 1
Foreman/supervisor 2   ASK Q156
Other type of employee 3   GO TO Q158

ASK IF MANAGER/FOREMAN
Q156 **How many employees worked in the establishment?**

                                                                 0

1-2 1
3-24 2
25-99 3
100-999 4
1000 or more 5
Don't know 6

IF RESPONDENT WAS EMPLOYEE, NOW GO TO Q158 ON P46

ASK IF SELF-EMPLOYED AT Q154

Q157 Did you employ any other people? How many?

                                                    (11)
          1-5 employees 1
          6-24 employees 2
          25 or more employees 3
          No employees 4

OFFICE USE ONLY: SOCIAL CLASS OF RESPONDENT TO BE CODED HERE	0

ASK ALL

Q158 Now I'd like to ask some questions about the head of your household. First of all I need to check if you are the head of the household, or if it is somebody else. The head of the household is normally the person who owns or rents the accommodation.

NB USE STANDARD MARKET RESEARCH DEFINITION OF HEAD OF HOUSEHOLD AND CHECK CAREFULLY BEFORE CODING.

                                                    0
Respondent is head of household 1   GO TO Q191, P53
Somebody else is head of household 2   ASK Q159

ASK IF RESPONDENT IS NOT HEAD OF HOUSEHOLD

Q159 What relation is the head of the household to you?

                                                    0
Husband/partner 1
Parent or parent-in-law 2
Son/daughter or son-in-law/daughter-in-law 3
Other relation (WRITE IN & CODE 4)

          4
Head of household is not related (eg flatsharer/landlady) 5

Q160 ASK OR RECORD GENDER OF HEAD OF HOUSEHOLD

                                                    0
Female 1
Male 2

Q161 What age is the head of your household?

GET ESTIMATE IF NECESSARY. WRITE IN BOXES BELOW.

          ☐☐ YEARS
          (23)(24)
Don't know . . . . Y

Q162   Was he/she in paid employment or self-employed in the week ending last Saturday?

PROBE TO FIND OUT WHICH.   CODE YES IF EMPLOYED/SELF-EMPLOYED FOR ANY NUMBER OF HOURS.

PAID EMPLOYMENT INCLUDES: SATURDAY JOBS; CASUAL WORK EG BABYSITTING; PEOPLE BEING PAID BY THEIR EMPLOYER TO ATTEND AN EDUCATIONAL ESTABLISHMENT; WIVES/HUSBANDS WORKING UNPAID IN A BUSINESS BELONGING TO THEIR SPOUSE, PROVIDED THEY WORK FOR 15 HRS OR MORE A WEEK; PEOPLE WORKING IN A FRIEND'S OR RELATIVE'S BUSINESS AS LONG AS THEY RECEIVE PAY OR A SHARE OF THE PROFITS; PEOPLE WORKING FOR EMPLOYERS ON GOVERNMENT TRAINING SCHEMES; PEOPLE ABSENT BECAUSE OF MATERNITY LEAVE, HOLIDAY, STRIKE, SICKNESS, TEMPORARY LAY-OFF OR ANY SIMILAR REASON PROVIDED THE HAVE A JOB TO RETURN TO WITH THE SAME EMPLOYER.

		0	
Yes:			
Employed	. . .	1	
Self-employed	. . .	2	ASK
Government training scheme	. . .	3	Q163
No	. . .	4	GO TO Q171, P49
Don't know	. . .	5	

ASK IF YES AT Q162 (OTHERS GO TO Q171, P49)

Q163   Was he/she working full-time or part-time?

FULL-TIME = MORE THAN 30 HRS PER WEEK; PART-TIME = 30 HOURS OR LESS

	0
Full-time	. . . 1
Part-time	. . . 2
Don't know	. . . 3

Q164   What is the name or title of his/her job?

PROBE FOR GRADE IF NECESSARY.   WRITE IN

. . . .
Don't know . . . . Y

Q165   What industry does he/she work in? WRITE IN

. . . .
Don't know . . . . Y

Q166   What kind of work does he/she do most of the time? WRITE IN

. . . .
Don't know . . . . Y

Q167 **Does he/she have any special training or qualifications for that job, or does he/she use any machinery or special skills?** IF YES: **What are these?** WRITE IN

. . . .

. . . .

Don't know . . . . Y

ASK IF EMPLOYED OR ON GOVT SCHEME AT Q162 (SELF-EMPLOYED GO TO Q170 BELOW)

Q168 **Is he/she a manager or a foreman or supervisor, or not?**

0

Manager 1

Foreman/supervisor 2   ASK Q169

Other type of employee 3   GO TO Q191 P53

Don't know 4

ASK IF MANAGER/FOREMAN

Q169 **How many employees work in the establishment?**

0

1-2 5

3-24 6

25-99 7

100-999 8

1000 or more 9

Don't know 0

IF HEAD OF HOUSEHOLD IS EMPLOYEE, NOW GO TO Q191 ON P53

ASK IF SELF-EMPLOYED (CODE 2 AT Q162)

Q170 **Does he/she employ any other people? How many?**

0

1-5 employees 1

6-24 employees 2

25 or more employees 3

No employees 4   (67)

Don't know 5

IF HEAD OF HOUSEHOLD SELF-EMPLOYED, NOW GO TO Q191,P53

ASK IF NO AT Q162
Q171 **Last week was he/she...**

READ OUT. CODE FIRST THAT APPLIES

Waiting to take up a job that he/she had already obtained? . 1   GO TO Q172, P50

THIS MEANS PEOPLE WHO HAVE A JOB FIXED UP BUT HAVEN'T STARTED WORK IN IT

Looking for work? 2   GO TO Q173, P50

THIS MEANS PEOPLE OUT OF EMPLOYMENT BUT ACTIVELY SEEKING WORK; INCLUDE PEOPLE DOING VOLUNTARY WORK IF THEY ARE ALSO SEEKING PAID WORK

Intending to look for work but prevented by temporary
  sickness or injury? 3   GO TO Q173, P50

EXCLUDE ANYONE WHOSE TEMPORARY SICKNESS/INJURY HAS ALREADY LASTED LONGER THAN 28 DAYS (IE 4 WEEKS) - THESE PEOPLE SHOULD BE CODED AS 'DOING SOMETHING ELSE', CODE 8

Going to school or college full-time? 4   GO TO Q173, P50

THIS APPLIES ONLY TO STUDENTS, NOT TEACHERS/LECTURERS. USE THIS CODE ONLY FOR PEOPLE AGED 16-49 - OLDER PEOPLE WHO ARE STUDENTS SHOULD BE CODED 8, BELOW

Permanently unable to work because of long-term
  sickness or disability? 5   GO TO Q173, P50

USE THIS CODE ONLY FOR MEN AGED 16-64 OR WOMEN AGED 16-59 - IF OUTSIDE THIS AGE RANGE, CODE 8 BELOW

Retired? 6   GO TO Q183, P51

FOR WOMEN, CHECK THE AGE AT WHICH THEY STOPPED WORK - ONLY USE THIS CODE IF THEY STOPPED WORK AT AGE 50 OR OLDER

Looking after the home or family? 7   GO TO Q173, P50

THIS INCLUDES WOMEN WHO STOPPED PAID WORK BEFORE AGE 50

Or was he/she doing something else?

THIS CODE COVERS ALL THOSE WHO COULD NOT BE CODED ABOVE

  (WRITE IN AND CODE 8) . . . .

  8   GO TO Q173, P54

Don't know 9   GO TO Q173, P54

ASK IF WAITING TO TAKE UP A JOB (CODE 1 AT Q171)
Q172 Apart from the job he/she are waiting to take up, has he/she ever been in paid employment?

	0	
Yes 1	GO TO Q174 BELOW
No 2	GO TO Q191, P53
Don't know 3	

ASK IF CODES 2-5 OR 7,8 AT Q171 (NOT CURRENTLY WORKING BUT NOT RETIRED)
Q173 Has he/she ever been in paid employment?

	0	
Yes 1	GO TO Q174 BELOW
No 2	GO TO Q191, P53

ASK IF YES AT Q172 OR Q173
Q174 In his/her last paid job or paid work, what was the name or title of his/her job?

(PROBE GRADE IF NECESSARY) WRITE IN

....
Don't know .... Y

Q175 What industry did he/she work in? WRITE IN

....
Don't know .... Y

Q176 What kind of work did he/she do most of the time? WRITE IN

....
Don't know .... Y

Q177 Did he/she have any special training or qualifications for that job, or did you use any machinery or special skills? IF YES : What were these? WRITE IN

....
....
Don't know .... Y

Q178 Was he/she an employee or self-employed?

	0	
Employee 1	ASK Q179
Self-employed 2	GO TO Q181, P51

ASK IF EMPLOYEE AT Q178
Q179 **Was he/she a manager or a foreman or supervisor, or not?**

                                                              0

Manager 1

Foreman/supervisor 2   ASK Q180

Other type of employee 3   NOW SEE

Don't know 4   Q182 BELOW

ASK IF MANAGER/FOREMAN
Q180 **How many employees worked in the establishment?**

                                                      0

1-2 1

3-24 2

25-99 3

100-999 4

1000 or more 5

Don't know 6   NOW SEE Q182 BELOW

ASK IF SELF-EMPLOYED AT Q178
Q181 **Did he/she employ any other people? How many?**

                                           (11)

1-5 employees 1

6-24 employees 2

25 or more employees 3

No employees 4

Don't know 5   NOW SEE Q182 BELOW

NOW CHECK Q171:
      ASK Q182 IF HEAD OF HOUSEHOLD CODED 1, 2 OR 3 AT Q171
      IF HEAD OF HOUSEHOLD CODED 4, 5, 7 OR 8, GO TO Q191, P53
      (IF CODE 6 - RETIRED - GO TO Q183 BELOW)

ASK IF HEAD OF HOUSEHOLD UNEMPLOYED LAST WEEK (CODE 1, 2 OR 3 AT Q171)
Q182 **How long altogether had he/she been out of employment but wanting work, in this current period of unemployment?**

READ OUT IF NECESSARY

                                                     0

Less than 6 months 1

6 months but less than 12 months 2

12 months but less than 2 years 3

2 years or more 4

Don't know 5   NOW GO TO Q191, P53

ASK IF RETIRED (CODE 6 AT Q171)
Q183 **In the main job he/she did before he/she retired, what was the name or title of his/her job?**

(PROBE GRADE IF NECESSARY) WRITE IN

....

Don't know .... Y

Q184 What industry did he/she work in? WRITE IN

. . . .
Don't know . . . . Y

Q185 What kind of work did he/she do most of the time? WRITE IN

. . . .
Don't know . . . . Y

Q186 Did he/she have any special training or qualifications for that job, or did he/she use any machinery or special skills? IF YES: What were these? WRITE IN

. . . .
. . . .
Don't know . . . . Y

Q187 Was he/she an employee or self-employed?

0
Employee 1   ASK Q188
Self-employed 2   GO TO Q190

ASK IF EMPLOYEE AT Q187
Q188 Was he/she a manager or a foreman or supervisor, or not?

0
Manager 1
Foreman/supervisor 2   ASK Q189
Other type of employee 3   GO TO Q191
Don't know 4

ASK IF MANAGER/FOREMAN AT Q188
Q189 How many employees worked in the establishment?

0
1-2 1
3-24 2
25-99 3
100-999 4
1000 or more 5
Don't know 6

IF HOH WAS EMPLOYEE, NOW GO TO Q191 ON P53

ASK IF SELF-EMPLOYED AT Q187
Q190 **Did he/she employ any other people? How many?**

                                                                    (11)
              1-5 employees 1
              6-24 employees 2
              25 or more employees 3
              No employees 4
              Don't know 5

| OFFICE USE ONLY: SOCIAL CLASS OF HEAD OF HOUSEHOLD TO BE CODED HERE | 0 |

ASK ALL
Q191 **Now for some different kinds of questions about your household. Does this household own this accommodation or do you rent it?**

        IF OWNED, PROBE TO FIND OUT IF CODE 1, 2 OR 3

                                                                    (21)
        Owned outright 1
        Owned/being bought on mortgage 2
        Bought from Council/under Right-to-Buy 3
        Rented from Council 4
        Rented from housing association 5
        Rented from private landlord 6
        Other (WRITE IN & CODE '7')

              7   (21)

Q192 **Do you personally own a car or have use of a car or van?**

                                                                    (32)
              Own car 1
              Use of car (eg company car) 2
              No car 3   (32)

Q193 **In what country were you born?**

                                                                    (36)
        West Indies/Jamaica, Trinidad etc/Guyana 1   ASK Q194
        England, Wales, Scotland, Northern Ireland 2   GO TO Q195
        Any other country (WRITE IN & CODE 3)

              3   ASK Q194

ASK THOSE NOT BORN IN THE UK AT Q193 (OTHERS GO TO Q195)
Q194 How old were you when you came to live in the UK?

RECORD IN BOXES. USE LEADING ZEROS IF NECESSARY

☐☐   years

(23)(24)   (23-24)

Don't know . . . . Y   NOW GO TO Q197, BELOW

ASK IF BORN IN UK AT Q193
Q195 And In what country was your mother born?

Q196 And In what country was your father born?

	Q195	Q196
	0	0
West Indies/Jamaica, Trinidad etc/Guyana	1	1
England, Wales, Scotland, Northern Ireland	2	2
Any other country (WRITE IN & CODE 3)		

. . . . 3

. . . . 3

ASK ALL
Q197 How would you describe your race or ethnic origin?

DO NOT PROMPT. CODE BELOW

                                                                    (34)

| Black British . . . . 1 |
| African-Caribbean . . . . 2 |
| West Indian (including Jamaican, Trinidadian). . . . . 3 |
| Guyanese. . . . . 4 |
| Other ethnic group (WRITE IN & CODE '5') |

. . . . 5

Don't know/refused 6   (34)

(SKIP QQ198-204)

ASK THOSE NOT BORN IN UK AT Q193 (OTHERS GO TO Q207)
Q205 Did you ever attend school?

                                                                    0
Yes   1   ASK Q
No   2   GO TO Q

ASK IF YES AT Q205
Q206 What was the highest level you achieved at school?

                                                                    0
. . . . 1
. . . . 2
. . . . 3
. . . . 4
. . . . 5

Q207 SHOWCARD   Now I'd like to ask you about your educational qualifications. Please look at this card and tell me whether you have passed any of the qualifications listed. Look down the list and tell me the first one you come to that you have passed.

READ OUT SHOWCARD ITEMS IF NECESSARY. CODE FIRST THAT APPLIES

(18)

Degree (or degree level qualifications) 1

Teaching qualification 2
HNC/HND, BEC/TEC Higher, BTEC Higher 2
City and Guilds Full Technological Certificate 2
Nursing qualifications (SRN, SCM, RGN, RM, RHV, Midwife) . . 2

'A' levels/SCE higher 3
ONC/OND/BEC/TEC **not** higher 3
City and Guilds Advanced/Final level 3

'O'level passes (Grade A-C if after 1975) 4
GCSE (grades (A-C) 4
CSE Grade 1 4
SCE Ordinary (Bands A-C) 4
Standard Grade (Level 1-3) 4
SLC Lower 4
SUPE Lower or Ordinary 4
School Certificate or Matric 4
City and Guilds Craft/Ordinary Level 4

CSE Grades 2-5 5
GCE 'O' level (Grades D and E if after 1975) 5
GCSE (Grades D,E,F,G) 5
SCE Ordinary (Bands D and E) 5
Standard Grade (Level 4,5) 5
Clerical or Commercial qualifications 5
Apprenticeship 5

CSE ungraded 6
Other qualifications (WRITE IN AND CODE 7)

. . . . 7

No qualifications 8

Q208　What is your religion or church?

	( )
Baptist	1
Buddhism	2
Islam	3
Sikhism	4
Hinduism	5
Church of England/Wales/Scotland/Ireland	6
Roman Catholic	7
Methodist	8
Seventh Day Adventist	9
Jehovah's Witness	0
Pentecostal/Church of God/Church of Christ	X
Cherubim and Seraphim	Y
	( )
Rastafarian	1
Other (WRITE IN & CODE '2')	
....	2
None	3
Don't know	4

Q209　Do you (and your husband/wife/partner) receive any of these benefits?

READ OUT. ROTATE ORDER. TICK START

		Yes	No	Don't know
☐	**Income support or social security** .... 1 .... 2 3
☐	**Family Credit** .... 1 .... 2 3
☐	**Housing benefit** .... 1 .... 2 3

INTERVIEWER PLEASE RECORD LANGUAGE IN WHICH INTERVIEW WAS CONDUCTED:

	0
English	1
Bengali/Sylheti	2
Gujerati	3
Punjabi (Sikh)	4
Punjabi (Pakistani)	5
Urdu	6
Other (WRITE IN & CODE 7)	
....	7

INTERVIEWER PLEASE RECORD HOW WELL RESPONDENT WAS ABLE TO READ SHOWCARDS:

	0
Respondent could read all showcards without any help from me	1
Respondent could read most things but needed a little help	2
Respondent could read a little and needed a lot of help	3
Respondent could not read showcards at all - I had	
to read everything out to him/her	4

INTERVIEWER PLEASE RECORD AMOUNT OF PRIVACY DURING INTERVIEW:

                                                                    0
    We were able to do the interview in total privacy 1
    There was someone else present during part of the interview . 2
    There was someone else present for most or all of the interview 3

IF SOMEONE ELSE WAS PRESENT DURING INTERVIEW, PLEASE CODE:

a)   Gender

                                                                    0
    The other person/people present were of the same
      gender as the respondent 1
    The other person/people present were of the opposite
      gender to the respondent 2
    There were both males and females present
      during the interview 3

b)   Relationship with respondent

                                                                    0
    The other person/people present were members of the
      respondent's household/family 1
    The other person/people present were friends or other
      visitors 2
    Both   3

INTERVIEWER PLEASE RECORD LENGTH OF INTERVIEW:

☐☐☐ MINUTES

Bibliography

Allied Dunbar National Fitness Survey (1992) Health Education Authority and Sports Council, London.

Balarajan, R. and Raleigh, V.S. (1993) *Ethnicity and health: a guide for the NHS*. Department of Health, London.

Balarajan, R. and Raleigh, V.S. (1997) 'Patterns of mortality among Bangladeshis in England and Wales', *Ethnicity and Health* 2(1/2): 5–12.

Bedi, R. (1996) 'Betel-quid and tobacco chewing among the United Kingdom Bangladeshi Community', *British Journal of Cancer* 674 Supplement XXIX: S73–7.

Bennett, N., Dodd, T. and Flatley, J., *et al.* (1995) *Health Survey for England*. Office of Population Censuses and Surveys, London.

Bhachu, P. (1985) *Twice migrants: East African Sikh settlers in Britain*. Tavistock, London.

Bhopal, R.S. (1990) 'Future research on the health of ethnic minorities: back to basics', *Ethnic Minorities Health: A Current Awareness Bulletin* 1(3): 1–3.

Blaxter, M. (1985) 'Self-definition of health status and consultation rates in primary care', *Quarterly Journal of Social Affairs*, 1: 131.

Blaxter, M. (1990) *Health and lifestyles*. Routledge, London.

Bowling, A. (1991) *Measuring health: a review of quality of life measurement scales*. Open University Press, Buckingham.

Brown, C. (1984) *Black and white Britain*. Policy Studies Institute, London.

Burke, G.L., Bild, D.E., Hilner, J.E., Folsom, A.R., Wagenknecht, L.E. and Sidney, S. (1997) 'Differences in weight gain in relation to race, gender, age and education in young adults: the CARDIA study', *Ethnicity and Health* 1(4): 327–35.

Calman, K. (1992) *On the state of the public health: the annual report of the Chief Medical Officer of the Department of Health for the Year 1991*. HMSO, London.

Colhoun, H. *et al.* (1996) *Health Survey for England, 1994*. HMSO, London. (Also referenced as Health Survey for England or HSE.)

Cox, D., Huppert, F. and Whichelow, M. (1993). *The Health and Lifestyle Survey: seven years on*. Dartmouth Publishing, Aldershot.

Cross, M., Johnson, M. and Cox, B. (1988) *Black welfare and local government*. Centre for Research in Ethnic Relations, University of Warwick, Coventry.

Currer, C. (1986) 'Concepts of mental well- and ill-being: the case of Pathan mothers in Britain', in Currer, C. and Stacey, M. (1986) *Concepts of health illness and disease: a comparative perspective*. Berg, Leamington Spa.

Department of Health (1992) *The health of the nation: a strategy for health in England*. HMSO, London.

Department of Health (1994) *Nutritional aspects of cardiovascular disease: report of the Cardiovascular Review Group, Committee on Medical Aspects of Food Policy*. HMSO, London.

Dodge, J.S. (1969) *The fieldworker in immigrant health*. Staples Press.

Edwards, C.R.W. and Bouchier, I.A.D. (1991) *Davidson's principles and practice of medicine*, 16th edn. Churchill Livingstone, London.

Farrell, S.W., Kohl, H.W. and Rogers, T. (1987) 'The independent effect of ethnicity on cardiovascular fitness', *Human Biology* 59(4): 657–66.

Fitzgerald, J.T., Singleton, S.P., Neale, A.V., Prasad, A.S. and Hess, J.W. (1994) 'Activity levels, fitness status, exercise knowledge and exercise beliefs among healthy older African American and white women', *Journal of Aging and Health* 6(3): 296–313.

Fitzgerald, M. and Hale, C. (1996) *Ethnic minorities: victimisation and racial harassment*. Research Study 154, Home Office, London.

Fleming, S. (1991) 'Sport, solidarity and Asian male youth culture'; 30–57, in Jarvie, G. (ed) (1991) *Sport, racism and ethnicity*. Falmer Press, London.

Gasperino, J. (1997) 'Ethnic differences in body composition and their relation to health and disease in women', *Ethnicity and Health* 1(4): 337–47.

Green, A.E. (1997) 'Patterns of ethnic minority employment in the context of industrial and occupational growth and decline', in Karn, V. (ed.) *Ethnicity in the 1991 Census*: vol. 4, *Employment, among the ethnic education and housing minority population of Great Britain*. HMSO, London.

Hansbro, J., Bridgwood, A., Morgan, A. and Hickman, M. (1997) *Health in England, 1996*. Health Education Monitoring Survey, Office of National Statistics and Health Education Authority, London.

Health Education Authority (1991) *Nutrition in minority ethnic groups: Asians and African-Caribbeans in the United Kingdom*. Health Education Authority, London.

Imtiaz, S. and Johnson, M. (1993) *Health care provision and the Kashmiri population of Peterborough*. NorthWest Anglia Health Authority, Peterborough.

Johnson, M.R.D. (1987) 'Towards racial equality in health and welfare: what progress?', *New Community* 15(1): 128–35.

Johnson, M.R.D. and Cross, M. (1984) *Surveying service users in multi-ethnic areas*. Centre for Research in Ethnic Relations, Warwick University, Coventry.

Johnson, M.R.D. and Verma, C. (1998) *It's our health too: Asian men's health perspectives*. Research Paper in Ethnic Relations 26, Centre for Research in Ethnic Relations, Warwick University, Coventry.

Joint Health Surveys Unit, Social and Community Planning Research/ Department of Epidemiology and Public Health, University College, London (1996) *Health Survey for England, 1994*. HMSO, London. (1996), *Health Survey for England*. (See also Colhoun *et al.*)

Keen, H. *et al.* (1994) *Blood pressure and diabetes: everyone's concern*. Report of a working party. RR Associates for Zeneca Pharma UK, Chineham, Hants.

Kish, L. (1965) *Survey sampling*. John Wiley, Chichester.

Lee, G.L. and Wrench, J. (1980) 'Accident-prone immigrants: an assumption challenged', *Sociology* 14(4): 551–66.

Mamdani, M. (1973) *From citizen to refugee: Ugandan Asians come to Britain*. Frances Pinter, London.

McKeigue, P.M., Miller, G. and Marmot, M.G. (1989) 'Coronary heart disease in South Asians overseas: a review', *Journal of Clinical Epidemiology* 42(7): 597–609.

McKeigue, P.M., Shah, B. and Marmot, M.G. (1991) 'Relation of central obesity and insulin resistance with high diabetes prevalence and cardiovascular risk in South Asians', *Lancet* 337: 382–6.

McKenzie, K.J. and Crowcroft, N.S. (1994) 'Race, ethnicity, culture and science', *British Medical Journal* 309: 286–7.

Modood, T. *et al.* (1997) *Ethnic minorities in Britain: diversity and disadvantage*. Policy Studies Institute, London.

Nazroo, J.Y. (1997) *The health of Britain's ethnic minorities*. Policy Studies Institute, London.

OPCS (1996) *Living in Britain, 1994: results from the 1994 General Household Survey*. HMSO, London.

Owen, D. (1993a) *Ethnic minorities in Great Britain: economic characteristics*. NEMDA 1991 Census Statistical Paper 3, Centre for Research in Ethnic Relations, University of Warwick, Coventry.

Owen, D.W. (1993b) *Ethnic minorities in Great Britain: housing and family characteristics*. NEMDA 1991 Census Statistical Paper 4, Centre for Research in Ethnic Relations, University of Warwick, Coventry.

Owen, D.W. (1997) 'Labour force participation rates, self-employment and unemployment', in Karn, V. (ed.) *Ethnicity in the 1991 Census: vol. 4: Employment, education and housing among the ethnic minority population of Great Britain*. HMSO, London.

Parmar, A. (1997) *An equal right to safety*. Discussion Paper, Royal Society for the Prevention of Accidents, Birmingham.

Physical Activity Task Force (1995) *More people more active more often*. Department of Health, London.

Ratcliffe, P. (ed.) *Ethnicity in the 1991 Census: vol 4: Geographical spread, spatial concentration and internal migration*. ONS, London.

Rudat, K. (1994) *Health and lifestyles: black and minority ethnic groups in England*. Health Education Authority, London.

Samanta, A., Burden, A.C. and Jagger, C. (1991) 'A comparison of the clinical features and vascular complications of diabetes between migrant Asians and Caucasians in Leicester', *Diabetes Research Clinical Practice* 14(3): 205–13.

Schoeller, D.A. and Kushner, R.F. (1997) 'Expert review: increased rates of obesity among African Americans confirmed', *Ethnicity and Health* 1(4): 313–15.

Senior, P.A. and Bhopal, R. (1994) 'Ethnicity as a variable in epidemiological research', *British Medical Journal* 309: 327–30.

Shaper, A.G., Wannamethree, S.G. and Walker, M. (1997) 'Body weight: implications for the prevention of coronary heart disease, stroke and diabetes mellitus in a cohort study of middle aged men', *British Medical Journal* 314: 1311–17.

Sinha, D.P. (1995) *Food nutrition and health in the Caribbean*. Caribbean Food and Nutrition Institute, Kingston, Jamaica.

Smaje, C. (1995) *Health, 'race' and ethnicity*. King's Fund Institute, London.

Sports Council (1994) *Black and ethnic minorities and sport*. Sports Council, London.

Sprotson, K. *et al* (1999) *Health and lifestyles of the Chinese population in England*. Health Education Authority, London.

Stevens, A. and Raftery, J. (1994) *Health care needs assessment*, vol. 1. Radcliffe Medical Press, Oxford.

Stubbs, M. (ed.) (1985) *The other languages of England: the linguistic minorities project*. Institute of Education/Routledge, London.